HOME CARE
FOR THE
High-Risk Infant

A FAMILY-CENTERED APPROACH

Second Edition

Elizabeth Ahmann, ScD, RN

An Aspen Publication®
Aspen Publishers, Inc.
Gaithersburg, Maryland
1996

Editorial Resources: Lenda P. Hill

Library of Congress Cataloging-in-Publication Data

Home care for the high-risk infant : a family-centered approach / edited by Elizabeth
   Ahmann. — 2nd ed.
      p.   cm.
   Rev. ed. of: Home care for the high risk infant / by Elizabeth Ahmann. 1986.
   Includes bibliographical references and index.
   ISBN 0-8342-0750-8 (alk. paper)
   1. Infants (Premature)—Home care.   2. Infants (Premature)—Diseases.
I. Ahmann, Elizabeth.
   [DNLM: 1. Infant, Premature, Diseases.   2. Home Care Services.
WS 410H765 1996]
RJ250.H58   1996
618.92'011—dc20
DNLM/DLC
for Library of Congress   96-7422
                                                                                 CIP

The authors have made every effort to ensure the accuracy of the information
herein, particularly with regard to drug selection and dose. However, appropriate information sources should be consulted, especially for new or unfamiliar
drugs or procedures. It is the responsibility of every practitioner to evaluate
the appropriateness of a particular opinion in the context of actual clinical
situations and with due consideration to new developments. Authors, editors,
and the publisher cannot be held responsible for any typographical or other
errors found in this book.

Library of Congress Catalog Card Number: 96—7422
ISBN 0-8342-0750-8 (loose leaf)

Printed in the United States of America

1 2 3 4 5

Table of Contents

Preface

When this book was originally published in 1986, home care of prematurely born infants remaining dependent on medical technology was a relatively young but growing field. Since that time, several factors have contributed to the continued high numbers of technology-dependent infants cared for in the home. These include improved survival of smaller, younger infants due to continuing advances in medical technology and the aggressive use of multisystem therapies; the higher incidence of morbidity associated with lower birth weights; the financial climate of health care, which results in earlier hospital discharge; and generally favorable experience with home care for this population.

As changes in health care financing have led to more rapid discharge of hospitalized patients, infants and children with complex care requirements are discharged earlier than thought possible several years ago. Because of this, some families are having to learn their child's care while they are still adjusting to the diagnosis and remain uncertain about the prognosis. In certain instances, portions of the "discharge" teaching are done only once the infant is at home. These factors place a heavy responsibility on the home care nurse both for collaborating with other health care providers and for developing a thorough and conscientious approach to assessment, teaching and care provision in the home setting. In conjunction with these changes, the need for appropriate documentation has never been greater.

Since the original edition of this book, new or modified technologies augment the home care of infants and young children with serious medical problems. Among these, car-

diorespiratory monitors with "memory" chips, more portable respiratory equipment, pulse oximetry, tracheostomy speaking valves, and parenteral nutrition are used in the home more frequently than in the past. At the same time, increased fiscal constraints may make it difficult for some families to obtain certain supplies and services that would ease some of the burdens of home care.

Since 1986, our understanding of the complex interplay between growth, development, and health status in the population of high-risk premature infants has increased. New research acknowledges the benefits of breastfeeding the preterm infant. Other recent studies have shed light on long-term sequelae of prematurity. Federal legislation has paved the way for more accessible developmental intervention services for at-risk infants and young children.

The problems of human immunodeficiency virus (HIV) and acquired immune deficiency syndrome (AIDS) have become epidemic. Some of the same factors that pose a risk for preterm birth are also associated with the population at risk for HIV exposure. Infants born both prematurely and HIV positive pose special challenges for health care providers and families. These infants, and the generally higher acuity level of infants and children discharged from the hospital, make the possibility of death in the home an eventuality for which home care nurses must be prepared.

Research and clinical experience have improved our understanding of the challenges families face and the strengths they bring to bear in successfully providing home care for their infants and young children with special needs.

The willingness of nurses and other professionals to acknowledge the central role of the family in the care of infants and children with chronic illness and disability has led to developing models and augmenting skills for parent–professional collaboration. Increasingly, cultural competence and family-centered care are considered best practice. These new approaches may present challenges and opportunities for nurses in terms of the nursing role and in relation to certain ethical and legal considerations. Nowhere are these issues more prominent than in the home care setting.

This new, revised, and expanded edition of *Home Care for the High-risk Infant: A Family-Centered Approach* (originally entitled *Home Care for the High-risk Infant: A Holistic Guide to Using Technology*) will prepare nurses to provide the comprehensive discharge preparation and home nursing care that is needed both for infants dependent on medical technology in the home and for their families.

The text's strong foundation in a collaborative, family-centered approach to care will contribute to the best practice of community health or home care nurses, whether providing intermittent home visits or hourly nursing care for the technology-dependent infant or young child in the home.

Updated, expanded, and new chapters on clinical topics will give the community health or home care nurse a framework for care on each home visit and will guide the nurse by detailing information and skills required for assessment, teaching, and provision of care. Sample care plans, assessment sheets, instruction sheets, and numerous tables and exhibits in each chapter will assist the nurse providing or supervising care in the home.

New features in this edition of the book include "Special Issues," which highlight a variety of topics of concern to the home care nurse. Included in each section of the book, Special Issues address matters such as working with substance-abusing mothers, suspected abuse and neglect in home care, breastfeeding the premature infant, parent perspectives, and so forth.

Chapter 1 of the book reviews the latest research and clinical implications for the health and developmental outcomes of infants born prematurely.

Part I, on family issues and family-centered care, consists of a new chapter addressing both the challenges home care poses to families and the strengths and resources families bring to bear; an expanded chapter on sibling concerns; and a new chapter on strategies for implementing family-centered care in a home care practice. Special Issues address ethical concerns and work with substance-abusing mothers.

Part II, addressing the transition to home care, includes an updated chapter on discharge planning for the infant or child with complex care needs; an updated, expanded chapter on the nursing intake process and the plan of care; a revised chapter on community resources, containing an extensive list of publications and resource organizations; and an expanded chapter on promoting health maintenance for the high-risk premature infant. Special Issues address standards of care, alternatives to home care, and suspected abuse and neglect.

The expanded Part III, on nutrition and feeding, consists of a thorough overview of nutrition and feeding, including assessment and intervention; an updated, expanded enteral feeding chapter; a new chapter on short bowel syndrome and home parenteral nutrition; and Special Issues on breastfeeding the premature infant and failure to thrive.

The updated Part IV, addressing respiratory concerns, includes a chapter providing an overview of bronchopulmonary dysplasia, including descriptions of common adventitious lung sounds and the components of a thorough respiratory assessment; and chapters with detailed approaches to assessment, teaching, and care for the infant or young child with a cardiorespiratory monitor, oxygen, tracheostomy, and/or ventilator. Special Issues offer an overview of cleaning equipment and supplies and a parent's perspective on home care.

Part V, on neurological concerns, includes a Special Issue featuring a parent's perspective on hydrocephalus; an updated chapter on home care of the infant with seizures, including expanded sections on the recognition, documentation, and management of seizures; and a revised chapter on hydrocephalus with both updated information and an expanded discussion of ongoing concerns families face.

Developmental and sensory concerns, in Part VI, are addressed in greater depth in this edition of the book. A Special Issue describes federally mandated early intervention services under Part H. A second Special Issue, written to parents, details approaches to normalization. An updated, expanded overview of development in the high-risk premature infant is provided, accompanied by a new chapter detailing the process of developmental assessment and intervention for this population. Updated chapters on hearing loss, speech and language development, and visual impairment complete the section.

Part VII of the text addresses additional concerns. A Special Issue discusses death in the home, and new chapters provide a detailed overview of home care for the infant or child who is HIV positive and an in-depth examination of genetic concerns for the home care professional.

Pediatric home care has never posed more challenges to nurses and families. Nurses play a pivotal role in any home care program through providing direct care, assessment, instruction, support, screening, referral, and case management. Each family plays a central role in caring for their child, as well as other family members, across many dimensions. It is my sincere hope that this edition of *Home Care for the High-risk Infant* will help smooth the path both to clinical competence and confidence for nurses caring for this population and to successful home care for families and children.

Elizabeth Ahmann, ScD, RN

Acknowledgments and Reviewers

Special thanks are due to my mother Margaret C. Ahmann, MLS, for her reference assistance; friends and neighbors Bob Sabbath and Ed Spivey for their assistance with computer diskettes; and Sheila Kelley for typing assistance on short notice; to my children, Sarah and Micah, for respecting "mommy's work time"; and, most of all, my husband, Richard Saviet, for his love, support & partnership that make it all possible.

I also wish to thank the following people who generously shared their time and expertise by reviewing one or more chapters for this second edition of the book:

Dolores Arroyo, OTR/L
Occupational Therapist
Mt. Ranier, Maryland

Anne M. Davis, MS, RD, CNSD
Assistant Professor of Pediatrics
Medical University of South Carolina Children's Hospital
Charleston, South Carolina

Elizabeth Grady, RRT
Clinical Specialist
Pediatric Home Ventilator Program
University of Michigan Medical Center
Ann Arbor, Michigan

Ruth Klug, MS, RN, PNP
Pediatric Nurse Practitioner
Vienna Pediatrics
Vienna, Virginia

Marie C. McCormick, MD, ScD
Professor and Chair
Department of Maternal and Child Health
Harvard School of Public Health
Professor of Pediatrics
Harvard Medical School
Cambridge, Massachusetts

Robert G. Meny, MD
Chief, SIDS Clinical Unit
Department of Pediatrics
University of Maryland Medical School
Baltimore, Maryland

Amy Purdy, RD, LD
Clinical Dietitian
Children's National Medical Center
Washington, DC

Jennifer Smith Stepanek
Parent of four children needing specialized medical care
and
Family-Professional Resource Specialist
Association for the Care of Children's Health
Bethesda, Maryland

Alicia Ward, MA, CCC-SLP
Speech-Language Pathologist
Hearing and Speech Center
Children's National Medical Center
Washington, DC

Ralph C. "Worth" Worthington, PhD
Associate Professor
Director, Division of Educational Development
Department of Family Medicine
School of Medicine
East Carolina University
Greenville, North Carolina

List of Contributors

Elizabeth Ahmann, ScD, RN
Consultant in Child and Family Health
Washington, District of Columbia
Senior Lecturer
Columbia University School of Nursing
New York, New York

Brenda Bird, RN, MSN
Department of Education
Children's Hospital of the King's Daughter
Norfolk, Virginia

Rachel Blinkoff, MA
Infant Educator
Children's National Medical Center
Center for Child Development
Washington, DC

Virginia L. Combs, RN, BSN
Nurse Manager
MCH Department
VNA of South Middlesex
Framingham, Massachusetts

B. Patrick Cox, PhD, CCC-A
Professor and Director
Graduate Studies in Audiology
Gallaudet University
Department of Audiology and Speech-Language Pathology
Washington, DC

Margaret W. Cox, RN, BSN, CCC-A
Associate Director of Home Care/Discharge Planning
Children's Home Health Care Services
Children's National Medical Center
Washington, DC

Karen Dixon
Parent
Washington, DC

Pamela L. Donaldson, RNC, MS, ARNP
Family Nurse Practitioner
Operation PAR, Inc.
St. Petersburg, Florida

Collette Duncliffe Driscoll, RN
Certified Pediatric Nurse
Children's Home Health Care Services
Children's National Medical Center
Washington, DC

Margie Farrar-Simpson, RN, MSN, CPNP
Private Pediatric Practice
Washington, DC

Christina Floyd, RN, BSN
Manager, Performance Improvement and Education
Children's Home Health Care Services
Children's National Medical Center
Washington, DC

Virginia C. Gebus, RN, MSN
Clinical Specialist for Nutrition Support
Children's National Medical Center
Washington, DC

Penny Glass, PhD
Developmental Psychologist
Director, Center for Child Development
Children's National Medical Center
Associate Professor of Pediatrics
The George Washington University Medical School
Children's National Medical Center
Washington, DC

Kathi Huddleston, RN, MSN
Pediatric Clinical Nursing Specialist
Consultant
Norfolk, Virginia

Lyn Ingersoll, MLS
Family Librarian
Children's National Medical Center
Washington, DC

Deirdre F. Jackson, MSN, CCRN, CPN
Pediatric Rehabilitation Clinical Nurse Specialist
Children's Specialized Hospital
Mountainside, New Jersey

Angela Jerome-Ebel, MSN, RN
Pediatric Clinical Nurse Specialist
Children's Home Health
Children's Hospital of the King's Daughters
Norfolk, Virginia

Kathleen Lipsi Klockenbrink, MA, EdS
Infant Educator/Consultant
St. Ismier, France

Ruth Klug, MS, RN, CPNP
Pediatric Nurse Practitioner
Vienna Pediatrics
Vienna, Virginia

Marian J. Kolodgie, MSN, CPNP
Department of Neurology
Children's National Medical Center
Washington, DC

Belinda Ledbetter, BA
Child Life Supervisor
Johns Hopkins Children's Center
Child Life Department
Baltimore, Maryland

Connie Lierman, RN, MSN
Nurse Team Leader
Children's Home Health Care Services
Children's National Medical Center
Washington, DC

Barbara L. Marino, RN, PhD
Nurse Researcher
Children's Hospital
Boston, Massachusetts

Nancy P. Miller, RNCS, MSN, PNP
Coordinator Special Care Infant Follow-up Program
Morristown Memorial Hospital
Center for Human Development
Morristown, New Jersey
Preceptor, PNP Students
Seton Hall University
South Orange, New Jersey

Doris Mitnick, MSN, ACSW, CCM
Department of Social Work
Children's Hospital of the King's Daughter
Norfolk, Virginia

Dorothy Page, MSN, RN-C
Pediatric Pulmonary and Cystic Fibrosis Center
University of Massachusetts Medical Center
Worchester, Massachusetts

Mary Rathlev, MSN
Program Manager/Educator
Project CHAMP
Children's National Medical Center
Washington, DC

Judy Rollins, MS, RN
Consultant
Rollins & Associates, Inc.
Georgetown University Medical Center
Washington, DC

Cindy Hylton Rushton, DNSc, RN, FAAN
Assistant Professor of Nursing
The Johns Hopkins University
Clinical Nurse Specialist in Ethics
The Johns Hopkins Children's Center
Baltimore, Maryland

Karen Patt Sachse, MSN, RN
Nurse Educator
Project CHAMP
Children's National Medical Center
Washington, DC

Barbara D. Schraeder, PhD, RN, FAAN
Assistant Nursing Director for Research and Evaluation
Thomas Jefferson University Hospital
Jefferson Medical College
Philadelphia, Pennsylvania

Ann Sher, ACSW, LICSW
Department of Social Work
Children's National Medical Center
Washington, DC

Jennifer Smith Stepanek
Parent of four children needing specialized medical care
   and
Family-Professional Resource Specialist
Association for the Care of Children's Health
Bethesda, Maryland

Janice Miller Theil, RN, BSN
Director of Clinical Services
Children's Home Health Care Services
Children's National Medical Center
Washington, DC

Margaret Wilson, MS, OT-R
(formerly) Occupational Therapist
Children's National Medical Center
Washington, DC

Lynette Wright, MN, RN
Clinical Nurse Specialist
Certified Genetics Counselor
Richlyn Associates
Assistant Professor
Emory University School of Nursing
Atlanta, Georgia

Contributors to the First Edition

The following authors contributed chapters to the first edition of this book, which have been revised by others for the current edition. The titles for revised chapters, when changed, are indicated in parentheses.

Elizabeth Ahmann, RN, MS, FNP contributed the following chapters: The Nursing Intake Process, Interviewing and Documentation (The Nursing Intake Process and the Plan of Care); Nutrition and Feeding of the High-risk Infant (Nutrition and Feeding of the Chronically Ill Infant); Home Care of the Infant Requiring Tube Feeding (Home Care of the Infant or Child Requiring Tube Feeding); Home Care of the Infant with Respiratory Compromise; Home Care of the Infant on an Apnea Monitor (Home Care of the Infant on a Cardiorespiratory Monitor); Home Care of the Infant Requiring Oxygen Therapy; Home Care of the Infant with a Tracheostomy (Home Care of the Infant or Child with a Tracheostomy); Home Care of the Infant Requiring Mechanical Ventilation; and Visual Impairment in the High-risk Infant (Visual Impairment in the Preterm Infant).

B. Patrick Cox, PhD and Elizabeth Ahmann, RN, MS, FNP contributed the chapter Hearing Impairment in the High-risk Infant (Hearing Loss in the High-risk Infant).

Jeannie O'Connor Egan, RN, MSN and Connie Jo Lierman, RN, MSN contributed the chapter Home Care of the Infant with Seizures.

Janice George, MSW, ACSW and Elizabeth Ahmann, RN, MS, FNP contributed the chapter Community Resources for the Family of the High-risk Infant.

Rebecca Ichord, MD contributed the following chapters: Profile of the High-risk Infant (Profile of the High-risk Premature Infant) and Developmental Issues in Care of the High-risk Infant (Overview of Developmental Issues).

Connie Jo Lierman, RN, MSN and Jeannie O'Connor Egan, RN, MSN contributed the chapter Home Care of the Infant with Hydrocephalus (Home Care of the Infant and Young Child with Hydrocephalus).

Sally McCarthy, MSN, RN contributed the chapter Discharge Planning for the High-risk Infant.

Teri Peck, BSN, CPNP contributed the chapter Siblings of Chronically Ill Children (Siblings of Children with Chronic Conditions).

Bonnie M. Simon, MA, CCC-SP contributed the chapter Speech and Language Development in the High-risk Infant (Speech and Language Development in the Chronically Ill Preterm Infant).

Additionally, Nancy Weinstock, MSW, ACSW contributed a chapter titled The Family of the High-risk Infant, which is not included in the second edition of the book.

Profile of the High-risk Premature Infant

Revised by Elizabeth Ahmann, ScD, RN

Rapid advances in neonatal intensive care have dramatically improved the survival rates of ever smaller premature infants. Before the 1980s, few infants with birth weights below 750 g were actively treated. Now, however, treatment of infants with birth weights of at least 500 g, or those born at 24 or more weeks gestation, or both, is accepted practice in North America (Hack et al., 1994). Improved survival has been effected through the use of aggressive, multisystem therapies requiring prolonged hospital stays. While survival rates have improved, the population of infants with ever-lower birth weights has an ever-higher incidence of neonatal morbidity and neurodevelopmental impairment during childhood. When these preterm infants are "ready" for discharge, parents frequently face complex home care demands for a multitude of medical and developmental concerns.

This chapter provides a profile of the high-risk premature infant. The discussion begins with a description of the infant population at risk for multiple long-term medical problems, and then proceeds to a review, system by system, of the most common chronic medical problems of prematurity.

DESCRIPTION OF THE POPULATION

Prematurity is defined as a gestational age of less than 37 weeks. Low birth weight (LBW) refers to a weight of less than 2,500 g—approximately 5½ lb—at birth. Very low birth weight (VLBW) premature infants weigh less than 1,500 g at birth, and extremely low birth weight (ELBW)

prematures weigh less than 1,000 g at birth. Some infants experience growth retardation during gestation and are called small for gestational age (SGA) at birth. Gestational age, rather than birth weight alone, is a better indicator of the medical problems an infant may face since these problems are directly related to the immaturity of various organ systems. However, various methods of determining gestational age can be in significant disagreement at early gestational ages (Hack et al., 1991).

The magnitude of the problem of prematurity can best be appreciated by considering its relative contribution to infant mortality and morbidity. In the United States, only 7% of all live-born infants are less than 2,500 g at birth (Statistical Abstract, 1993a). However, LBW infants account for an extremely high percentage of neonatal deaths, and VLBW itself accounts for the majority of neonatal deaths. The mortality risk increases directly as gestational age decreases: the mortality rate for infants born at less than 751 g, and surviving to neonatal intensive care unit (NICU) admission, is over 300% that of infants in general in the United States (Hack et al., 1991).

Nonetheless, advances in neonatal care have led to a steady improvement in the survival of premature infants. In 1960, the lower limit of viability was a birth weight of 1,000 g; now this figure is 500 g. In one recent study, based on NICU admissions (and excluding delivery room deaths), the survival rate was as follows: 34% for birth weights less than 750 g; 66% at 751 through 1,000 g; 87% at 1,001 through 1,250 g; and 93% at 1,251 through 1,500 g (Hack et al., 1991). Survival rates, if delivery room deaths were included, would be lower.

Morbidity is another indicator of the problems associated with this population. While the rates of many complications of prematurity vary from one institution to another, as a group, VLBW and ELBW infants require long periods of hospitalization, particularly if they have significant lung disease. During their first year of life, LBW infants are hospitalized twice as often, and VLBW infants four and one-half times as often as normal birth weight infants (Goldman & Goldman, 1992). Other measures of health and developmental morbidity persist into the school years, especially for VLBW and ELBW infants (Hack et al., 1992, 1993, 1994; Hille et al., 1994; McCormick, Brooks-Gunn, Workman-Daniels, Turner, & Peckham, 1992; McCormick, Gortmacker, & Sobol, 1990; Robertson, Etches, Goldson, & Kyle, 1992; Saigal et al., 1994a, 1994b; Saigal, Rosenblum, Szatmari, & Campbell, 1991). Among VLBW infants, the overall incidence of disability, including major and minor disability, has been estimated at 25% (Escobar, Littenberg, & Pettiti, 1991).

The impact of premature birth is unevenly distributed among groups of the United States population. For example, the incidence of LBW is much greater in blacks than whites (13.3% vs. 5.7%; Statistical Abstract, 1993b). In 1991, VLBW rates among blacks were three times that of whites (2.96% compared with 0.96%; U.S. Department of Health and Human Services, 1994). Teenage pregnancy, a low level of maternal education, a lack of prenatal care, and an abnormal obstetric history are other factors associated with an increased incidence of LBW. These socioeconomic factors translate into hard, cold reality for those planning and implementing home care services for this population. Plans for home care must take into account the infant's needs in the context of the home environment and the familial or parental resources and motivation to provide complex and demanding care.

MEDICAL DISORDERS OF PREMATURITY

The medical disorders of the premature infant occur because of both the immaturity of a multiplicity of organ systems and the invasive treatment technologies necessary to maintain the infant's viability. Problems may be encountered with every organ system at one time or another. In most cases, the dominant problems relate to respiratory disease and neurologic, gastrointestinal, and nutritional disorders. Some of these problems interact in complex ways, exacerbating chronic conditions. Table 1–1 summarizes the common medical disorders of the premature infant. It classifies the problems of each major organ system according to acute and chronic forms. It is by no means an exhaustive list. Rather, like the following discussion, it highlights the

Table 1–1 Common Medical Disorders of the Premature Infant

Organ system	Disorders	
	Acute	Chronic
Respiratory system	Respiratory distress syndrome Apnea of prematurity Pneumonia	Bronchopulmonary dysplasia Apnea of prematurity Tracheostomy Subglottic stenosis Croup syndromes Frequent respiratory infections
Cardiovascular system	Patent ductus arteriosus Cor pulmonale	Cor pulmonale
Central nervous system	Hypoxic brain damage Intraventricular hemorrhage Seizures	Neurodevelopmental disorders Hydrocephalus Seizures
Gastrointestinal system	Necrotizing enterocolitis Jaundice	Malabsorption syndrome Malnutrition Growth retardation
Hematologic system	Anemia	Anemia
Other	— Sepsis Meningitis Pneumonia	Hernias Retinopathy of prematurity Sepsis Recurrent respiratory and gastrointestinal infections

most common disorders that have a long-term impact on the infant's health care needs.

Respiratory Disorders

Acute Disease

The most common medical disorder related to prematurity is respiratory disease. The immature lung does not have the mechanical or biochemical characteristics necessary to provide for adequate exchange of oxygen and carbon dioxide. Because of this, hyaline membrane disease (HMD) or respiratory distress syndrome (RDS) develops shortly after birth, and treatment with supplemental oxygen and, frequently, mechanical ventilation becomes necessary. In a recent study of seven medical centers, 90% of infants born at 750 g to 1,000 g required assisted ventilation (Hack et al., 1991). Although these treatment measures are life-saving, their use is associated with occasional pneumothorax, tissue injury, and altered physiologic responses in the lung. Since approximately 1990, exogenous surfactant treatments have been used on some neonates to reduce the incidence of RDS (Horbar, Wright, Onstad, & the NKHD Neonatal Research Network, 1993).

Chronic Disease

When RDS is acute, the syndrome may evolve into a chronic picture of respiratory insufficiency called *bronchopulmonary dysplasia* (BPD). Infants with BPD have problems with excessive bronchial secretions, narrowed airways, and inefficient oxygen and carbon dioxide exchange. (See also Chapter 12.) In its most severe form, BPD necessitates continued mechanical ventilation. In less severe forms, it causes dependence on supplemental oxygen, decreased exercise tolerance, increased work of breathing, and increased susceptibility to infection. The impact of BPD on other organ systems is difficult to measure. However, it certainly alters the energy economy of the infant as a whole, with wide-ranging implications for feeding, nutrition, growth, cardiovascular function, behavior, and possibly neurodevelopmental status.

Most infants with BPD slowly grow out of their worst symptoms of chronic lung disease through a careful balance of several treatment strategies. These strategies aim to maintain adequate nutrition, minimize cardiac decompensation, and prevent respiratory infection. With time, for most infants, the healing of damaged tissue occurs more rapidly than does continued tissue damage, and healthy new lung tissue develops. However, in a small minority of infants, the respiratory insufficiency is so severe, and so compromises cardiac function, that a steady downhill progression occurs, typically ending in death.

Lung disease in the premature infant affects respiratory function in other ways also. Prolonged and repeated endotracheal intubations may injure the upper airway, leading to subglottic stenosis (narrowing or constriction). This problem may not be manifested until a viral infection is superimposed, causing a croup-like syndrome that can be life threatening. Some infants showing a prolonged dependence on mechanical ventilation will require a tracheostomy both to provide for maximal control of the airway and to avoid permanent upper airway damage. The small lower airways, or bronchioles, may also be damaged, giving rise to a disorder that closely resembles asthma. Symptoms of reactive airways disease may be present all the time in more severe cases or only intermittently in less severe cases. Current data suggest that reactive airways disease will occur in 15% to 20% of VLBW/ELBW survivors (McCormick et al., 1992). Symptoms are precipitated by viral infection, exercise, or exposure to irritants such as cigarette smoke in the air.

Respiratory disorders involving the large or small airways may have their onset at variable times, beginning in the nursery or not appearing until months after discharge. These disorders differ from the croup and asthma syndromes in normal children in that they generally occur at a younger age, are more severe and more frequent, and last longer. Although the majority of survivors of prematurity-related lung diseases do not develop the most severe forms of these late-onset respiratory complications, they do have a greatly increased vulnerability. Some studies suggest that some survivors have abnormalities of respiratory function, such as evidence of obstructive airway changes, persisting into adolescence (Unwin, 1993). More common is the well-documented susceptibility of VLBW children to severe symptoms with respiratory syncytial virus (RSV)-bronchitis in the first year or so of life.

Cardiovascular Disorders

Acute Disorder

Disorders of the cardiovascular system are closely linked to respiratory disorders in the premature infant. In the transition from intrauterine to extrauterine life, the cardiovascular system rapidly adapts to channel blood flow appropriately to lung and systemic circuits. This channeling requires closure of the ductus arteriosus, a vessel that connects the two circuits in utero. In the premature infant, because of lung immaturity, respiratory physiology is abnormal, and this vessel remains patent; that is, it is a patent ductus arteriosus (PDA). In one recent study, symptomatic PDA was noted in 25% of VLBW infants (Hack et al., 1991). PDA increases the workload of the heart and exacerbates respiratory insufficiency already imposed by the immature pulmonary mechanisms. In some infants, treatment can be effected medically. In others, PDA ligation, a very safe and effective surgical procedure, may be required.

Chronic Disorder

A more difficult management problem is posed by the chronic cardiac insufficiency, cor pulmonale, or congestive heart failure caused by chronic lung disease (see Chapter 12). When cor pulmonale occurs, the heart becomes enlarged, pumps less efficiently, and causes total body fluid build-up. The infant can then tolerate less fluid intake and frequently develops metabolic disturbances owing to fluid imbalances and necessary diuretic drug therapy. The cardiac dysfunction and both fluid and metabolic imbalances in turn further compromise pulmonary function. Additionally, both congestive heart failure and the medications used in its management have implications for nutritional management of the preterm infant. In infants with chronic cardiac insufficiency, recovery of normal cardiac function parallels recovery of pulmonary function.

Apnea

Acute and Chronic Condition

One of the most common cardiorespiratory disorders in this population is apnea of prematurity. This type of apnea (described in Chapter 13) has many causes, all of which relate to immaturity and ineffectiveness of the brain's respiratory control centers. Apnea may occur independently of other heart or lung disease, or it may be the presenting symptom of a correctable condition, such as anemia or sepsis. In the absence of a treatable cause, apnea is attributed to brain immaturity. When apnea occurs, a transient decrease in blood oxygen levels results, frequently accompanied by bradycardia, or slowing of the heart beat. Although episodes of apnea are sometimes self-limited, in many premature infants some intervention is needed. Intervention ranges from light tactile stimulation, to vigorous stimulation, to oxygen administration, to use of bag and mask. In most cases, the infant eventually outgrows apnea. While there is substantial debate on the utility of home monitoring for apnea, some centers encourage continuous cardiorespiratory monitoring in conjunction with a readiness on the part of the caregivers to provide immediate intervention, including cardiopulmonary resuscitation (CPR), if needed.

Neurologic and Neurodevelopmental Disorders

Acute Disorders

Acute disorders include intraventricular hemorrhage, hypoxic brain damage, and brain infections or meningitis.

Intraventricular hemorrhage (IVH) refers to bleeding in the brain. IVH arises from fragile immature blood vessels whose integrity has been disturbed by some other disorder of prematurity, such as hypoxia, low blood pressure, or infection. The incidence of IVH has decreased since the 1970s and is estimated at 30% to 50% among preterm infants born less than 1,500 g birth weight or earlier than 32 weeks gestational age (Minarcik & Beachy, 1989). The acute manifestations of IVH are highly variable, ranging from clinically "silent" episodes to a sudden, life-threatening syndrome of hemorrhagic shock, seizures, and coma. IVH also ranges in severity according to the extent of brain substance involved and is graded as I or II (mild), III (moderate), or IV (severe). Ultrasound diagnostic scanning can be used to pinpoint the exact location and severity of the bleed and to monitor its resolution. In a recent study, at least 45% of VLBW infants were found to have evidence of IVH on head ultrasound (Hack et al., 1991). The incidence increases with decreasing birth weight. However, only a very small percentage of VLBW infants with IVH have severe bleeds, and less severe bleeds are rarely associated with long-term sequelae. Fewer than 10% of cases of mild IVH result in hydrocephalus; however, with grade IV IVH, 50% to 60% of preterm infants die, and 65% to 100% of survivors develop hydrocephalus (Minarcik & Beachy, 1989).

More recent research suggests that neonatal disorders of the white matter of the brain, noted as echodensities or echolucencies on ultrasound, may be more predictive of long-term sequelae such as cerebral palsy than is IVH (McCormick, personal communication, May 30, 1995).

Hypoxic brain damage, also called *asphyxial brain damage*, can occur as a result of fetal distress during labor or delivery, lung disease, or cardiovascular instability, among other factors. Hypoxic brain injury is much more difficult to quantify than hemorrhage, partly because there are no discrete laboratory or radiologic indicators, and partly because the premature infant's neurologic system responds in nonspecific and global ways to brain injury.

Chronic Disorders

The chronic forms of brain disorders in premature infants include hydrocephalus, microcephaly, seizure disorders, cerebral palsy, and other neurodevelopmental handicaps. The symptoms of chronic brain disorders may be subtle and diffuse, including poor feeding, irritability or drowsiness, altered muscle tone and movements, delayed acquisition of developmental skills, and poor school functioning.

Treatment for hydrocephalus often begins with aggressive medical management, through the use of drugs that decrease brain fluid production or through the use of ventricular or spinal taps. If ventricles continue to enlarge, surgical treatment—the placement of a ventriculoperitoneal shunt—may be required (Gardner & Hagedorn, 1992; see also Chapter 18 in this book.) In either case, therapy requires close monitoring for effectiveness and complications. Similarly, therapy for seizure disorders must be closely monitored (see Chapter 17).

Assessment for neurodevelopmental handicaps (see Chapters 19 and 20) begins in the intensive care nursery and helps to define the starting point for the infant as normal, suspect, or abnormal for gestational age. Perhaps most salient for home care of the infant is the transient, symmetric hypertonia experienced in the first 12 to 18 months. This hypertonia has implications for the aquisition of early motor skills as well as the timing of the assessment of more permanent sequelae (McCormick, personal communication, May 30, 1995).

Other chronic neurosensory impairments include blindness, hearing impairment, and the more common disorders of refraction and eye muscles. (Visual and auditory concerns are addressed in detail in Chapters 23 and 21, respectively.)

Gastrointestinal Disorders

Acute Disorders

VLBW premature infants are also susceptible to gastrointestinal (GI) diseases. Immaturity of the digestive system, combined with an increased vulnerability to tissue injury imposed by cardiorespiratory instabilities, can lead to necrotizing enterocolitis (NEC). NEC is a destructive infection of the small bowel, which can be associated with signs of severe illness, such as excessive bleeding, cardiovascular collapse, or respiratory decompensation. In a recent study, 6% of VLBW infants developed NEC (Hack et al., 1991). In milder forms, NEC can be managed with medications and supportive measures; in the severe forms, however, surgery to remove the most damaged portions of the bowel is required. According to the data of Hack and colleagues (1991), surgery may be required in up to 46% of affected VLBW infants. Such surgery usually leads to a temporary interruption of the intestinal passage by way of an ileostomy, a surgically created connection through the abdominal wall. After some months of healing and growth, another surgical procedure can usually be performed to restore a normal passageway through the colon and rectum.

Chronic Disorders

Whether or not intestine is removed, the infant with NEC will lose permanently some length of functional intestine; this can have an impact on the infant in several ways. First, during the acute phase, intravenous feeding, also called *total parenteral nutrition* (TPN), is necessary for a variable period of time. Second, it may take much longer than normal to advance the amount and/or frequency of formula feedings to a point that sustains growth. In the chronic stage, the infant is highly susceptible to symptoms of malabsorption, such as diarrhea and abdominal discomfort, which are triggered more easily by dietary changes or intestinal infections. All of these factors combined may contribute to feeding disorders and delayed physical growth. Failure to thrive may be seen commonly associated with short bowel syndrome, resulting from surgery to remove tissue damaged by NEC (Gardner & Hagedorn, 1991). Long-term use of TPN may be required in some cases (see Chapter 11).

Another gastrointestinal disorder common preterm infants with bronchopulmonary dysplasia chronic cardiac insufficiency (CHF), or neurologic ab malities is gastroespohageal reflux. In addition to compr mising nutritional intake, this condition may compromise marginal pulmonary function in some infants with BPD and has been associated with laryngospasm/bronchospasm leading to apnea and death.

Perhaps the most common problems compromising feeding of the VLBW infant at home are easy fatiguability and poor state regulation. These problems affect the length and frequency of feeding required and result in the expenditure of a great deal of parental effort to ensure adequate caloric intake. Chapter 9 discusses nutrition and feeding in detail.

As with chronic lung disease, the minor diseases of normal infancy can lead to major setbacks for the infant with chronic GI sequelae of prematurity. An intestinal virus that would cause a few days of vomiting in a normal infant may, in the premature infant with a history of NEC, lead to a rapid and severe dehydration, rehospitalization, and prolonged recovery time to reach an acceptable feeding regimen and growth rate.

Infections

Acute and Chronic

Infections constitute another group of diseases to which the premature infant is highly susceptible. Every aspect of the infant's immunologic system is immature, including antibody production, cellular immune defenses, and even the integrity of simple barrier defenses such as skin and mucous membranes. Superimposed is the dramatically increased exposure to infectious agents necessitated by the use of invasive treatment devices such as umbilical vessel catheters, endotracheal tubes, and chest tubes. When infections do occur in the unstable neonate, they tend to be serious systemic infections of the blood (sepsis), the brain (meningitis), or the lungs (pneumonia). Sepsis occurs in approximately 17% of VLBW infants and meningitis in 2% (Hack et al., 1991). Thus, infections can prolong the neonatal hospital stay by virtue of both the symptoms they produce and the treatment they require. Once at home, the prematurely born infant with chronic disease may suffer more profound and lasting effects than a healthy term infant from intercurrent infections such as bronchiolitis and pneumonia (Hagedorn & Gardner, 1989).

Hematologic Disorders

Acute and Chronic

Premature infants suffer from a variety of hematologic disorders. These include both inadequate numbers and the cellular components of the white blood cells, and platelets. in red blood cells are most com- . Anemia may be caused by mul- w iron stores due to premature d bone marrow due to other dis- ....r hemorrhage or necessary labo- ...v.y studies, infections, and poor nutrition. The symptoms will vary according to the infant's other problems. There may be unexplained lethargy, irritability, an exacerbation of underlying cardiac or lung disease, or even no symptoms. Most premature infants will require some iron supplementation after discharge from the nursery. Chronic disorders involving other components of the blood system are infrequent and are not further discussed here.

Other Disorders

Premature infants as a group have a disproportionate prevalence of congenital defects. These various defects can pose challenges for health and development, and may create additional stressors for families (Ballard, 1988). Although a less global concern, premature infants have, for unknown reasons, a very high prevalence of inguinal hernias. In many cases, these require surgical repair, which usually proceeds without complication. Ideally, surgery is planned through close cooperation between medical and surgical experts in order to minimize the surgical risks resulting from such chronic sequelae of prematurity as malnutrition and lung disease.

In addition, premature infants can suffer from a unique eye disorder called *retinopathy of prematurity* (ROP), also known as *retrolental fibroplasia* (RLF). The severity ranges from mild abnormalities in eye structure, causing near-sightedness, to more severe damage to the retina, causing severe visual impairment or even blindness. Routine medical care should thus include timely screening for ROP in all premature infants exposed to supplemental oxygen (see Chapter 23). Strabismus is also more common in the low birth weight population.

LONG-TERM CHRONIC SEQUELAE OF PREMATURITY

Most of the research in neonatal medicine focuses on disease processes occurring within the intensive care nursery setting. Unfortunately, the hazards of prematurity do not end at the time of discharge. While many individual and composite measures suggest that the quality of life for ELBW and VLBW survivors is less favorable than for term infants of normal birth weight, the majority of survivors do have a quite acceptable quality of life. This section describes the impact of chronic neonatal disorders among survivors at school age.

Several difficulties arise in attempting to present general data on chronic morbidity for preterm infants. First, reports from a single study or institution may have limited generalizability due to variations in treatment approaches among institutions and geographic regions (Hack et al., 1991; McCormick, 1994). Second, metaanalyses (analyses of numerous studies and reports) suffer from lack of consistency in definitions of terms and conditions across studies. Third, practice changes in neonatology change the frontiers of survival so that by the time research is published, it may be outdated (McCormick, 1989). Fourth, much of the outcomes research has been limited to children under 2 years of age, an age at which many dimensions of functioning cannot accurately be assessed or predicted (McCormick, 1989). School-age outcomes reported in recent research are based on survivors of neonatal intensive care technologies of 5 to 10 years ago; outcomes may be more optimistic for current survivors (Saigal et al., 1994a). Additionally, substantial heterogeneity in outcomes suggests that factors other than birth weight or gestational age influence health status (McCormick, 1989); socioeconomic disadvantage is a primary concern. Finally, early intervention programs have been shown to have beneficial effects on the outcomes for at least some premature infants (McCormick, 1993).

Despite limitations in obtaining and presenting data on chronic morbidity for survivors of prematurity, the information is of great interest to clinicians and families. McCormick (1989) reviewed studies published since 1970 to examine long-term outcomes of VLBW infants across a number of dimensions. More recently, several researchers have presented regional data on school-age outcomes in children born ELBW and VLBW, in some cases comparing findings to term normal birth weight (NBW) control groups. These various sources will be summarized here; however, for reasons detailed above, the data should be considered indicative, but not prescriptive, of chronic problem areas among VLBW and ELBW survivors.

Pulmonary Morbidity

Surviving premature infants who develop BPD are at the greatest risk of later pulmonary problems. While symptoms of overt distress may resolve during the first 2 years of life, high rates of respiratory illness may persist into later life. Bader and colleagues (1987) reported persistent respiratory symptoms in 8 of 10 ten-year-olds who had a previous diagnosis of BPD. Other studies have reported a substantially higher prevalence of respiratory conditions in the first 8 to 10 years of life of ELBW and VLBW survivors as compared to NBW groups (Hack et al., 1993; McCormick et al., 1992).

Physical Growth

Chronic gastrointestinal disorders diminish in severity in the first several years of life. As gastrointestinal and pulmonary problems lessen in severity, improved growth can be seen.

VLBW children may achieve normal head circumference by late infancy, but studies at 3, 4, 8, and 10 years indicate they remain small for age in measures of height and weight (McCormick, 1989; Hack et al., 1993). Significantly more ELBW than VLBW children are small in head circumference, weight, and height at school age than normal birth weight controls (Hack et al., 1994).

Neurological Impairment

Premature LBW infants experience higher rates of neurological and neurosensory impairments than NBW infants. While major neurological sequelae are substantially less common than minor sequelae, birth weight is associated with the prevalence of each. One study of 8 to 10-year-old children reported neurological sequelae (including epilepsy, hydrocephalus, cerebral palsy, and mental retardation) in the following ranges: 4.5% among NBW, 6% among LBW, 17% among VLBW, and 20% among ELBW infants (McCormick et al., 1992). Sensorineural problems were reported in approximately 20% of NBW, 24% of LBW, 23% of VLBW, and 41% of ELBW infants (McCormick et al., 1992).

Among older surviving children, the percentage with severe impairment may be in the relatively low range. Hack and colleagues (1994) reported that 15% of ELBW children and 8% of VLBW children had major neurosensory impairments at school age. Rates of cerebral palsy are quite low: less than 10% of VLBW infants, 10% of ELBW, and 20% of infants born less than 800 g (McCormick, personal communication, May 30, 1995). Minor neurological findings in older children may be associated with learning and behavior disorders.

Functional Status

Functional status, measured by limitations in activities of daily living (ADLs), is one measure of long-term morbidity. McCormick, Stemmler, Bernbaum, and Farran (1986) found that 35% of surviving VLBW children were reported as limited in one or more ADLs during the preschool period. In a more recent study, McCormick and colleagues (1992) found that LBW was also associated with limitations in ADL among 8 to 10-year-olds. Almost half of ELBW, 34% of VLBW, 26% of LBW, and 17% of NBW infants had limitations in one or more ADLs.

Utilizing a measure of quality of life based on functional limitations in multiple health attributes, Saigal and colleagues (1994a, 1994b) have reported that, at 8 years of age, ELBW children have a great variability in quality of life and lower mean scores for quality of life than children born at NBW, and only 14% of ELBW survivors have perfect health as compared to 50% of NBW children.

Educational Achievement

In general, intelligence quotients (IQs) of VLBW children, measured by standard tests, fall within the normal range but slightly lower than controls of NBW (McCormick, 1989). However, the risk of an IQ lower than 85 is significant for VLBW and ELBW infants; almost half of all ELBW infants have an IQ less than 85 (McCormick et al., 1992).

School problems occur at higher rates than among NBW children; reported rates vary from 24% to 58%, depending on the definition of the term. Significantly more VLBW and ELBW children require special education placements than full-term NBW children. VLBW birth seems to have independent effects on school performance (Hack et al., 1992; Saigal et al., 1991). Other related factors include major discrepancies on subscale scores of the IQ test (McCormick, 1989); hyperactivity (McCormick et al., 1990; Saigal et al., 1991); temperament (Schraeder, Heverly, & Rappoport, 1990); and, perhaps most importantly, socioeconomic disadvantage (Hack et al., 1992; McCormick et al., 1992; Saigal et al., 1991).

When compared with children born at term, ELBW infants have significantly poorer scores on numerous measures, including tests in the following areas: cognitive ability; language; fine motor, gross motor, and visual motor skills; memory; attention; and academic achievement and performance (Hack et al., 1994). In many areas, ELBW infants also score significantly lower than VLBW infants. Studies are not in agreement regarding whether differences in measures of learning disorders and academic achievement remain significant when children with neurologic compromise and subnormal intelligence are excluded from the comparison (Hack et al., 1994; Saigal et al., 1991; Saigal et al., 1994a).

Behavioral/Mental Health

Behavioral and mental health outcomes in VLBW survivors have received little research attention. However, reports of alterations in VLBW infant social interactions and an increased risk of certain behavior problems in infancy and at 5 years among LBW infants suggest reason for concern (Golding & Butler, 1986; Hoy, Bill, & Sykes, 1988). Recently, Hack and colleagues (1994) found scores on measures of behavior and social skills to be significantly lower among ELBW than VLBW or term infants; severe behavior problems were also more prevalent among ELBW than VLBW or term infants. McCormick and colleagues (1992) found that significantly more behavior problems were reported by parents of VLBW and ELBW infants than NBW controls. However, no differences were found in affective health (depression and anxiety).

CONCLUSION

The full impact of higher rates of mortality and morbidity among preterm infants has not been measured. It is reasonable to expect that for the infant's family, family functioning in general, and adaptation to the premature infant's special needs in particular, would be a great challenge. The potential certainly exists for timely and competent home-based intervention to reduce the disproportionate burden related to both illness and death among these infants and to stress among their families.

The success of the field of home care for the high-risk infant will be enhanced by linking service to research. Experienced practitioners should be encouraged to ask critical questions and to document the results of their interventions so that their contribution to the total service network can be appropriately recognized. One of the greatest current challenges in neonatal medicine is posed by the explosion of knowledge and treatment technology. For example, newer methods of treating lung disease of premature infants such as extracorporeal membrane oxygenation (ECMO) are being used, intrauterine surgery for life-threatening birth defects is being attempted, and organ transplantation for malformations such as congenital heart disease or renal failure is being performed in younger infants than ever before. As increasingly sophisticated technology promotes survival from more severe illness, so too must the long-term care of the survivors be supported.

In relation to these technologies, more and more infants will require specialized, long-term, multidisciplinary supportive care and monitoring. Paradoxically, the development of these technologies occurs in an era of shrinking health dollars and a transfer of care from expensive acute care facilities to more cost-effective ambulatory and home care settings. The long-term success of new medical technologies will depend in part on the extension of specialized knowledge and skills to settings such as the home.

REFERENCES

Bader, D., Kamos, A.D., Lew, C.D., Platzker, A.C.G., Stabile, M.W., & Keens, T.G. (1987). Childhood sequelae of infant lung disease: Exercise and pulmonary function abnormalities after bronchopulmonary dysplasia. *Journal of Pediatrics, 110,* 693–699.

Ballard, R.A. (1988). *Pediatric care of the ICN graduate.* Philadelphia, PA: W.B. Saunders.

Escobar, G.J., Littenberg, B., & Pettiti, D.B. (1991). Outcome among surviving very low birthweight infants: A meta analysis. *Archives of Disease in Childhood, 66,* 204–211.

Gardner, S.L., & Hagedorn, M.I. (1991). Physiologic sequelae of prematurity: The nurse practitioner's role. Part V. Feeding difficulties and growth failure. *Journal of Pediatric Health Care, 5*(3), 122–134.

Gardner, S.L., & Hagedorn, M.I. (1992). Physiologic sequelae of prematurity: The nurse practitioner's role. Part VII. Neurologic conditions. *Journal of Pediatric Health Care, 6*(5), 263–270.

Golding, J., & Butler, N.R. (1986). The end of the beginning. In N.R. Butler & J. Golding (Eds.), *From birth to five: A study of the health and behavior of Britain's 5-year olds.* Elmsford, NY: Pergamon Press.

Goldman, D.J., & Goldman, S.L. (1992). Prematurity. In P.L. Jackson & J.A. Vessey (Eds.), *Primary care of the child with a chronic condition.* St. Louis, MO: Mosby-Year Book.

Hack, M., Breslau, N., Aram, D., Weissman, B., Klein, N., & Borawski-Clark, E. (1992). The effect of very low birthweight and social risk on neurocognitive abilities at school age. *Developmental and Behavioral Pediatrics, 13*(6), 412–420.

Hack, M., Horbar, J.D., Malloy, M.H., Tyson, J.E., Wright, E., & Wright, L. (1991). Very low birth weight outcomes of National Institute of Child Health and Development Neonatal Network. *Pediatrics, 87*(5), 587–597.

Hack, M., Taylor, H.G., Klein, N., Eiben, R., Schatschneider, C., & Mercuri-Minich, N. (1994). School-age outcomes in children with birth weights under 750 g. *The New England Journal of Medicine, 331*(12), 753–759.

Hack, M., Weissman, B., Breslau, N., Klein, N., Borawski-Clark & Fanaroff, A.A. (1993). Health of very low birthweight children during their first eight years. *The Journal of Pediatrics, 122*(6), 887–892.

Hagedorn, M.I., & Gardner, S. (1989). Physiologic sequelae of prematurity: The nurse practitioner's role. Part I. Respiratory issues. *Journal of Pediatric Health Care, 3*(6), 288–297.

Hille, E.T.M., den Ouden, A.L., Bauer, L., van den Oudenrijn, C., Brand, R., & Verloove-Vanhorick, S.P. (1994). School performance at nine years of age in very premature and very low birthweight infants: Perinatal risk factors and predictors at five years of age. *Journal of Pediatrics, 125*(2), 426–434.

Horbar, J.D., Wright, E.C., Onstad, L., & the NICHD Neonatal Research Network. (1993). Decreasing mortality associated with the introduction of surfactant therapy: An observational study of neonates weighing 601 to 1300 grams at birth. *Pediatrics, 92*(2), 191–196.

Hoy, E.A., Bill, S.J., & Sykes, D.H. (1988). Very low birthweight: A long term developmental impairment? *International Journal of Behavioral Development, 11,* 37–67.

McCormick, M.C. (1989). Long-term follow-up of infants discharged from neonatal intensive care units. *JAMA, 261*(12), 1,767–1,772.

McCormick, M.C. (1993). Has the prevalence of handicapped infants increased with improved survival of the very low birthweight infant? *Clinics in Perinatology 20*(1), 263–277.

McCormick, M.C. (1994). Survival of very tiny babies: Good news and bad news [Editorial]. *New England Journal of Medicine, 331*(12), 802–803.

McCormick, M.C., Brooks-Gunn, J., Workman-Daniels, K., Turner, J., & Peckham, G.J. (1992). The health and developmental status of very low-birth weight children at school age. *JAMA, 267*(16), 2,204–2,208.

McCormick, M.C., Gortmacker, S.L., & Sobol, A.M. (1990). Very low birth weight children: Behavior problems and school difficulty in a national sample. *Journal of Pediatrics, 117,* 687–693.

McCormick, M.C., Stemmler, M.M., Bernbaum, J.C., & Farran, A.C. (1986). The very low birth weight transport goes home: Impact on the family. *Pediatrics, 7,* 217–223.

Minarcik, C.J., & Beachy, P. (1989). Neurologic disorders. In G.B. Merenstein & S.L. Gardner (Eds.), *Handbook of neonatal intensive care* (2nd ed.). St. Louis, MO: C.V. Mosby.

Robertson, C.M.T., Etches, P.C., Goldson, E., & Kyle, J.M. (1992). Eight year school performance, neurodevelopmental, and growth outcomes of neonates with bronchopulmonary dysplasia: A comparative study. *Pediatrics, 89*(3), 365–372.

Saigal, S., Feny, D., Furlong, W., Rosenbaum, P., Burrows, E., & Torance, G. (1994a). Comparison of the health-related quality of life of extremely low birthweight children and a reference group of children at age eight years. *Journal of Pediatrics, 125,* 418–425.

Saigal, S., Rosenblum, P., Stoskopf, B., Hoult, L., Furlong, W., Feeny, D., Burrows, E., & Torance, G. (1994b). Comprehensive assessment of the health status of extremely low birthweight children at eight years of age: Comparison with a reference group. *Journal of Pediatrics, 125,* 411–417.

Saigal, S., Rosenblum, P., Szatmari, P., & Campbell, D. (1991). Learning disabilities and school problems in a regional cohort of extremely low birthweight (< 1000 G) children: A comparison with term controls. *Developmental and Behavioral Pediatrics, 12*(5), 294–299.

Schraeder, B.D., Heverly, M.A., & Rappoport, J. (1990). Temperament, behavior problems, and learning skills in very low birth weight preschoolers. *Research in Nursing and Health, 13*(1), 27–34.

(1993a). Table 102, Low birthweight and births to teenage mothers and births to unmarried women: States, 1980 and 1990. Statistical Abstract of the United States (113th ed.). Lanham, MD: Bernan Press.

(1993b). Table 98, Live births by race and type of Hispanic origin: Selected characteristics: 1985 & 1990. Statistical Abstract of the United States (113th ed.). Lanham, MD: Bernan Press.

Unwin, J.F. (1993). Long term sequelae of bronchopulmonary dysplasia: A review of the literature. *Physiotherapy, 79*(9), 633–636.

U.S. Department of Health and Human Services. (1994). *Health United States 1993*. (DHHS Publication No. PHS 94-1232). Hyattsville, MD: Author.

Part I

Family Issues and Family-Centered Care

Ethical Issues in Home Care

Cindy Hylton Rushton, DNSc, RN, FAAN

Caring for children in their homes may create unique ethical challenges for nurses and other providers. Home care providers may struggle with various conflicting values as they attempt to benefit patients and families while avoiding undue burden, particularly when their values are different from the child's or parents'. Providers may also struggle with issues of confidentiality and privacy as they attempt to create therapeutic relationships in a home setting. Issues of noncompliance or child abuse or neglect may also generate ethical tensions. In today's health care environment, there may be conflicts about access and financing of certain services. As nurses and others assume the role of case managers, many will experience with greater intensity the tension that results between advocating what is best for the patient from a clinical standpoint versus what is best for the institution and the bottom line.

Home care professionals must be proactive in identifying and developing mechanisms to address current and future ethical issues. Becoming knowledgeable about the nature of the ethical tensions and striving to articulate ethically sound justifications for nursing actions will be essential.

ADVOCACY AS A FRAMEWORK

Addressing ethical concerns begins with a robust understanding of the advocacy role of professionals. Advocacy means assisting patients or, in the case of children, their surrogates, to make informed choices and to act in the child's best interest. Advocacy is not acting instead of someone else, and it should not be confused with "rescuing" someone. (At times, providers become confused about the boundaries of their advocacy role. They may begin to make decisions for the patient instead of with the patient. This paternalistic approach usurps patients', or their surrogates', authority to act for themselves.) The appropriate advocacy role involves advising, sharing specific information, and offering recommendations to enable patients to make their own decisions. It embodies an authentic model of shared decision making that presumes equal power and authority.

The goal of advocacy is to enable the patient, family, and significant others to adjust to the changes in health of their loved one in their own unique way. Nursing actions are directed toward maximizing the control exerted by the patient and family while assisting them in this process (Rushton & Reigle, 1993). In this way, the nurse advances the sense of personhood, self-worth, and dignity of the child and family, consistent with a family-centered philosophy of care. Successful advocacy demands that nurses be engaged in trusting relationships with patients and families and appreciate their unique values and life goals within the context of the their culture, religion, and belief system.

DEVELOPING MORAL SENSITIVITY

Moral sensitivity refers to the individual's ability to recognize that a moral problem or conflict exists. In the broadest sense, it means being attuned to the moral dimensions of the situation: being able to recognize what is morally significant in the context of a particular situation. Such attunement can be enhanced by paying attention to one's emotional barometer and intuitions and using such information to articulate the moral tensions and questions.

Clarifying personal and professional values and societal norms is a related and essential prerequisite for sound ethical deliberations. Values clarification involves a process of examining one's personal and professional values. It includes examining the origin of certain values and testing their application in various clinical situations. Nurses should engage in an ongoing process of self-reflection and assessment of their values regarding life, death, disability, relationships, and the like.

ETHICAL PRINCIPLES

Ethical theories and principles provide a foundation for ethical analysis and moral reasoning. Theories that focus on consequences (such as utilitarian or virtue theories) or on duties (such as deontologic theories) each guide the reasoning process. Ethical principles, such as beneficence (doing good), nonmaleficence (avoiding or minimizing harm), veracity (telling the truth), justice (ensuring fairness or equality), fidelity (keeping promises), or autonomy (deciding for oneself) are commonly applied to clinical situations. Principles provide an organizing framework by offering a guide for organizing and understanding ethically relevant information in a troubling situation. They also suggest direction, propose how to resolve competing claims, and often supply the reasons for justifying moral action. Ethical principles are universal in nature, but they are not absolute: even these principles have exceptions in certain situations.

A moral framework for decision making involving children includes the principles of beneficence and its corollary nonmaleficence, respect for persons, and justice. Based on the principles of beneficence and nonmaleficence, health care professionals seek to promote the well-being of their patients and to reduce or alleviate harm. Choices among alternative treatments should benefit the infant or child, and clearly outweigh the associated burdens and harms. Even though children are not autonomous or self-determining, respect for persons is still required in decisions about their care since the lives of children have unique meaning. To treat children with respect is to acknowledge and value who they are outside of a medical context, rather than to treat them only according to how professional goals and values are advanced. Justice demands that individual patients be treated fairly and that decisions are not made based on subjective criteria such as race, age, sex, diagnosis, or socioeconomic status.

Decisions about what will benefit individual patients should be separated from decisions about how society will allocate its health care resources generally. While nurses have a moral mandate to be involved individually and collectively to promote efforts to meet the health needs of groups of patients and of society generally (American Nurses Association, 1985, 1991; Fowler, 1989), such decisions are not suited for the bedside but, rather, belong within the context of a larger societal debate. However, when marginally beneficial treatments are considered, health care providers have a responsibility to allocate resources in a fair, fiscally responsible manner (Rushton & Glover, 1990).

IMPLEMENTING MORAL DECISIONS

The nurse must give priority to moral values and then carry out moral decisions. This is often the most difficult dimension of the process. Often, the actions of nurses are not discrete actions to solve the problem but rather take the form of facilitating, educating, advocating, communicating, and understanding the values, preferences, and goals of others. Effective advocacy, therefore, must be viewed as an evolving process rather than an isolated event.

INSTITUTIONAL SUPPORT FOR ADVOCACY

Nurses must be the catalysts for creating an environment where advocacy is expected and nurses are encouraged to bring ethical issues to the forefront (Levine-Ariff & Groh, 1990). Opportunities for nurses to gain expertise in ethical decision making should be incorporated into orientation and continuing education offerings. Nurses, physicians, and administrators must share responsibility for formulating policies and practices that support the role of the nurse as patient advocate. Nurses must have direct access to ethics consultants and to ethics committee consultation in order to be effective patient advocates. The Joint Commission on Accreditation of Healthcare Organizations (Joint Commission), for example, has developed standards for home care (Joint Commission, 1995). Like hospitals, home care agencies must establish formal mechanisms to address ethical concerns.

REFERENCES

American Nurses Association. (1985). *Code for nurses with interpretive statements.* Kansas City, MO: American Nurses Publishing.

American Nurses Association. (1991). *Nursing's agenda for health care reform.* Kansas City, MO: American Nurses Publishing.

Fowler, M. (1989). Social advocacy. *Heart and Lung, 18,* 97–99.

Joint Commission on Accreditation of Healthcare Organizations. (1995). *Accreditation manual for home care.* Oakbrook Terrace, IL: Author.

Levine-Ariff, J., & Groh, D. (1990). *Creating an ethical environment.* Baltimore, MD: Williams & Wilkins.

Rushton, C.H., & Glover, J. (1990). Involving parents in decisions to forego life-sustaining treatment for critically ill infants and children. *AACN Clinical Issues in Critical Care Nursing, 1*(1), 206–214.

Rushton, C.H., & Reigle, J. (1993). Ethical issues in critical care nursing. In M. Kinney, D. Packa, & S. Dunbar (Eds.), *AACN's clinical reference for critical-care nursing* (8–27). St. Louis, MO: Mosby.

Caring for Substance-Abusing Mothers and Their Infants

Pamela A. Donaldson, RNC, MS, ARNP

From a public health standpoint, perinatal substance abuse is in epidemic proportions, the results of which are devastating to families and totally preventable. A recent National Institute on Drug Abuse survey estimates that 5.5% of women used some illicit drug during pregnancy (Leshner, 1994). In addition, 18.8% of women used alcohol, and 20.4% smoked cigarettes at some time during pregnancy. Rates of illicit drug use were higher in women who were not married, had less than 16 years of formal education, and relied on some public source of funding to pay for their hospital stay. Rates of cocaine use during pregnancy were highest among African-American women, while alcohol and cigarette use were highest among Caucasian women. Because of their specialized training and willingness to work in homes and communities, nurses provide a significant contribution to public health by proper identification, referral, and treatment of perinatal substance abuse.

Ideally, the process of identification, intervention, referral, and treatment of a mother's substance abuse problem begins prenatally with a goal of intervention in the substance abuse problem for the current or subsequent pregnancies. Unfortunately, the reality is that if substance-abusing mothers are identified, identification often occurs postnatally, via positive urine drug screens or self-report, after the birth of a substance-exposed newborn. At that time, hospital and child protection policies are enacted. Often, the infant is sent home with a close relative, sometimes to a foster home, and sometimes with the parents. History and type of drug use, family support, and mother's willingness to seek drug treatment are generally determining factors in the infant's placement.

Even if the infant is sent home with a relative instead of the mother, the mother may actually live in the same household. This can create a disturbing and threatening environment for the infant. Therefore, recognizing unsafe and undesirable living conditions due to a current drug or alcohol problem in the home is an important nursing intervention. Signs of concern may include the following:

- an unkempt house
- little or no food in the refrigerator
- signs of illicit drug paraphernalia, alcohol and tobacco use
- signs of personal hygiene neglect
- signs of maternal depression: flat affect, excessive sleeping, crying, etc.
- harsh or derogatory language when talking to or referring to one's infant
- lack of attention to the infant's needs
- poor maternal–infant interaction.

The approach to working with substance-abusing mothers should be three-pronged: (1) support the mother and assist in referring her for treatment; (2) identify special needs of the infant; (3) provide special training and support to caregivers as needed. (Note: Excellent protocols developed by The Center for Substance Abuse Treatment [U.S. Department of Health and Human Services, 1993a, 1993c] are available free of charge from the National Clearinghouse for Drug and Alcohol Information, P.O. Box 2345, Rockville, MD 20852-2345, 800-729-6686.)

First, the mother needs support and guidance from non-judgmental health care providers. While the mother is in the throes of addiction, she will be unable to care properly for her infant. However, a safe and nurturing environment can be provided for the infant if drug/alcohol treatment, family support, and quality nursing care are put in place.

Referral to an appropriate drug/alcohol treatment program is essential and can be accomplished by the nurse familiarizing herself with community programs. Both public and private programs may be available. Options include inpatient hospital detoxification, day-treatment, outpatient, and residential programs. For communities without a drug treatment program, a referral can be made to Alcoholics or Narcotics Anonymous. In this way, the client has a support system for her continued sobriety.

While the mother is receiving help from drug and alcohol treatment specialists, home health nurses can do much in the area of fostering infant well-being. Perinatal drug use can result in either fetal loss or preterm birth. In both prematurely born and term infants, withdrawal from depressant drugs may occur (U.S. Department of Health and Human Services, 1992). Medical complications related to drug use during pregnancy are wide ranging. Substance-exposed infants are at higher risk for congenital birth defects, low birth weight, respiratory difficulties, sudden infant death syndrome, and developmental delays (Bauchner & Zuckerman, 1990; Suguihara & Bancalari, 1991; U.S. Department of Health and Human Services, 1993b).

Other areas of concern related to infant care include poor feeding ability, frantic sucking, inability to self-console, irritability, and sleep disturbances (Redding & Selleck, 1993). Nurses can assist caregivers with these behaviors. While research on long-term effects to infants of prenatal drug exposure are inconclusive, ongoing research suggests early intervention postnatally can significantly improve infant growth and development outcomes (Coletti et al., 1992; U.S. Department of Health and Human Services, 1993c; Weiner & Morse, 1994).

Third, recent research on teaching mothers of cocaine-exposed infants cardiopulmonary resuscitation has shown that mothers can learn this life-saving skill and increase in self-esteem as a result (Messmer, Meehan, Gillam, White, & Donaldson, 1993). Additionally, parenting strategies teaching comforting techniques for irritable substance-exposed newborns may decrease the child abuse potential of mothers lacking coping strategies and improve maternal–infant interaction (Donaldson, 1991; Freier, Griffith, & Chasnoff, 1991; Redding & Selleck, 1993).

Problems of substance-abusing women and their infants are complex and challenging. Based on the most recent National Institute on Drug Abuse prevalence survey, the odds are increasing for home care nurses to encounter perinatally addicted women (Leshner, 1994). With two lives at stake, it becomes even more important for nurses to develop expertise in this area.

REFERENCES

Bauchner, H., & Zuckerman, B. (1990). Cocaine, SIDS, and home monitoring. *Journal of Pediatrics, 117,* 904–906.

Coletti, S.C., Hughes, P.H., Landress, H.J., Neri, R.L., Sicilian, D.M., Williams, K.M., Urmann, C.F., & Anthony, J.C. (1992). PAR village: Specialized intervention for cocaine abusing women and their children. *Journal of Florida Medical Association, 79,* (10), 701–705.

Donaldson, P.L. (1991). *Improving interactions of cocaine using mothers and their prenatally cocaine-exposed infants by using comforting techniques.* Unpublished master's thesis, University of South Florida, Tampa.

Freier, M.C., Griffith, D.R., & Chasnoff, I.J. (1991). In utero drug exposure: Developmental follow-up and maternal–infant interaction. *Seminars in Perinatology, 15*(4), 310–316.

Leshner, A. (1994, September). *Drug addiction research and the health of women.* Paper presented at the meeting of the National Institute on Drug Abuse, National Institute of Health, Tyson's Corner, VA.

Messmer, P., Meehan, R., Gillam, N., White, S., & Donaldson, P. (1993). Teaching infant CPR to mothers of cocaine positive infants. *Journal of Continuing Education in Nursing, 24,* 217–220.

Redding, B.A., & Selleck, C.S. (1993). Perinatal substance abuse: Assessment and management of the pregnant woman and her children. *Nurse Practitioner Forum, 4*(4), 216–223.

Suguihara, C., & Bucalari, E. (1991). Substance abuse during pregnancy: Effects on respiratory function in the infant. *Seminars in Perinatology, 15*(4), 302–309.

U.S. Department of Health and Human Services. (1992). *Maternal drug abuse and drug exposed children: Understanding the problem* (DHHS Publication No. ADM 92-1949). Washington, DC: U.S. Government Printing Office.

U.S. Department of Health and Human Services, Public Health Service, Substance Abuse and Mental Health Services Administration, Center for Substance Abuse Treatment. (1993a). *Improving treatment for drug-exposed infants: Treatment improvement protocol (TIP) series* (DHHS Publication No. SMA 93-2011). Rockville, MD: Author.

U.S. Department of Health and Human Services, Public Health Service, Substance Abuse and Mental Health Services Administration, Center for Substance Abuse Prevention. (1993b) *Pregnancy and exposure to alcohol and other drug use* (DHHS Publication. No. ADM 93-2040). Rockville, MD: Author.

U.S. Department of Health and Human Services, Public Health Service, Substance Abuse and Mental Health Services Administration, Center for Substance Abuse Treatment. (1993c). *Pregnant, substance-using women: Treatment improvement protocol (TIP) series* (DHHS Publication No. SMA 93-1998). Rockville, MD: Author.

Weiner, L., & Morse, B.A. (1994). Intervention and the child with FAS. *Alcohol Health and Research World. 18*(1), 67–73.

Chapter 2

The Family and Home Care: Common Challenges and Resources

Elizabeth Ahmann, ScD, RN

Parenthood is challenging. Balancing the needs of children and parents, juggling the demands of keeping employment and running a household: even in the best of circumstances, a tremendous amount of energy is required both to manage daily life and to guide the children and family toward a satisfactory future. Sailtross (1986) describes the hospital discharge of a "healthy" preterm infant as being highly stressful for families. The family of the infant with multiple ongoing problems faces many additional and special challenges. This chapter provides an overview both of these challenges and of the strengths and resources families can utilize in meeting the challenges.

CHALLENGES FACED BY FAMILIES

Each family is unique: their hopes, dreams, values, needs, and strengths are uniquely theirs. For this reason, families will vary in how they adjust to and manage home care of their infant or child with special needs. Cultural factors, family structure, family values, economic factors, and personal resources are among the many factors that can shape the experience. The complexity of the child's care requirements and the technology utilized also influence family impact (Fleming et al., 1994). Chapter 4 will provide a framework for collaboration with families in individualizing care.

At the same time, families who face chronic illness or disability in a child often face many similar challenges. Understanding common challenges families face when providing home care for their children is important for several reasons. Assisting families in assessing their needs is more effective when nurses have a context for understanding common needs and challenges. Effective anticipatory guidance is based on understanding common issues families face. Similarly, while care plans must be individualized, providing education, information, referrals, and support are facilitated by awareness of the array of challenges a family may face. Nurses who are aware of the themes and experiences common to families providing home care are better poised to assist families in this endeavor.

Adjustment to the Preterm Birth

Even before a family brings their infant with special needs home, they have faced many challenges. Shock and distress are common reactions to preterm birth. Without preparation, seeing the infant and the neonatal intensive care unit (NICU) can be frightening and overwhelming. Preterm and very low birth weight newborns look very different from healthy term newborns. Furthermore, the tubes, machines, lights, and isolettes are foreign to most parents.

Many types of responses to the birth of an infant with a disabling condition have been identified in the literature. Twenty years ago, Drotar and colleagues (1975) described seven stages in the grief reaction following the birth of such an infant: (1) shock, (2) denial, (3) sadness, (4) anger, (5) anxiety, (6) adaptation, and (7) reorganization. Intertwined with these stages are times of ambivalence, numbness, disbelief, bereavement, a search for hope, intense reexperiencing of expectations for the idealized child, and a final stage of acceptance of and commitment to the infant. Even earlier, Olshansky (1962) described an experience of chronic sorrow that parents face after the birth of a mentally retarded child. Current research and clinical experience confirms that even well-functioning families of children with special needs, developmental delay, or chronic medical problems can experience chronic or recurrent sorrow (Clubb, 1991).

The NICU Experience

In a study of families of ventilator-dependent children, 82% of families had concerns related to the hospitalization experience (Aday, Aitken, & Wegener, 1988). In the NICU, families face concerns about their infants' survival. Parents with little or no prior experience with the health care system may be faced both with a great deal of overwhelming information and the need to make life and death decisions. They must learn to negotiate the maze of health care providers in the NICU and to somehow carve out a role for themselves. Neither becoming nor being a parent in the NICU setting is an easy experience.

Preparation for Home Care

As the infant stabilizes, parents are expected to participate increasingly in initially learning and then providing the infant's care in preparation for eventual transition home. The amount of information, the number of skills, and the degree of judgment that parents must acquire is immense. For most parents, this occurs while balancing the many other demands of employment, marriage, a household, other children, and transportation.

The parents' emotional responses to the experience should not be underestimated. Parental reactions to the idea of home care may vary. Almost 3 out of 10 families (27%) in a study of children dependent on mechanical ventilation spontaneously expressed concerns about their ability to provide home care for the child (Aday et al., 1988).

Initial Adjustment to Home Care

Research on families of infants on home apnea monitors suggests that the first 4 to 6 weeks on a home monitor may be the most stressful to a family (Ahmann, 1992). Clinical experience suggests that families of children with complex care needs or other technologies also face a stressful transition and adjustment period (Lewis, Alford-Winston, Billy-Kornas, McCaustland, & Tachman, 1992). As one mother said, "It was a big adjustment to realize that the doctor wasn't just outside the door if a problem arose. I had to find out I was capable of taking care of him with no one at home to help. The first month I thought I'd never be able to do it. The first few weeks were chaos—then I got it down to a system" (Ahmann 1986, p. 3).

The length of the adjustment period may vary based on the child's condition(s), stability, the family's preparedness and flexibility, and supportive resources in the community. For the first 4 to 6 weeks after hospital discharge, frequent home visits, 24-hour availability of a nurse by telephone, and/or additional hourly nursing may be instrumental in assisting families with the transition to home care.

The Child's Health and Development

Several studies suggest that even after discharge from the hospital, the child's health and development continue to be areas of great concern for parents (Aday et al., 1988; Diehl, Moffitt, & Wade, 1991). Specific concerns include uncertainty about diagnoses and prognosis, equipment functioning, medication schedules, infant interactions, feeding, developmental intervention, long-term development, educational placements, and rehospitalizations. The unpredictable and intense medical crises that can arise and uncertain long-term prognoses can be particularly challenging and can lead to a feeling of loss of control over daily life (Jessop & Stein, 1985). As one father said, "No matter what training you've had, there is always the unexpected" (Ahmann, 1986, p. 11).

To some extent, nursing interventions, such as parent education, anticipatory guidance, and referrals to specialists or community services, may assist parents in addressing these concerns. Both parent-to-parent networking and the use of stress-management skills can support parents as they deal with the daily and long-term uncertainty of caring for their child with special needs.

Family Structure and Functioning

Children with complex care needs require a great deal of their parents' time and energy. The intensity of their care needs has a reverberating effect on all family members. Diehl and colleagues (1991) conducted focus group interviews of 80 caregivers of 98 medically complex/technology-dependent children. These families were concerned about the deterioration they experienced in family life. One father stated, "To be honest, I feel I lost my wife somewhere down the line. Because of [our son's] health problems, our relationship has fallen off track" (Ahmann, 1986, p. 11).

Families report that the lack of ability to function spontaneously as a family unit affects family life in arenas as diverse as grocery shopping and taking vacations. Little time as a couple, sibling jealousy and embarrassment, lack of public acceptance, and lack of respite care are frequently mentioned concerns (Ahmann, 1986; Diehl et al., 1991; Thorpe, 1987). Quint, Chesterman, Crain, Winkleby, and

Boyce (1990) report that family closeness may be affected in families who have cared for a ventilator-dependent child for 2 or more years. Family impact may also be affected by family finances, the social and physical environment of the family, and the comprehensiveness of the child's discharge plan (Wegener & Aday, 1989).

Nurses can play an important role in reducing the stress experienced by families by advocating with insurance companies and health maintenance organizations (HMOs) for adequate home care coverage; by finding or creating sources of respite care in the community; and by training family friends or relatives to provide occasional care for the child, thereby giving parents a much-needed break.

Isolation

Caring for a child with complex medical problems and/or dependence on medical technology can be an isolating experience for a family (Baley, Hancharik, & Rivers, 1988; Klein-Berndt, 1991; Perrin, Shayne, & Bloom, 1993). Few friends are likely to have shared a similar experience. Extended family members and friends may be reluctant to visit the home because of fears or anxiety related to the medical equipment. Babysitters or respite care can be difficult to locate for a child with special needs (Diehl et al., 1991). Parents understandably may be hesitant to leave the child with anyone but a nurse. Additionally, taking the child with an unstable condition or cumbersome equipment on outings may be unmanageable for many families. Aday and colleagues (1988) report that 18% of families in their study mentioned feeling either trapped or unable to leave their home. Six percent mentioned feeling isolated and alienated from the outside world. The majority of mothers in Thorpe's (1987) study reported, simply, "We don't go out."

While support groups have been cited by families as helpful (Diehl et al., 1991), difficulty finding an appropriate support group and difficulty finding babysitting often limit attendance (Diehl et al., 1991; Perrin et al., 1993). An often-overlooked avenue for support is the use of parent support networks to make one-to-one links between experienced families and families with a newly diagnosed child (Worthington, 1992). If nurses can help families to find these connections, families may not have to be deprived of the rich instrumental and emotional benefits of a social support network.

Managing Time

The demands of providing and orchestrating the care of a child with multiple or complex medical problems are extraordinary. Many parents have described the challenge of time management involved in providing for the child's needs around the clock and attending to personal and family needs. Families have expressed this concern in the following ways:

- "The hardest thing is getting up around the clock to suction him, do what I need to do to take care of him" (Sterling, 1990, p. 58).
- "You have to be very planned and organized" (Diehl et al., 1991, p. 177).
- "Physicians make these kinds of schedules and they don't take into account what it does to the rest of the family" (Diehl, et al., 1991, p. 176).

Based on their research, Leonard, Johnson, and Brust (1993) report an association between the time devoted to a disabled child's care and the perception by caregiving parents that they needed more help or could not manage much longer. While many of the demands of care are inevitable, in some situations nurses can assist families to normalize care requirements and adjust schedules for medication and care procedures to reduce unnecessary burden.

Family Member Health

Family members' sleep may be disrupted by many factors, including the immature sleep patterns of the preterm infant, machine alarms, the schedule for medications and care, anxiety about the child's breathing, and the frequent lack of nighttime nursing coverage. As one mother put it, "You never do sleep well" (Thorpe, 1987, p. 125).

A related issue is the experience of symptoms of depression that may result from sleep deprivation, the burden of care, isolation, and/or unresolved feelings about the child's health status. Poor health among mothers of infants on apnea monitors and with other conditions has also been reported (Ahmann, Meny, Wulff, & Fink, 1993).

Nurses should encourage mothers to seek appropriate care for any health or mental health concerns. Assisting families in normalizing schedules, especially in reducing or eliminating night-time doses of medication when possible, can also promote better sleep. Nursing care, respite care, household help, and other efforts to reduce the burden on the primary caregiver can be helpful as well.

Privacy

One mother of a ventilator-dependent child described feeling invaded by the help she knows her son needs:

> I quit work when Chris was born. I got used to being home all day by myself. Then all of a sudden [when he came home] the nurses were here. Therapists four times a week. Ventilator company one time a week and other people in and out. I have no time anymore for nothing. It's hard to accept no time all day I'd be alone. Sometimes it gets on your nerves. Sometimes I get so aggravated. (Ahmann, 1986, p. 5)

There is a lack of agreement in two studies reporting data on the issue of privacy. In a study of pediatric home care, Quint and colleagues (1990) found that 12 of 17 families they interviewed (71%) experienced a lack of privacy with their spouse, and 7 (41%) reported a lack of privacy with their children. However, Aday and colleagues (1988) report that only 6% of families had concerns about privacy. Privacy concerns were attributed to having nurses in the home.

Thomas's research (1986) identified several family concerns and preferences regarding privacy. These include having care providers respect confidentiality of data and communications, respect (without criticism) family lifestyles, remove themselves from matters unrelated to the child's direct care, and respect a family's right to define private areas of the home. As Thomas explains, "Families simply wish to function, to the extent possible, as normal families within the confines of their refuge, the home" (Thomas, 1987, p. 50). Chapter 4 addresses these issues in greater detail, providing suggestions and guidance for nurses working with families in the home.

Financial Burden

Financial concerns are a challenge facing many families (Leonard et al., 1993; Quint et al., 1990; Sterling, 1990; Wegener & Aday, 1989). Quint and colleagues (1990) surveyed 18 northern California families with ventilator-dependent children and found that every family described extra out-of-pocket expenses related to home health care. Fifteen of them spent $1,000 or more for essential home care needs in the 12 months preceding the survey. Wegener and Aday (1989) found that for 138 families of ventilator-assisted children, family finances were the most powerful predictor of family impact and caregiver stress. Stress was high among families who viewed their present financial situation as a serious problem and among those with a large number of out-of-pocket expenses remaining from the hospital stay. One parent explained it simply: "Money—our finances are terrible. We have a hard time paying for everything" (Sterling, 1990, p. 58).

In the case management role, nurses can help families advocate for improved coverage of home care expenses and can direct families to other potential sources of financial assistance when appropriate. Chapter 7 reviews both strategies and resources that can help ease financial concerns for many families.

Long-term Care and Concerns

In a study of families with children dependent on home mechanical ventilation, Quint and colleagues (1990) found that the primary caregiving parents who had provided home care for longer than 2 years had significantly lower scores on a scale measuring coping than did caregivers providing care for 2 years or less. The authors suggest several explanations: the sustained caregiver role, a long-term vision of dependency, uncertainty about the child's future, and exhaustion. Chronic or recurrent sorrow also affects many families of children with special needs (Clubb, 1991).

STRENGTHS AND CAPABILITIES

There is no doubt that caring for medically fragile children is challenging to families, but families also utilize a great wealth of resources, strengths, and capabilities in meeting the challenges. Based on a study of families with infants on home apnea monitors, Ahmann, Wulff, and Meny (1992) concluded that the "majority of families in supportive monitoring programs . . . cope well with the demands and stresses of home monitoring and . . . function capably in many aspects of family life" (p. 72).

Home care nurses can assist families to recognize their own strengths and build on them. Families can utilize their strengths to promote successful adaptation, to engage in effective problem-solving, and to provide for the best possible care for their child and the family unit as a whole. Recognizing and utilizing strengths are key to empowerment and success. Many strengths and capabilities that promote family coping will be reviewed here.

Family Beliefs about the Value of Home Care

Families have reported that their beliefs about and commitment to home care make a substantial difference in the success of a home care plan. In their comprehensive study of children who were ventilator-assisted or had severe respiratory disabilities, Aday and colleagues (1988) found the following:

- 32% of families felt their own beliefs about home care were their best preparation for the challenges of home care;
- 21% felt the caregiver's inner strength and personal commitment to having the child home were the best preparation;
- 20% mentioned the belief that home care was a better and more normal environment for the child;
- 10% of families felt that their love for the child was their best preparation for providing home care. (p. 276)

Internal Family Strengths

Families draw on their internal family strengths in successfully managing home care. Preexisting family or marital cohesion predicts positive family adaptation to caring for a chronically ill or technology-dependent child (Ahmann et al., 1993; Desmarez, Blum, Montauk, & Kahn, 1987). Youngblut, Brennan, and Swegart (1994) interviewed families of medically fragile children and found that, despite the tendency to worry about many things, a number of family strengths were supportive. These included trust in each other, shared values and beliefs, few conflicts, ability to express feelings, family pride, family loyalty, and the belief that things work out well for them. In addition, single parents having a child with multiple medical problems must have a great deal of personal inner strength as well as a supportive network of relatives, friends, and service providers (Clements, Copeland, & Loftus, 1990). Regardless of family structure, nurses can help families recognize and build on their inherent strengths.

Intimate Knowledge of the Child and Family

It is essential to recognize that the family is the center and the constant in the child's world, while professionals move in and out of that world (Shelton & Stepanek, 1994). The family's intimate knowledge of the child is critical to the development of a successful home care plan (Bishop, Woll, & Arango, 1993). Several studies have indicated parental frustration that health care providers fail to incorporate parental observations in the plan of care (Diehl et al., 1991; McNeil, 1992).

Like other parents, the parents of a child who is chronically ill or disabled care not only for the child's medical problems, but for the totality of the child's "well being, happiness and progress" (Leff & Walizer, 1992, p. 30). Similarly, the family is most intimately aware of the needs of all family members and how these must be balanced for home care to be successful. Parents bring this information and expertise to collaborative partnerships with nurses and other professionals.

Knowledge and Skill

Parental ability to care for the child at home is based on acquiring the necessary knowledge and skills. Parents, themselves, cite the importance of this process (Sterling, 1990). Aday and colleagues (1988) report that 42% of families felt that an excellent discharge training process was their best preparation for home care. Observation and participation in care prior to discharge was cited as most important by 28%, and the specific aspects of care learned (e.g., trach care, cardiopulmonary resuscitation [CPR], etc.) were cited by 26%.

Several studies point to a desire by families to have more information about their child's medical problems (42%), treatment prescribed (28%), available programs and services (56%), community resources (61%), and information

related to home care and future expectations (Walker, Epstein, Taylor, Crocker, & Tuttle, 1989; Diehl et al., 1991).

Providing information is a key role of the home care nurse and an essential step in empowering families. Nurses can also assist family members in developing the skills required to obtain successfully the type(s) of information they wish to gather from physicians and other professionals.

Social Support

Social support, both instrumental (physical) and emotional, has been repeatedly identified in the literature as an important feature moderating the effects of stressful events and challenging experiences (Crnic et al., 1983; Crnic, Greenberg, & Slough, 1986; Dunst, Trivette, & Cross, 1986). This seems to hold true for families having children with chronic illness. Ahmann and colleagues (1993) found that low satisfaction with available social support predicted poor family functioning among families of infants on home apnea monitors. Conversely, high satisfaction with social support predicted better family outcomes. The five areas of family life affected were (1) parental health, (2) parental role restriction, (3) relationship with spouse, (4) marital satisfaction, and (5) social isolation. In another study, mothers of chronically ill infants identified both physical and psychological aspects of social support as an important resource (Sterling, 1990).

Nurses can help families identify and effectively utilize their personal and professional support networks. Because most families have little experience managing as complex a situation as they face when providing home care, parents may welcome suggestions regarding both how they could involve friends or relatives in helping the family and what assistance they can expect from various professional resources. Nurses can also facilitate parental efforts to build networks for parent-to-parent support.

Flexibility and Adaptability

Because of the many and changing demands of caring for a medically fragile child, a family's ability to adapt lifestyle choices and alter family member roles contributes to the success of home care (Knafl & Deatrick, 1990). Physical changes in the family's home are often required as well, varying from simple rearrangements of furniture to accommodate equipment and supplies to remodeling the house itself. Some families move to be closer to a major medical center.

At the same time, some families of children with chronic illness or disability face major limitations on important choices. For example, because many health insurance plans do not cover preexisting conditions, parental career opportunities may be limited. Additionally, because many families organize a network of care providers that includes the extended family, the family may be reluctant to move and disrupt the network (R.C. Worthington, personal communication, November 17, 1994).

Values and Meaning

Cultural traditions give families "a sense of stability and support from which they draw comfort, guidance, and a means of coping with the problems of daily life" (McCubbin, Thompson, Thompson, McCubbin, & Kaston, 1993, p. 1,063). These traditions may become even more important to families having a child with a serious illness or disability. Cultural traditions, culturally determined child-rearing values and methods, and culturally derived responses to illness are strengths that families draw upon in the care of their children (Adams, 1990; Ahmann, 1994).

Family values and beliefs may be central in successful coping (Able-Boone & Stevens, 1994). Some parents of disabled children draw on their faith for support. Others must reconsider their beliefs in order to find meaning in the experience of the child and family. For example, Affleck and Tennen (1991) report that mothers who actively sought meaning for the NICU experience were less distressed.

A family's own traditions and beliefs should be a central part of the plan of care. Nurses can elicit family concerns and preferences regarding the child's care and can encourage family involvement in the process of assessment and planning, intervention, and evaluation of the home care plan. (See Chapter 4.)

Coping Strategies

Lazarus and Folkman (1984) define coping as "constantly changing cognitive and behavioral efforts to manage specific external and/or internal demands that are appraised as taxing or exceeding the resources of the person" (p. 141). Coping abilities may wax and wane over time in relation to the child's condition and other factors affecting the family.

Coping strategies take many forms. Sterling's (1990) research on mothers of chronically ill infants indicates that mothers felt that coping strategies related to stress reduction were important to them. Ray and colleagues (1993) report that coping mechanisms most useful to parents of technology-dependent children included maintaining family strength, maintaining an optimistic outlook, and getting tasks done. Youngblut and colleagues (1994) identified a number of commonly used coping strategies of families with medically fragile children (see Exhibit 2–1).

Coping strategies are important in that they promote successful adaptation to the challenges of chronic illness (Patterson & Geber, 1991). When necessary, over time or in response to specific challenges or stressors, new coping strategies can be learned by families (Knafl & Deatrick, 1990). When appropriate, nurses can facilitate a family's

---

Exhibit 2–1 Coping Strategies of Families with Medically Fragile Children

1. Internal strengths
   Knowing that we have the power to solve major problems
   Accepting that difficulties occur unexpectedly
   Showing that we are strong
   Knowing that we have the strength to solve our problems
   Having faith in God
2. Social support strategies
   Sharing difficulties with a relative
   Seeking advice from relatives
   Seeking encouragement and support from friends
   Asking neighbors for favors and assistance
   Seeking information and advice from families who faced similar problems
3. Professional support strategies
   Seeking information and advice from family physician
   Seeking advice from a member of the clergy
   Seeking professional counseling and help
   Seeking assistance from community agencies

Source: Adapted from *Pediatric Nursing,* Vol. 20, No. 5, p. 467, with permission of Jannetti Publication, Inc., Pitman, New Jersey, © 1994.

---

identification of its coping skills and the acquisition of new skills as necessary.

CONCLUSION

Home care poses many challenges to families. Several studies suggest that the greatest stress is experienced by families with the greatest caregiving burden (Fleming et al., 1994; Ray et al., 1993). Nonetheless, most families cope successfully with the challenges of home care, utilizing a range of intra- and interpersonal strengths and a variety of coping mechanisms.

Nurses can assist families when necessary to understand the challenges they face and ways they can apply their strengths to promote successful adaptation. Nurses can empower families by acknowledging family strengths and coping mechanisms (Pokorni, 1992). Through education, support, and referral to community resources, nurses can help families build their skills and best meet the needs of the child and family. A family-centered approach to home care nursing, described in detail in Chapter 4, encourages the family's central role in the care of the child and builds models of parent–professional collaboration that can foster successful home care.

REFERENCES

Able-Boone, H., & Stevens, E. (1994). After the intensive care nursery experience: Families' perceptions of their well being. *Children's Health Care, 23*(2), 99–114.

Adams, E.V. (1990). *Policy planning for culturally comprehensive special health care services.* Washington, DC: Bureau of Maternal and Child Health, U.S. Department of Health and Human Services. Also available from: CEDEN Family Resource Center, 1208 E. 7th St., Austin, TX 78702.

Aday, L.A., Aitken, M.J., & Wegener, D.H. (1988). *Pediatric home care: Results of a national evaluation of programs for ventilator assisted children*. Chicago, IL: Pluribus Press.

Affleck, G., & Tennen, H. (1991). The effect of newborn intensive care on parents' psychological well being. *Children's Health Care, 20,* 6–14.

Ahmann, E. (1986). *"It's a whole new world": Home care of a medically fragile child: The perspective of three families*. Unpublished manuscript. The Johns Hopkins University School of Hygiene and Public Health.

Ahmann, E. (1992). Family impact of home apnea monitoring: An overview of research and its clinical implications. *Pediatric Nursing, 18*(6), 611–616.

Ahmann, E. (1994). "Chunky stew": Appreciating cultural diversity while providing health care for children. *Pediatric Nursing, 20*(3), 320–324.

Ahmann, E., Meny, R.G., Wulff, L., & Fink, R.J. (1993). Home apnea monitoring and risk factors for poor family functioning. *Journal of Perinatology, 13*(4), 310–318.

Ahmann, E., Wulff, L., and Meny, R. (1992). Home apnea monitoring and disruptions in family life: A multidimensional controlled study. *American Journal of Public Health, 82*(5), 719–722.

Baley, J.E., Hancharik, S.M., & Rivers, A. (1988). Observations of a support group for parents of children with severe bronchopulmonary dysplasia. *Developmental and Behavioral Pediatrics, 9*(1), 19–24.

Bishop, K.K., Woll, J., & Arango, P. (1993). *Family/professional collaboration for children with special health needs and their families*. Burlington, VT: Department of Social Work, University of Vermont.

Clements, D., Copeland, L., & Loftus, M. (1990). Critical times for families with a chronically ill child. *Pediatric Nursing, 16*(2), 157–161, 224.

Clubb, R. (1991). Chronic sorrow: Adaptation of parents with chronically ill children. *Pediatric Nursing, 17*(5), 461–466.

Crnic, K.A., Greenberg, M.T., Ragozin, A.S., Robinson, N.M., & Basham, R.B. (1983). Effects of stress and social support on mothers and preterm infants. *Child Development, 54,* 209–217.

Crnic, K.A., Greenberg, M.T., & Slough, N.M. (1986). Early stress and social support influences on mothers and high risk infants functioning in late infancy. *Infant Mental Health Journal, 7,* 19–33.

Desmarez, C., Blum, D., Montauk, L., & Kahn, A. (1987). Impact of home monitoring for sudden infant death syndrome on family life. *European Journal of Pediatrics, 146,* 159–161.

Diehl, S.F., Moffitt, K.A., & Wade, S.M. (1991). Focus group interview with parents of children with medically complex needs: An intimate look at their perceptions and feelings. *Children's Health Care, 20*(3), 170–178.

Drotar, D., Baskiewicz, A., Irvin, N., Kennell, J., & Klaus, M. (1975). The adaptation of parents to the birth of an infant with a congenital malformation. *Pediatrics, 56,* 710–716.

Dunst, C.J., Trivette, C.M., & Cross, A.H. (1986). Mediating influences of social support: Personal, family and child outcomes. *American Journal of Mental Deficiency, 90,* 403–417.

Fleming, J., Challela, M., Eland, J., Hornick, R., Johnson, P., Martinson, I., Nativio, D., Nokes, K., Riddle, I., Steele, N., Sudela, K., Thomas, R., Turner, Q., Wheeler, B., & Young, A. (1994). Impact on the family of children who are technology dependent and cared for in the home. *Pediatric Nursing, 20*(4), 379–388.

Jessop, D.J., & Stein, R.E.K. (1985). Uncertainty and its relation to the psychological and social correlates of chronic illness in children. *Social Science and Medicine, 20,* 993–999.

Klein-Berndt, S. (1991). Bronchopulmonary dysplasia in the family: A longitudinal case study. *Pediatric Nursing, 17*(6), 607–611.

Knafl, K.A., & Deatrick, J.A. (1990). Family management style: Concept analysis and development. *Journal of Pediatric Nursing, 5*(1), 4–14.

Lazarus, R.S., & Folkman, S. (1984). *Stress, appraisal and coping*. Springer Publishing.

Leff, P.T., & Walizer, E.H. (1992). *The healing partnership: Parents, professionals & children with chronic illness and disabilities*. Cambridge, MA: Brookline Books.

Leonard, B.J., Johnson, A.L., & Brust, J.D. (1993). Caregivers of children with disabilities: A comparison of those doing "OK" and those needing more help. *Children's Health Care, 22*(2), 93–105.

Lewis, C.C., Alford-Winston, A., Billy-Kornas, M., McCaustland, M.D., & Tachman, C.P. (1992). Care management for children who are medically fragile/technology-dependent. *Issues in Comprehensive Pediatric Nursing, 15,* 73–91.

McCubbin, H.I., Thompson, E.A., Thompson, A.I., McCubbin, M., & Kaston, A.J. (1993). Culture, ethnicity, and the family: Critical factors in childhood chronic illness and disabilities. *Pediatrics, 91*(5), 1,063–1,070.

McNeil, D. (1992, March). *Uncertainty, waiting and possibilities: Becoming a mother in the NICU*. Paper presented at the National Association of Neonatal Nurses' Preconference Research Symposium, Washington, DC.

Olshansky, S. (1962). Chronic sorrow: A response to having a mentally defective child. *Social Casework, 43,* 190–193.

Patterson, J.M., & Geber, G. (1991). Preventing mental health problems in children with chronic illness or disability. *Children's Health Care, 20*(3), 150–161.

Perrin, J.M., Shayne, M.W., & Bloom, S.R. (1993). *Home and Community Care for Chronically Ill Children*. New York, NY: Oxford University Press.

Pokorni, J. (1992). *Promoting Family Collaboration* [Videotape and study guide]. Lawrence, KS: Learner Managed Designs.

Quint, R.D., Chesterman, E., Crain, L.S., Winkleby, M., & Boyce, T. (1990). Home care for ventilator-dependent children: Psychosocial impact on the family. *American Journal of Diseases of Children, 144,* 1,238–1,241.

Ray, L., et al. (1993). Caring for chronically ill children at home: Factors that influence parents' coping. *Journal of Pediatric Nursing, 8*(4), 217–225.

Sailtross, P. (1986). Transitional infant care: A bridge to home for high risk infants. *Neonatal Network, 4*(4), 35–41.

Shelton, T.L., & Stepanek, J.S. (1994). *Family-centered care for children needing specialized health and developmental services*. Bethesda, MD: Association for the Care of Children's Health.

Sterling, Y.M. (1990). Resource needs of mothers managing chronically ill infants at home. *Neonatal Network, 9*(1), 55–59.

Thomas, R.B. (1986). *Ventilator dependency consequences for child and family*. Doctoral dissertation, University of Washington School of Nursing, Seattle, WA.

Thomas, R.B. (1987). Family adaptation to the child with a chronic condition. In M.H. Rose & R.B. Thomas (Eds.), *Children with chronic conditions: Nursing in a family and community context*. Orlando, FL: Grune & Stratton.

Thorpe, E.K. (1987). *Mothers' coping with home care of severe chronic respiratory disabled children requiring medical technology assistance*. Doctoral dissertation, School of Education and Development, George Washington University, Washington, DC.

Walker, D.K., Epstein, S.G., Taylor, A.B., Crocker, A.C., & Tuttle, G.A. (1989). Perceived needs of families of children who have chronic health conditions. *Children's Health Care, 18,* 196–201.

Wegener, D.H., & Aday, L.A. (1989). Home care for ventilator-assisted children: Predicting family stress. *Pediatric Nursing, 15,* 371–376.

Worthington, R.C. (1992). Family support networks: Help for families of children with special needs. *Family Medicine, 24,* 41–44.

Youngblut, J.M., Brennan, P.F., & Swegart, L.A. (1994). Families with medically fragile children: An exploratory study. *Pediatric Nursing, 20*(5), 463–469.

Chapter 3

Siblings of Children with Chronic Conditions

Revised by Judy Rollins, MS, RN

Living with a child with a chronic or disabling condition can be both challenging and rewarding for all members of the family. Because of the intensity and intimacy of the sibling relationship, brothers and sisters can be affected in unique and sometimes profound ways.

A review of research reveals that the effects on siblings can be negative, positive, or absent (Gallo, Breitmayer, Knafl, & Zoeller, 1992). Findings from earlier studies reported heavily on negative effects, citing behavioral problems and somatic complaints such as poor academic performance, increased social withdrawal, deprivation of parental attention, attention-seeking behavior, and feelings of isolation. Findings from later studies, which used more reliable methods, demonstrated less dramatic rates of sibling maladjustment and, in some cases, no severe adjustment problems.

As with any sibling relationship, having a brother or sister with special health care needs can have negative aspects, but the experience can also provide rich opportunities for both personal and family growth. Parents and professionals who recognize the special role siblings play in one another's health and development can provide the support needed to strengthen this role.

THE SIBLING EXPERIENCE

A child with a chronic or disabling condition can place many demands on a family. Parents may, by necessity, spend a great deal of time taking the child to physician or clinic appointments, staying with the child when he or she is hospitalized, and providing care and treatments in the home.

Siblings' routines are often disrupted or become nonexistent. The child's condition may require parents to cancel plans to attend the siblings' activities and may interfere with other long-awaited holiday celebrations, vacations, or special events. Williams, Lorenzo, and Borja (1993) reported a significant increase in siblings' household activities, including both housekeeping and well-sibling caretaking, with an accompanying decrease in school and social activities.

Finances frequently become an issue as medical and related costs mount. Siblings may have to go without items they want, or in some cases, items they need. With less money available, activities the family previously enjoyed may no longer be possible.

Changes in the Sibling Relationship

Some of the problems that brothers and sisters encounter stem from the fact that they are brothers and sisters. For example, children learn to share, compete, and give and take with others through their interactions with a brother or sister. When a child is chronically ill or disabled, the equal status that is shared among brothers and sisters is lost, at least for a time.

Because siblings identify with each other, when a brother or sister has a chronic condition, siblings sometimes think that they, too, will "catch" what their brother or sister has.

Previous experiences, such as passing around colds or the chicken pox, serve to reinforce this notion.

Feelings

Most siblings experience a range of mixed and sometimes conflicting emotions (Rollins, 1992b). Brothers and sisters often feel *left out* and *concerned* about the changes that are occurring in the family. They may feel *sad* when their brother or sister is unable to participate in an activity the rest of the family members can enjoy. Some siblings may feel *guilty* that they are healthy and escaped their brother's or sister's fate.

Having a brother or sister who is ill, disfigured, or disabled marks the family as "different" from the norm (Gallo, Breitmayer, Knafl, & Zoeller, 1991). Because of the stigma that sometimes accompanies such circumstances, siblings may feel *embarrassed* and not reveal their brother's or sister's condition to others. This may lead to feelings of *shame,* which only increase feelings of guilt.

Fear is a common emotion. In addition to fear of "catching" what their brother or sister has and fear of how their friends will react, siblings may also worry about their brother's or sister's future. As they get older, some siblings worry that their own children may have the child's condition.

As in all sibling relationships, siblings are sometimes *resentful* or *jealous* of their brother or sister. The child may receive more attention or preferential treatment from parents and other adults. Older siblings may resent being called upon to take on additional responsibilities, such as babysitting or performing household chores.

Feeling *angry* is not unusual. Siblings can feel angry toward their parents for not giving them attention. When siblings are not clear about the cause of their brother's or sister's condition, they may be angry at their parents for not protecting the child. A younger sibling may thread together certain unrelated events and decide that their parents are responsible for the child's condition. An older sibling may be angry with parents, wondering if the situation would have been different if the parents had taken their brother or sister to the physician sooner. Insensitive friends or classmates may also be targets of sibling anger.

However, not all of the feelings siblings experience are negative. They are often very *proud* of themselves for their contribution to the family. Often overlooked is the *positive caring* that develops between brothers and sisters who share in the *joy* and *excitement* about each other's accomplishments and genuine *love* for each other.

BEHAVIORS

The stress a sibling experiences may be reflected in behavior changes that may go unnoticed by preoccupied parents and health care professionals. Siblings having trouble adjusting react in various ways. In general, younger children usually become irritable and withdrawn; older siblings tend to act out (Rollins, 1992a).

In some children, jealousy and anger can lead to aggressive behaviors against playmates, pets, the ill child, or themselves. Guilt, as well as the concern that "I may be next," leads other children to become withdrawn and uncommunicative; they attempt to avoid any behaviors that may draw punishment and, therefore, as they perceive cause and effect, illness. The concerns of some children with a brother or sister who is chronically ill may also generate excessive somatic complaints over minor illnesses and injuries. Separation anxiety often leads to regressive behavior such as bed wetting or thumb sucking. Sleep disturbances and fear of the dark can also occur, often as a result of misconceptions about the illness or disability.

It is important to remember that stress is a normal aspect of life for all children. Siblings of children with chronic conditions are not immune to everyday stresses that other children experience. Some may have more stressors than others or may be more vulnerable to stress than other children. Some stress may be related to the continuous change children experience while proceeding through various stages of individual and family development. Therefore, effective help for siblings considers all of the stressors that may be occurring in children's lives (Rollins, 1992b). The knowledgeable and observant nurse can assist parents in noticing and understanding behavior changes and in planning purposeful interventions to mitigate problems that arise.

RISK FACTORS

No two children, even children in the same family, will experience having a brother or sister with a chronic or disabling condition in the same way. However, certain factors seem related to sibling adjustment (Lobato, 1990; Powell & Gallagher, 1993):

- *Ease of understanding and predictability of the condition.* Siblings of children with conditions that are easier to understand and disorders that are predictable tend to adapt more easily than siblings of children with disorders that are more difficult to understand.
- *Family size.* Siblings in larger families tend to adjust better than those from two-child families.
- *Sibling spacing.* Siblings with a larger age gap tend to adjust better than those close in age to, or younger than, the child with a chronic or disabling condition.
- *Type of disability.* Siblings of children with mental disabilities tend to adjust better, have a higher self-concept, and get along better socially than siblings of children with physical or sensory disabilities or siblings of children with milder disabling conditions.

- *Age of the children.* The older the child with the chronic or disabling condition, the more behavior problems are reported in the siblings. Younger brothers or older sisters tend to experience more difficulties.
- *Parents' level of acceptance.* Siblings are more likely to have adjustment problems when parents are unaccepting of the child with special needs.

CRITICAL TIMES

There are certain times during the family life cycle that seem to be more stressful for siblings. Powell and Gallagher (1993) suggest that stress may be greatest at the following times:

- Another child is born.
- The child with special needs enters school.
- The (older) sibling starts to date.
- Friends reject the child.
- Friends ask questions about the child.
- The child becomes critically ill.
- Problems related to the child are handled in secrecy.
- Parents die.
- Siblings marry.

Lack of information and/or communication between the parents and siblings during these times are believed to be the significant factors. The nurse can help families through these periods by encouraging parents to recognize potential problems and to discuss the problems and possible solutions openly among family members.

MEETING SIBLING NEEDS

Although every sibling's situation is unique, certain basic needs are common among all brothers and sisters of children with chronic conditions. These needs must be readdressed as siblings enter each developmental stage and encounter new situations or concerns.

Siblings require special attention, understanding, and support. Paramount is the need to be recognized for one's own strengths, talents, and unique contributions to the family (Rollins, 1992b).

Respect and Understanding

Siblings need their parents to recognize their own unique identities, without either positive or negative comparisons to other brothers and sisters. They need their parents' time, attention, and understanding that their lives are different from those of other children. Even though their special concerns and feelings may not be shared by parents, these concerns and feelings need to be acknowledged as legitimate and normal.

Ideally, parents should spend time alone with each child, even if for only 1 or 2 hours a week. They can also help each sibling identify someone who can offer special support and help meet the sibling's practical needs when parents are unavailable.

Siblings often feel excluded when their brother or sister is hospitalized. Efforts are needed to help retain contact among all family members. Children unable to visit their brother or sister in the hospital can be encouraged to find other methods of staying in touch, such as regular telephone calls or letters.

Information

Siblings need honest, direct, and age-appropriate information. The nurse can encourage parents to provide the information siblings need to understand the child's condition, their family, themselves, school, special services, guardianship, treatment, or other special concerns. In some cases, parents may want the nurse present to help clarify information and provide support.

The nurse can offer age-appropriate suggestions for communicating information. For instance, to a young sibling of a child with a tracheostomy, a parent can explain, "It was hard for your sister to breathe through her nose the way you and I breathe through ours. We took her to the doctors, and they helped her breathe this way instead." Similarly, oxygen can be described simply as "extra air," and a ventilator as a "special breathing machine." Children will need reassurance that the same problems will not happen to them: "You weren't born too early like your sister was; you won't need this special equipment."

Opportunities to Express Concerns and Feelings

The nurse can encourage parents to help children discuss fears and other feelings. Brothers and sisters need to understand that they have no blame for the illness of their brother or sister. Likewise, parents should assure and reassure children that they will not "catch" the condition or disability (if this is true), and tell them that it is permissible to sometimes feel angry or frightened, just as the parents sometimes feel. In this connection, parents may need to be reminded that verbalizing these ideas will not put such thoughts into a child's mind. Rather, it will only acknowledge what the child already thinks, as well as correct any misconceptions.

Children often act out their daily concerns in their play and can be encouraged to use this comfortable medium to express their feelings and fears. In a therapeutically orchestrated play session, many of the sibling's fears and misconceptions will become apparent and can be mitigated. A sound knowledge of child development and an understanding of common fears and misconceptions are essential for facilitating this process. Pediatric mental health professionals are often experts at using play therapy. Nurses and parents can also develop some skills in the techniques (see resources in Exhibit 3–1).

Support

It is often helpful for siblings to share their experiences, feelings, and fears with the nurse or a trained counselor. Parents may also enroll their children in sibling support groups, available through hospitals, agencies, or associations.

Many health care professionals, recognizing the impact of the birth or diagnosis of a child with special needs on family members, recommend at least a few sessions of professional counseling for *all* families. Whether formal or informal, counseling can provide siblings the opportunity to learn effective ways to cope with the stresses in their lives. Some siblings may benefit from group sessions, whereas others may need individual sessions or a combination of both.

Training

One of the functions of a sibling relationship is interacting with and learning from one another. Siblings may want to help provide care for their brother or sister with special needs. Parents can facilitate this process by asking a child to perform simple tasks, such as bringing a diaper or holding the feeding tube. The home care nurse can dramatize with the other children special procedures done for their brother or sister. For instance, the nurse might encourage siblings to use a stethoscope on a doll, change a dressing on a doll, or weigh the doll.

Older siblings may require training in first aid or special skills to provide more sophisticated care. In some situations, siblings can benefit from simply learning how to interact and play with their brother or sister.

CONCLUSION

With understanding and appropriate support, growing up in a family with a child with a chronic condition can be a very positive experience for his or her brothers and sisters. Understanding the siblings' experience and their unique

Exhibit 3–1 Resources for Assisting Siblings

Sibling Organizations

Sibling Information Network
The A. J. Pappanikou Center on Special Education and
    Rehabilitation
991 Main Street
East Hartford, CT 06108
203-344-7500

Siblings for Significant Change
United Charities Building
105 East 22nd Street
New York, NY 10010
212-420-0776

Books on Play Therapy

Hart, R., Mather, P., Slack, J., & Powell, M. (1992). *Therapeutic play activities for hospitalized children.* St. Louis, MO: Mosby Year Book.

Petrillo, M., & Sanger, S. (1980). *Emotional care of hospitalized children.* Philadelphia, PA: Lippincott.

Rollins, J. (1991). Assisting with therapeutic play. In D. Smith, K. Nix, J. Kemper, R. Liguori, D. Brantly, J. Rollins, N. Stevens, & L. Clutter (Eds.), *Comprehensive child and family nursing skills.* St. Louis, MO: Mosby Year Book.

---

needs lays the foundation for nurses in planning purposeful interventions. The community health or home care nurse has the opportunity to observe sibling behavior and to assist parents in prevention, noting behavior changes, and planning interventions to alleviate problems that arise.

REFERENCES

Gallo, A., Breitmayer, B., Knafl, K., & Zoeller, L. (1991). Stigma in childhood chronic illness: A well sibling perspective. *Pediatric Nursing, 17*(1), 21–25.

Gallo, A., Breitmayer, B., Knafl, K., & Zoeller, L. (1992). Well siblings of children with chronic illness: Parents' reports of their psychologic adjustment. *Pediatric Nursing, 18*(1), 23–27.

Lobato, D. (1990). *Brothers, sisters, and special needs.* Baltimore, MD: Paul H. Brookes.

Powell, T., & Gallagher, P. (1993). *Brothers & sisters: A special part of exceptional families* (2nd ed.). Baltimore, MD: Paul H. Brookes.

Rollins, J. (1992a). *Brothers and sisters: A guide for families of children with epilepsy/Just for You!* Landover, MD: Epilepsy Foundation of America.

Rollins, J. (1992b). *Brothers & sisters: What affiliates can do.* Landover, MD: Epilepsy Foundation of America.

Williams, P., Lorenzo, F., & Borja, M. (1993). Pediatric chronic illness: Effects on siblings and mothers. *Maternal-Child Nursing Journal, 21*(4), 111–119.

Chapter 4

Family-Centered Home Care

Elizabeth Ahmann, ScD, RN

What is family? Although there are many definitions that could be used for the term *family,* there are exceptions to each definition (Kavanagh, 1994). The House Memorial 5 Task Force on Young Children and Families (1990) in New Mexico has proposed a broad and flexible definition of *family:* "Families are big, small, extended, nuclear, multigenerational, with one parent, two parents, and grandparents. We live under one roof or many. A family can be as temporary as a few weeks or as permanent as forever. We become part of a family by birth, adoption, marriage, or from a desire for mutual support . . ." (p. 1). This definition acknowledges that family means different things to different people. Families are self-defining.

However a family defines itself, research involving families of children who have special health and developmental needs demonstrates parental desires for family-centered approaches to care (Diehl, Moffit, & Wade, 1991; McNeil, 1992; Moeller, Coufal, & Hixon, 1990). Increasingly, family-centered care is being considered "best practice" in medical, mental health, and developmental arenas (Johnson, Jeppson, & Redburn, 1992). While relevant in all practice settings, a family-centered approach to nursing practice seems particularly fitting in the home care arena (Ahmann, 1994b).

THE PHILOSOPHY OF FAMILY-CENTERED CARE

Family-centered care is "based on the belief that all families are deeply caring and want to nurture their children"

(Edelman, 1991, p. 1). The foundation of this philosophy is the recognition that the family is central in a child's life and should be central to decision making in the plan of care. Unlike professionals who see a child only episodically, families know the child on a continuous basis, through different developmental stages, and in various settings; thus, they are the true "experts" on their children's overall needs and strengths within the family context. (Shelton & Stepanek, 1994).

Families have the ultimate responsibility for ensuring that a child's health and developmental, social, and emotional needs are met (Shelton & Stepanek, 1994). Parents must balance, in the short and long term, the various needs of the child with the needs of other family members and the resources of the family as a whole. As Shelton and Stepanek (1994) state, family-centered care takes parental "observations, recommendations and choices seriously" (p. 8).

Family-centered care embraces diversity in family structures, cultural backgrounds, choices, and strengths, as well as support, service, and information needs. A family-centered approach to care recognizes each family as unique and supports families by building on their own strengths and values, respecting their choices and their coping methods, and responding to their particular and unique needs.

The philosophy of family-centered care calls for partnerships between parents and professionals—partnerships that support parents in their central caring role. In a collaborative model, professionals respect the contribution family members make in the child's care and, in fact, view parental input in the plan of care as the "cornerstone" of quality in service provision (Shelton & Stepanek, 1994, p. 8). Through collaboration, parents and professionals share information and strategies with the goal of developing the best possible plan of care for the child and family.

Developing a new understanding of the role of the nurse and both learning and practicing new family-centered skills are essential to implementing family-centered care. Each of the eight elements of family-centered care listed in Exhibit 4–1 defines an important aspect of the practice of family-centered care. To support the practice of family-centered home care nursing, cultural competence, collaboration, communication issues, appropriate boundaries in the therapeutic relationship, and instrumental and emotional support will be discussed in this chapter. Other chapters of the book allude to and/or directly address additional key points of family-centered care.

Exhibit 4–1 The Key Elements of Family-centered Care

- Incorporating into policy and practice the recognition that the *family is the constant* in a child's life, while the service systems and support personnel within those systems fluctuate.
- Facilitating *family/professional collaboration* at all levels of hospital, home, and community care:
  —care of an individual child;
  —program development, implementation, evaluation, and evolution; and
  —policy formation.
- *Exchanging complete and unbiased information* between family members and professionals in a supportive manner at all times.
- Incorporating into policy and practice the recognition and *honoring of cultural diversity,* strengths, and individuality within and across all families, including *ethnic, racial, spiritual, social, economic, educational, and geographic diversity.*
- Recognizing and respecting *different methods of coping* and implementing comprehensive policies and programs that provide *developmental, educational, emotional, environmental, and financial supports* to meet the diverse needs of families.
- Encouraging and facilitating *family-to-family support* and networking.
- Ensuring that *home, hospital, and community service and support systems* for children needing specialized health and developmental care and their families are *flexible, accessible, and comprehensive* in responding to diverse family-identified needs.
- *Appreciating families as families* and children as children, recognizing that they possess a wide range of strengths, concerns, emotions, and aspirations beyond their need for specialized health and developmental services and support.

Source: Reprinted from *Family-Centered Care for Children Needing Specialized Health and Developmental Services* by T.L. Shelton and J.S. Stepanek. Association for the Care of Children's Health, 1994.

DEVELOPING CULTURAL COMPETENCE

The practices relevant to cultural competence are relevant to working with any family, even families of the same cultural background as the nurse, as they have at their core respect for others and appreciation of diversity. Culturally competent nursing care promotes the well-being of the child and family and should be a central component of providing family-centered home care services.

Cultural traditions give families "a sense of stability and support from which they draw comfort, guidance, and a means of coping with the problems of daily life" (McCubbin, Thompson, Thompson, McCubbin, & Kaston, 1993, p. 1,063). Cultural traditions may become even more important to families faced with a child's chronic illness or disability.

Certain ethnic and minority populations define and address chronic illness and disability differently from "mainstream" American culture (Groce & Zola, 1993). As an example, Anderson (1986) described problems faced by Chinese immigrants who did not share the dominant belief of Western health care providers in the "normalization" principles regarding child development.

When nurses or other health care providers perceive such differences as bad or wrong, insensitive patient care results (Chrisman & Kogood, no date). When, on the other hand, cultural or other family traditions and responses to illness can be seen as strengths rather than deficits, they can be drawn upon to enhance the care of the child (Adams, 1990).

Language barriers pose an obvious challenge in cross-cultural nursing practice. In communities with significant numbers of non-English-speaking residents, bilingual nurses or translators should be standard in a home care practice. Some guidelines for using an interpreter are included in Exhibit 4–2. However, even when language is not a barrier, cross-cultural communication can pose challenges.

The meaning of certain terms can have undesirable connotations in some cultures. For example, the term *family support* may be interpreted by some families as meaning that they are weak (Patterson & Blum, 1993). Styles of communication may vary as well. In some cultures, families do

Exhibit 4–2 Guidelines for Using an Interpreter

Obtain the family's permission for use of an interpreter.
Ensure that the interpreter understands confidentiality issues.
Inform the interpreter of the general nature of the interview.
Inquire of the interpreter whether there may be any cultural concerns related to the nature of the questions to be asked.
Introduce the interpreter to the family.
Look at family members while asking questions and listening to answers.
Avoid medical "jargon."
Arrange for the same interpreter for subsequent visits when possible.

not openly discuss certain topics; as a result, some parents may feel uncomfortable participating in discussions about their child's condition (Munet-Vilaro & Vessey, 1990). Displaying (or not displaying) grief, anxiety, fear, concern, and disagreement may also be culturally determined (Groce & Zola, 1993).

In communicating with families, particularly those of different cultures, three practices may be especially useful:

1. emphasizing careful listening with the goal of understanding the family's perspective
2. recognizing and resolving conflicts between practices stemming from the "mainstream" medical model and the family's cultural preferences (Patterson & Blum, 1993)
3. understanding and using the family's cultural perception of health and disease in discussions and in the plan of care (Brookins, 1993; McCubbin et al., 1993).

Effective care for children and families must be individualized, based on each family's own perceptions of illness, its meaning and relevance in their life, and their own conceptions of how healing can occur (Ahmann, 1994a). Awareness of the many ways in which culture can influence both belief and action can encourage a nurse to approach each family with an open mind, learn about a family's culture, and ask questions without implying judgment (Stone & Hoffman, 1993). When a family's preferences are understood, they can be made part of the plan of care.

Incorporating a family's preferences directly into the written plan of care can guide nurses and other providers who may be less familiar with the family in providing appropriate care. Interdisciplinary team meetings can also be used to enhance understanding and respect for the family's choices (Zagorsky, 1993).

COLLABORATION WITH FAMILIES

One of the key elements of family-centered care is family–professional collaboration or partnerships. Collaborative relationships are characterized by several features outlined in Exhibit 4–3. Parent–professional partnerships recognize that the family is the center of the provision of comprehensive care for a child (Leff & Walizer, 1992). "Family/professional collaboration promotes a relationship in which family members and professionals work together to ensure the best services for the child and family" (Bishop, Woll, & Arango, 1993, p. 15).

To implement a collaborative or partnership model, nurses must alter the traditional nursing process somewhat to include elements that can both "enable, empower and strengthen families as well as promote acquisition of the competencies necessary" to meet the needs of the child and family (Bond et al., 1994, p. 123).

Exhibit 4–3 Principles of Family–Professional Collaboration

Family/professional collaboration:
1. promotes a relationship in which family members and professionals work together to ensure the best services for the child and family;
2. recognizes and respects the knowledge, skills, and experience that families and professionals bring to the relationship;
3. acknowledges that the development of trust is an integral part of a collaborative relationship;
4. facilitates open communication so that families and professionals feel free to express themselves;
5. creates an atmosphere in which the cultural traditions, values, and diversity of families are honored;
6. recognizes that negotiation is essential in a collaborative relationship; and
7. brings to the relationship the mutual commitment of families, professionals, and communities to meet the needs of children with special health needs and their families.

Source: Reprinted from *Family/Professional Collaboration for Children with Special Health Needs and Their Families* by K.K. Bishop, J. Woll, and P. Arango, p. 15, with permission of the University of Vermont, Department of Social Work, © 1993.

Assessment Process

Parental participation in the assessment process is the first step. Assessment should include not only needs and problems but also strengths and resources (Bond et al., 1994). Areas of need may include information about the child's health and development, skills related to care of the child, financial assistance, assistance with arranging the home environment, strategies to improve communication with and among care providers, mobility concerns, time management, identification of community resources, access to a parent network, sibling issues, and the like.

Some family strengths and resources are discussed in Chapter 2 and include inter- and intrapersonal resources such as values, cultural identity, friends and relatives, churches, clubs, and other formal organizations (Dunst, Trivette, & Deal, 1988).

As a first step in collaborating with family members regarding the assessment process, the nurse can ask family members how they would like to participate (Rushton, 1990). Some families may want complete involvement in the process, whereas others may defer to professionals. The nurse can offer options to encourage family involvement. For example, family members could list observations, questions and concerns in writing; they could meet with one professional of their choice (e.g., the home care case manager or the primary care provider) to discuss these issues; or they could meet with an interdisciplinary team of professionals one or more times as part of the assessment process.

Nurses can facilitate family member identification of needs and resources by asking open-ended questions, using

Table 4–1 Measures to Help Families Identify Concerns, Priorities, Resources, and Sources of Support

Measure	Author(s)	Source
1. *Family Needs Survey, Revised Edition* (1990)	D. Bailey & R. Simeonsson	Frank Porter Graham Child Development Center; CB#180; University of North Carolina; Chapel Hill, NC 27599.
2. *How Can We Help?* (1988)	Child Development Resources	Child Development Resources; P.O. Box 299; Lightfoot, VA 23098.
3. *Parent Needs Survey* (1988)	B. Darling	Seligman, M., & Darling, B. (1989). *Ordinary families, special children: A systems approach to childhood disability.* New York: Guilford Press.
4. *Family Needs Scale* (1988)	C. Dunst, C. Cooper, J. Weeldreyer, K. Snyder, & J. Chase	Dunst, D., Trivette, C., & Deal, A. (1988). *Enabling and empowering families: Principles and guidelines for practice.* Cambridge, MA: Brookline Books.
5. *Family Support Scale* (1984)	C. Dunst, V. Jenkins, & C. Trivette	Dunst, D., Trivette, C., & Deal, A. (1988). *Enabling and empowering families: Principles and guidelines for practice.* Cambridge, MA: Brookline Books.
6. *Exercise: Social Support* (1985)	J. Summers, A. Turnbull, & M. Brotherson	Summers, J., Turnbull, A., & Brotherson, M. (1985). *Coping strategies for families with disabled children.* Unpublished manuscript, University of Kansas, Kansas University Affiliated Facility at Lawrence.
7. *Family Profile* (1993)	B. McCord	The Coordinating Center for Home and Community Care; 8258 Veterans Highway; Suite 13; Millersville, MD 21108.

Notes: 1–6 may be found in Appendix D of McGonigel, M., Kaufmann, R., Johnson, B. (Eds.). (1991) *Guidelines and recommended practices for the Individualized Family Service Plan* (2nd ed.). Bethesda, MD: Association for the Care of Children's Health. ACCH is located at 7910 Woodmont Avenue, Suite 300, Bethesda, MD 20814; (301) 654-6549. For more information regarding measure 7, contact the Coordinating Center for Home and Community Care; 8258 Veterans Highway; Suite 13; Millersville, MD 21108; (410) 987-1048.

Source: Reprinted from *Pediatric Nursing,* Vol. 20, No. 2 (March–April), p. 125, with permission of Jannetti Publications, Inc., Pitman, New Jersey © 1994.

parental self-report instruments (see Table 4–1), asking for clarification where necessary, and contributing observations (Bond et al., 1994). The nurse's contributions should be made in a neutral manner and without value judgment so that the family's central role in decision making is preserved.

Plan of Care

Developing the plan of care should also be a joint effort of family members and professionals (Ahmann & Bond, 1992). The family's goals and priorities should assume a central role in the development of the home care plan. The nurse can assist the family in clarifying their short- and long-term goals and breaking them into measurable objectives.

Intervention plans arise in relation to goals and objectives. Intervention plans should be developed in collaboration with the family. Attention should be paid to how the special care needs of the child can be provided in the context of a normal flow to family life. For example, developmental interventions need not occur in 1-hour blocks each day; they could instead be incorporated in small bits into the diaper change routine. Medication schedules should be arranged to allow parents a full night's sleep.

In circumstances where the family and nurse may disagree on priorities and goals, several steps can be taken. Ahmann and Bond (1992) suggest that the nurse can try the following strategies:

- work with the family's priorities and reevaluate as necessary over time;
- share the professional's perspective and explain why different priorities might be recommended;
- explain the risks or drawbacks, if any, if the priorities the family chooses are placed first;
- suggest another priority goal if the family agrees. (p. 402)

In the unusual event that the nurse has a liability concern (Hogue, 1992) resulting from implementing a family's priority (or not implementing a nurse's priority), this concern can be respectfully communicated with the family, and the conversation can be documented in the nursing notes. A case example illustrating the process is included in Exhibit 4–4. As part of developing the plan of care, the nurse can also assist the family in developing outcome measures that can be used as indicators in the evaluation process (Bond et al., 1994).

Implementation of the Plan

Cooperation and partnership in the implementation of the home care plan are critical to its success as well (Bond et al., 1994). Respecting the family's priorities and obtaining their ongoing feedback can help make this a reality. Defining

Exhibit 4–4 Case Example: Family Goals Conflict with Medical Management

> **Family's Goal:** Oral feeding for their 3-year-old child who is ventilator-dependent and is currently tube fed.
>
> **Conflict with medical management:** Child is at high risk of aspiration and already has compromised respiratory status.
>
> **Nursing actions:**
> 1. Acknowledge the family's expressed goal.
> 2. State concern of health team—risk of aspiration, possible pneumonia, difficulties that can arise in treating pneumonia given child's other diagnoses.
> 3. Suggest smaller incremental steps—for example, obtaining an oral motor assessment, and/or having speech therapist provide oral motor therapy program.
> 4. Involve parents in the oral motor therapy so they can develop understanding of child's progress or the unrealistic nature of their original goal.
> 5. Explore with parents the reason they desire oral feeding. Normalizing meal time and reducing parental burden of care in this case led to scheduling tube feeding during family meal times and teaching the child to assist in administration of the tube feeding with the goal of eventually taking over the responsibility completely.
>
> *Source:* Copyright © 1992, E. Ahmann and N. Bond.

roles and responsibilities for aspects of the child's care, equipment maintenance, and case management functions can ensure a smooth implementation of the plan of care.

At times, nurses may wonder about the boundaries between respecting parental choices about implementing care that differ from choices of the nurse and permitting inappropriate or unsafe nursing practice (Ahmann, 1994b). The Special Issue on suspected abuse and neglect addresses these and other concerns. As in the process of jointly developing a plan, disagreements about its implementation should be handled with honest, respectful communication and careful documentation when necessary. Case managers or nursing supervisors can be called on to assist in negotiating areas of disagreement.

Evaluation

Evaluation of the home care plan takes place both formally and informally and is an ongoing process. Evaluation forms that parents fill out can be a useful part of quality assurance. Meetings between parents and providers can occur on a scheduled basis to evaluate the need for changes in the plan of care as well as the process of planning and implementation. Because home care places great demands on the family, evaluation can provide an opportunity to celebrate their success (Bond et al., 1994).

COMMUNICATION

Good communication skills are essential in a family-centered practice model. The nurse who can communicate genuine interest in the well-being of the child and family, who promotes openness, and who is committed to honest communication will foster trust (Bishop et al., 1993). Trust develops over time out of openness and implies that both parties are willing to work together to meet the needs of the child and family in the best way possible. Trust is the foundation for honest dialogue and negotiation—important characteristics of collaboration.

Bishop and colleagues (1993) describe dialogue as a process involving active listening—"checking out with others your interpretation of their statements and listening beyond words to hear and understand concerns" (p. 27). Dialogue is a two-way street. An open mind and respect for the views of each party are necessary. In the process of dialogue, sharing and exchange of information and ideas can occur with the goal of finding solutions.

Similarly, skills in negotiation may be useful in collaborative relationships between families and professionals. The process of negotiation demands flexibility and requires setting aside power. It involves laying out the options, priorities, and preferences of each party and then focusing, together, on the best outcomes for the child and family (Bishop et al., 1993). Negotiation may be required for decisions that range from simple (such as scheduling a convenient time for a home visit) to complex (such as preferences in how certain aspects of care are provided or preferences in methods for nurse–parent communication).

The LEARN framework for communication gives attention to careful listening and acknowledges the potential for differing points of view. It can be a useful model for communication in a collaborative relationship (Berlin & Fowkes, 1983). The acronym LEARN stands for the following:

- *L*: Listen with sympathy and understanding to the family's perception of the problem.
- *E*: Explain your perception of the problem.
- *A*: Acknowledge and discuss differences and similarities.
- *R*: Recommend treatment.
- *N*: Negotiate agreement.

By working together the nurse(s) and family members can recognize the goal of all communication efforts in a collaborative process: to create the best solutions for the child and family (Bishop et al., 1993).

PROFESSIONAL BOUNDARIES

Family-centered nursing practice and collaborative relationships with families are critical in the home care setting.

However, collaborating with the family must be distinguished from becoming a part of the family system. In most instances, an optimal therapeutic relationship involves maintaining well-defined boundaries among the nurse, child, and family in order to empower the family in the care of the child (Barnsteiner & Gillis-Donovan, 1990).

Klug (1993) points out several factors that can make maintaining professional boundaries challenging in the home setting:

- informality of the home environment
- family participation in care

Exhibit 4–5 House Rules

	Comments
I. House Rules	
1. Parking: Where to park and community regulations.	_____
2. Access: Where to enter the home. Is knocking preferred or ringing the bell?	_____
3. Personal belongings: Where does the nurse store her coat, boots, etc. Does the family prefer slippers to shoes in the home?	_____
4. Meals: Where may the nurse store her food? Note: This is very important given cultural diversity of clients.	_____
5. Radio and Television: Identify preferences regarding the usage. Remember this may help nurses to remain awake at night.	_____
6. Patient Room: The nurse is responsible for the child's immediate environment. Maintaining a clean working area and cleaning the room up at the end of the shift is the nurse's responsibility.	_____
7. Telephone: Agency policy may dictate that all personal calls be limited to very brief time periods and be charged to the nurse making them. Note: Many nurses do need to check in with home at some interval during the evening.	_____
8. Visitors: Identify who may enter the home when the parents are away (that is, child's friends or grandparents). A list of names should be available.	_____
9. Privacy: Describe what parts of the home are off limits to the nurse and at what times.	_____
II. Child	
1. Routine: specify times for playtime, bathtime, and bedtime. What does the mother want to participate in regarding these routines?	_____
2. Mealtime: Specify where the family wants the child fed and if tube fed, specify a preference as to how and where it is done.	_____
3. Clothing: Identify who picks out the child's clothes. Identify where the laundry is and who is responsible for washing the sick child's clothing.	_____
4. Discipline: Discuss specific guidelines for discipline.	_____
5. Homework: Discuss when it should be done and who is responsible for it being completed.	_____
III. Siblings	
1. Discipline: Establish guidelines regarding how parents should be informed of siblings' conflicts and how discipline should be handled. Note: Parents or another caretaker must be in the home when siblings are home.	_____
2. Patient Care: Be specific regarding how children have helped with the child's care. Discuss any concerns regarding behavior that may compromise the child or siblings' safety.	_____
IV. Nursing	
1. Specify what information the family wishes to be aware of immediately and what can wait until they are home.	_____
2. Environment: Discuss the need to have adequate lighting and a comfortable working area.	_____

Source: Reprinted from *Pediatric Nursing,* Vol. 19, No. 4, July–August, p. 375, with permission of Jannetti Publications, Inc., Pitman, New Jersey, © 1993.

- tendency of some families to integrate the nurse into their lives to reduce the discomfort of having a stranger in the home
- nurse's need for a social outlet during the shift, in association with the unavailability of professional colleagues in the home setting.

Several strategies can assist the nurse's effort to maintain boundaries while working in the home. First, individual nurses can develop a network of colleagues practicing home care nursing. Members of the network can talk informally or even meet regularly to socialize, provide each other support, and assist each other in thinking clearly about boundary issues. Second, home care agencies can hold periodic in-service meetings, both to assist nurses in networking and to address specific boundary issues relevant to the role of the home care nurse.

Finally, the case manager should negotiate "house rules" with the family in order to promote the family's control of their environment and the care of the child (Klug, 1993). Examples of house rules are included in Exhibit 4–5. The family and all nurses and other professionals providing care in the home should receive copies of the rules.

INSTRUMENTAL AND EMOTIONAL SUPPORT

Thorough discharge teaching, followed by assessment and review as necessary in the home setting, is critical to developing family competence and confidence in providing home care. This teaching should occur over time and in various ways to give family members the opportunity to develop competence. Individual learning styles and attention spans should be respected. Parental questions should be encouraged and answered throughout the learning process both before and after discharge. Skills should be demonstrated, and parents should be allowed to provide a return demonstration until they feel confident and are competent in the care requirements. Chapter 5 and many chapters of this text address teaching issues in greater detail.

In addition to meeting parental education needs, nurses can assist families with instrumental support in various ways. Support should be targeted to needs identified by the family and can include the following:

- assuring competent care for the child
- providing information about the child's condition and care and therapeutic, educational, and community resources
- assisting with time organization and management skills
- advocating for improved insurance coverage and locating other sources of financial assistance
- developing programs in the community, such as respite care or medical day care.

Chapter 7 addresses community resources in some detail, and its appendixes include listings of both books and organizations that may be of interest to families.

Nurses can also provide critical emotional support to families. Knowledge of the challenges families face and the strengths they can use when providing home care for their medically fragile children (see Chapter 2) lays the groundwork for successful nursing interventions with families. Nurses must recognize and respect the central role of families in the lives of medically fragile children and can empower families by acknowledging family strengths and coping mechanisms (Pokorni, 1992). Nurses can teach new coping strategies when families identify a need (Knafl & Deatrick, 1990). Nurses can assist families when necessary to understand the challenges they face and how they can apply their strengths to promote successful adaptation.

Nurses also should recognize the irreplaceable value of family-to-family support and should facilitate the networking of families. Sometimes family support groups are valuable. However, not all families can or wish to attend such meetings. Telephone networks may be useful to some parents. Additionally, a number of the organizations listed in Appendix 7–A provide parent-to-parent networking.

CONCLUSION

Implementing a family-centered home care nursing practice can be challenging (Ahmann, 1994b). However, ultimately, a family-centered practice will be most effective and rewarding. When principles of family-centered care are incorporated into practice, families will be able to function better as their children's primary caregivers; nurses and other professionals will feel more effective; and most importantly, the "children . . . will benefit from the consistent and dedicated involvement of all their caregivers" (Pokorni, 1992).

REFERENCES

Adams, E.V. (1990). *Policy planning for culturally comprehensive special health services.* Washington, DC: Bureau of Maternal and Child Health, U.S. Department of Health and Human Services.

Ahmann, E. (1994a). "Chunky stew": Appreciating cultural diversity while providing health care for children. *Pediatric Nursing, 20*(3), 320–324.

Ahmann, E. (1994b). Thinking critically about family-centered home care nursing. *Pediatric Nursing, 20*(6), 588–590.

Ahmann, E., & Bond, N. (1992). Promoting normal development in school-age children and adolescents who are technology dependent: A family centered model. *Pediatric Nursing, 18*(4), 399–401.

Anderson, J. (1986). Ethnicity and illness experience: Ideological structures and the health care delivery system. *Social Science and Medicine, 22*(11), 1,277–1,283.

Barnsteiner, J., & Gillis-Donovan, J. (1990). Being related and separate: A standard for therapeutic relationships. *The American Journal of Maternal-Child Nursing, 15*(4), 223–228.

Berlin, E.A., & Fowkes, W.C. (1983). A teaching framework for cross-cultural health care. *The Western Journal of Medicine, 139*(6), 934–938.

Bishop, K.K., Woll, J., & Arango, P. (1993). *Family/professional collaboration for children with special health needs and their families.* Burlington, VT: Department of Social Work, University of Vermont.

Bond, N., Phillips, P., & Rollins, J. (1994). Family-centered care at home for families with children who are technology dependent. *Pediatric Nursing, 20*(2), 123–132.

Brookins, G.K. (1993). Culture, ethnicity, and bicultural competence: Implications for children with chronic illness and disability. *Pediatrics, 91*(5, Part V: Supplement), 1,065–1,062.

Chrisman, N., & Kogood, S.K. (no date). *Training in culturally sensitive health care: Whys and wherefores.* Bethesda, MD: Bridges in Organizations, Inc.

Diehl, S.F., Moffit, K.A., & Wade, S.M. (1991). Focus group interview with parents of children with medically complex needs: An intimate look at their perceptions and feelings. *Children's Health Care, 20*(3), 170–178.

Dunst, C., Trivette, C., & Deal, A. (1988). *Enabling and empowering families.* Cambridge, MA: Brookline Books.

Edelman, L. (Ed.). (1991). *Getting on board: Training activities to promote the practice of family-centered care.* Bethesda, MD: Association for the Care of Children's Health.

Groce, N.E., & Zola, I.K. (1993). Multiculturalism, chronic illness, and disability. *Pediatrics, 91*(5), 1,048–1,055.

Hogue, E. (1992). Parental noncompliance in home care. *Pediatric Nursing, 18*(6), 603–606.

House Memorial 5 Task Force on Young Children and Families. (1990, November 6). *First steps to a community-based coordinated continuum of care for New Mexico children and families.* (Available from Polly Arango, PO Box 338, Algodones, New Mexico 87001.)

Johnson, B., Jeppson, E., & Redburn, L. (1992). *Caring for children and families: Guidelines for hospitals.* Bethesda, MD: Association for the Care of Children's Health.

Kavanagh, K.H. (1994). Families: Is anything more diverse? *Pediatric Nursing, 20*(4), 423–426.

Klug, R.M. (1993). Clarifying roles and expectations in home care. *Pediatric Nursing, 19*(4), 374–376.

Knafl, K.A., & Deatrick, J.A. (1990). Family management style: Concept analysis and development. *Journal of Pediatric Nursing, 5*(1), 4–14.

Leff, P., & Walizer, E. (1992). *Building the healing partnership.* Cambridge, MA: Brookline Books.

McCubbin, H.I., Thompson, E.A., Thompson, A.I., McCubbin, M., & Kaston, A.J. (1993). Culture, ethnicity, and the family: Critical factors in childhood chronic illness and disabilities. *Pediatrics, 91*(5), 1,063–1,070.

McNeil, D. (1992, March). *Uncertainty, waiting, and possibilities: Becoming a mother in the NICU.* Paper presented at the National Association of Neonatal Nurses' Preconference Research Symposium, Washington, DC.

Moeller, M.P., Coufal, K., & Hixon, P. (1990). The efficacy of speech-language pathology intervention: Hearing impaired children. *Seminars in Speech and Language, 2*(4), 227–241.

Munet-Vilaro, F., & Vessey, J. (1990). Children's explanation of leukemia: A Hispanic perspective. *Journal of Pediatric Nursing, 5*(4), 274–282.

Patterson, J.M., & Blum, R.W. (1993). A conference on culture and chronic illness in childhood: Conference summary. *Pediatrics, 91*(5), 1,025–1,030.

Pokorni, J. (1992). *Promoting family collaboration* [Videotape and study guide]. Lawrence, KS: Learner Managed Designs, Inc.

Rushton, C. (1990). Family-centered care in the critical care setting: Myth or reality? *Children's Health Care, 19*(2), 68–78.

Shelton, T.L., & Stepanek, J.S. (1994). *Family-centered care for children needing specialized health and developmental services.* Bethesda, MD: Association for the Care of Children's Health.

Stone, M., & Hoffman, R. (1993, April 30). *Cultural understanding: How far do you go?* Paper presented at the ACCH Affiliates Conference, Caring for the quilt: Incorporating cultural awareness into pediatric health care, Washington, DC.

Zagorsky, E.S. (1993). Caring for families who follow alternative health practices. *Pediatric Nursing, 19*(1), 71–75.

Part II

Transition to Home Care

Standards of Care

Ruth Klug, MS, RN, CPNP

In any field, the purpose of standards is to define the criteria for accountability and to improve service. In nursing, standards additionally reflect the values and priorities of the profession, provide direction for practice, and offer a framework for evaluation of practice (Klug, 1994).

Many sources of standards and guidelines for care may influence the home care nurse. Some of these include the following:

- agency policies and procedures
- job descriptions and employment contracts
- certification criteria
- licensing by the state and federal governments
- agency accrediting bodies such as the Joint Commission on Accreditation of Healthcare Organizations (Joint Commission) and Community Health Accreditation Program (CHAP)
- implied or established standards of Medicaid and private insurers.

The American Nurses Association (ANA) has developed both *Standards of Home Health Nursing Practice* (1986b) and *Standards of Community Health Nursing Practice* (1986a) with which the home care nurse should become familiar. Exhibit A lists the 12 standards of home health nursing practice outlined by ANA. These documents represent the nursing process, which includes data collection, diagnosis, planning, implementation, and evaluation. The concepts of structure, process, and outcome, reflecting Donabedian's framework (Donabedian, 1980), are incorporated into the standards, making them useful for quality improvement, performance appraisal, client assessment, and development of care plans. *A Statement on the Scope of Home Health Nursing Practice* (American Nurses Association, 1992), the *Standards of Clinical Nursing Practice* (American Nurses Association, 1991), and the *Code for Nurses* (American Nurses Association, 1976) are additional resources that can be used in establishing standards in home care.

Accrediting bodies such as the Joint Commission and CHAP have developed standards of care as well. Nurses should be aware of these standards, but should not equate standards that comply with regulatory guidelines and standards that focus on quality of care provided.

Along with standards of care and standards of professional practice, there are guidelines that are developed to assist the nurse in taking action related to the nursing diagnosis or clinical situation. Practice guidelines are developed as a result of research and expert opinion and, unlike standards, are dynamic, changing with both the needs of the client and changes in health care practice. Practice guidelines can be found in agency policies and procedures statements, certification criteria, and the nursing literature.

The dilemma facing many home care agencies today is providing quality care efficiently and effectively in a managed care environment. Linking standards of care both to performance standards, based on guidelines for practice, and to nursing resources will be a critical step. Standards of care

Exhibit A American Nurses Association Standards of Home Health Nursing Practice

Standard I: Organization of Home Health Services
All home health services are planned, organized, and directed by a Master's-prepared professional nurse with experience in community health and administration.

Standard II: Theory
The nurse applies theoretical concepts as a basis for decisions in practice.

Standard III: Data Collection
The nurse continuously collects and records data that are comprehensive, accurate, and systematic.

Standard IV: Diagnosis
The nurse uses health assessment data to determine nursing diagnoses.

Standard V: Planning
The nurse develops care plans that establish goals. The care plan is based on nursing diagnoses and incorporates therapeutic, preventive, and rehabilitative nursing actions.

Standard VI: Intervention
The nurse, guided by the care plan, intervenes to provide comfort; to restore, improve, and promote health; to prevent complications and sequelae of illness; and effect rehabilitation.

Standard VII: Evaluation
The nurse continuously evaluates the client's and family's response to interventions in order to determine progress toward goal attainment and to revise the data base, nursing diagnoses, and plan of care.

Standard VIII: Continuity of Care
The nurse is responsible for the client's appropriate and uninterrupted care along the health care continuum, and therefore uses discharge planning, case, and coordination of community resources.

Standard IX: Interdisciplinary Collaboration
The nurse initiates and maintains a liaison relationship with all appropriate health care providers to assure that all efforts effectively complement one another.

Standard X: Professional Development
The nurse assumes responsibility for professional development and contributes to the professional growth of others.

Standard XI: Research
The nurse participates in research activities that contribute to the profession's continuing development of knowledge of home health care.

Standard XII: Ethics
The nurse uses the code for nurses established by the American Nurses Association as a guide for ethical decision making in practice.

Source: Reprinted with permission from *Standards of Home Health Nursing Practice,* © 1986, American Nurses Association, Washington, DC.

are the criteria for judging quality care; conversely, they are also the standard for judging negligence in malpractice liability (Northrop, 1986). Neither standards of care or standards of performance can be compromised if quality care is to be provided.

REFERENCES

American Nurses' Association. (1976). *Code for nurses.* Kansas City, MO: Author.

American Nurses' Association. (1986a). *Standards of community health nursing practice.* Kansas City, MO: Author.

American Nurses' Association. (1986b). *Standards of home health nursing practice.* Kansas City, MO: Author.

American Nurses' Association. (1991). *Standards of clinical nursing practice.* Kansas City, MO: Author.

American Nurses' Association. (1992). *A statement on the scope of home health nursing practice.* Kansas City, MO: Author.

Donabedian, A. (1980). *Explorations in quality assessment and monitoring* (Vol. 1). Ann Arbor, MI: Health Administration Press.

Klug, R.M. (1994). Setting home care standards. *Pediatric Nursing, 20*(4), 404–406.

Northrop, C. (1986). Malpractice and standards of care. *Nursing Outlook, 34*(3), 160.

Alternatives to Home Care for Medically Fragile Children

Elizabeth Ahmann, ScD, RN, and Ann E. Scher, LICSW

Most families successfully provide home care for their children with special needs. However, home care poses many challenges and can contribute to various hardships for families. For some families, home care is not possible or satisfactory. Reasons may include the unavailability of a parent, the availability of only one parent while two are required for medical management of the child, or parental inability to cope with home care of the child on a temporary or permanent basis (Yost & Hochstadt, 1987). Some families may recognize that home care will not work for them before the child is ready to leave the acute care setting; others will conclude this after a trial of home care.

What options are there for families in this situation? While options may vary from one location to another, the primary possibilities are three: (1) medical day care, (2) placement in a long-term care setting, or (3) medical or specialized foster care.

MEDICAL DAY CARE

While some regular day care settings have responded positively to the idea of enrolling children with specific chronic illnesses or disabilities, few actually enroll them (Crowley, 1990). The major impediments day care settings identify to enrolling disabled or chronically ill children are lack of resources and staffing to meet the children's special needs (Fewell, 1993). For much the same reasons, respite care services are frequently denied to families of children with more complex medical conditions (O'Connor, Van der Plaats, & Betz, 1992).

A recent and rapidly growing alternative or adjunct to home care services is prescribed child care, or medical day care. Prescribed child care centers are nonresidential programs that provide skilled nursing care, developmental programming, and parent education. Services are generally available Monday through Friday, during daytime hours. A physician's prescription may be required, although insurance coverage is variable. Because of a nurse-to-child ratio that is different from the home care setting, prescribed day care may realize a cost savings in comparison to home care services in the range of 17% to 37% (Stutts, 1994). At the same time, medical day care is more expensive than standard day care and may be beyond the financial reach of many needy families.

LONG-TERM/TRANSITIONAL CARE

Increasingly, tertiary care centers are reluctant to provide long-term hospitalizations for children with stabilized chronic illness, even if technology dependent. Once a child is medically stable, the hospital no longer receives compensation for the costly care it provides. Tertiary care settings are also not optimal long-term settings for the child; developmental, intellectual, emotional, and psychosocial needs are easily overlooked (Britton & Johnston, 1993). Few pediatric nursing homes exist across the country, and most adult nursing homes will not accept pediatric clients.

Across the country, a small number of specialized hospitals have been able to provide residential/transitional care for medically fragile children at a lower cost than the tertiary care centers. However, several factors are making it increasingly difficult to arrange placements for children in these facilities. First, many transitional facilities are revamping their programs to provide very specialized rehabilitative care. As a result, it is increasingly difficult to qualify for admission to these programs.

Second, these facilities are increasingly shifting their focus from a custodial model to a transitional focus. On a case-by-case basis, they may still consider accepting medically fragile children. However, it is easier to obtain placement for a transitional stay—until the child's medical condition stabilizes, less technology is required, or the family's confidence in their home care skills increases—than to arrange a long-term or lifetime placement.

Third, insurers are increasingly scrutinizing the appropriateness of transitional placements and will frequently deny placement if they feel the child's medical condition does not warrant it.

MEDICAL OR SPECIALIZED FOSTER CARE

Hill, Hayden, Lakin, Menke, & Amado (1990) examined data on foster care placements to determine the utilization of generic foster care as a long-term care placement for children and youth with handicapping conditions. They suggest that approximately 20% of children in foster care do have handicaps but that the handicap *per se* is seldom the reason for placement.

In some locations, unique programs offer specialized medical foster care. Gurdin and Anderson (1987), for example, report on acquired immune deficiency syndrome (AIDS)-specialized foster care homes in the New York City area. Recruiting foster families was described as a major challenge of the program, and a high reimbursement rate, as well as intensive medical and psychological support services are described as key to the success of the program. As another example, LaRabida Children's Hospital and the Children's Home and Aid Society of Illinois collaborated to develop foster care services for children who are medically fragile/technology dependent (Yost & Hochstadt, 1987). Specialized foster care parents must receive detailed information and training regarding the child's individualized care needs, as well as extensive ongoing support. For specialized

medical foster care to be successful, health care providers also need information about the relationship between agency staff, foster and biologic parents, and available resources (Schor, 1988).

CONCLUSION

Alternatives to home care for children with complex medical conditions are necessary for some families but often difficult to arrange. Programs and funding vary widely from one location to another. Community health nurses, discharge planners, and social workers may be most knowledgeable of the options available in any given locale.

Some communities may experience an increasing need to create options for families in this arena. Fewell (1993) suggests that when innovative and effective models or strategies for child care for children with special needs are examined, several factors can be noted. These include a strong, innovative leader, collaboration with families, and connection with a setting providing high-quality services to children and families. Nurses and families together can lead the way to making more alternatives available to families having children with complex medical problems.

REFERENCES

Britton, L.J., & Johnston, J.D. (1993). Dependent on technology: A child grows up hospitalized. *Pediatric Nursing, 19*(6), 579–584.

Crowley, A.A. (1990). Integrating handicapped and chronically ill into day care centers. *Pediatric Nursing, 16*(1), 39–44.

Fewell, R.R. (1993). Child care for children with special needs. *Pediatrics, 91*(1), 193–198.

Gurdin, P., & Anderson, G.R. (1987). Quality care for ill children: AIDS specialized foster family homes. *Child Welfare, LXVI*(4), 291–300.

Hill, B.K., Hayden, M.F., Lakin, K.C., Menke, J., & Amado, A.R.N. (1990). State-by-state data on children with handicaps in foster care. *Child Welfare, LXIX*(5), 447–462.

O'Connor, P., Van der Plaats, S., & Betz, C.L. (1992). Respite care services to caretakers of chronically ill children in California. *Journal of Pediatric Nursing, 7*(4), 269–275.

Schor, E.L. (1988). Foster care. *Pediatric Clinics of North America, 35*(6), 1,241–1,252.

Stutts, A.L. (1994). Selected outcomes of technology dependent children receiving home care and prescribed child care services. *Pediatric Nursing, 20*(5), 501–507.

Yost, D.M., & Hochstadt, N.J. (1987). Medical foster care for seriously medically ill children: A growing need. *Child and Adolescent Social Work, 4*(3&4), 142–302.

Suspected Abuse and Neglect in Home Care of the Child Who Is Technology Dependent

Elizabeth Ahmann, ScD, RN, and
Doris Mitnick, MSW, ACSW, CCM

A home care nurse and a parent may sometimes have different views of what constitutes appropriate care of the infant or child who is technology dependent. Differences may arise in the development of the overall goals of the plan of care or in specific arenas such as how to carry out certain procedures, how to discipline a child, and the degree to which siblings may be incorporated into the plan of care (Ahmann, 1994). Ahmann and Bond (1992) outline a process for negotiating agreement between the nurse and family members, suggesting that, in general, the nurse should respect the family's choices. Nurses should realize that, for some families, the appropriate goal will be to strive for minimal care standards, not necessarily ideal care. Klug (1993) also suggests that a parent's authority should be respected unless either risk or harm is posed to the child, or the written medical orders are not followed.

At the same time, Hogue (1992) suggests that nurses may have legal liability not only for their own actions but for parental "noncompliance" also. Agency policies will provide some guidance for the nurse in how to proceed when there is serious disagreement between the nurse and family regarding safe and appropriate care of the child. In general, honest, respectful communication with the family about the nurse's concerns should be accompanied by careful documentation of both the concerns and the discussion. The nurse, the case manager or nursing supervisor, the physician, and the family can also meet to discuss care preferences and safety concerns and to negotiate medical orders and care plan standards in areas where disagreement arises.

Some of what might be considered inappropriate care or medical neglect may result from factors such as the family feeling overwhelmed; family members not being fully informed about or trained to provide the proper care requirements; and/or denial about the diagnosis, prognosis, or complexities of the illness and care plan. As part of a comprehensive plan of care, the nurse and family should address these issues, and, as appropriate, the nurse should provide information, training, support, and referrals to respite, counseling, or other services so that the family can properly care for the child.

In most instances, the frequency and severity of "noncompliance" will affect the nurse's legal responsibility. For example, one missed medication dose may be appropriately handled by documentation and counseling. On the other hand, regularly missed doses or a single instance of turning off a ventilator alarm would require a more vigorous response (Hogue, 1992). The point at which such instances cross the line into reportable neglect or abuse depend in part on the definition of abuse and neglect in the state in which the services are provided. Physical abuse is generally more clear-cut than medical neglect. In any case, nurses should always inform a family when they feel they may have to report neglect or abuse and why.

The legal definitions of abuse and neglect vary from state to state. In the state of Virginia, the State Code on Suspected Child Abuse and Neglect (SCAN, Section 63.1–348 et. seq, Code of Virginia) defines the abused/neglected child as a person under age 18 whose parent/caregiver creates a situation that results in a substantial risk of death, disfigurement, or impairment of bodily or mental function. SCAN includes five categories:

1. sexual abuse
2. physical abuse/neglect
3. mental abuse/neglect
4. medical neglect
5. abandonment.

When reporting abuse or neglect, appropriate documentation consists of facts, not opinions, and can consist of evidence regarding the parent's success or failure in learning the appropriate care for the child. For example, the following statement of fact would be appropriate documentation of medical neglect concerns:

> 5/13/95   Arrived at the home, no answer at door. Waited 7 minutes and mother returned. Child with trach was unattended in the apartment. Mother stated, "I just ran to the store for a minute."

The following statement of opinion would not be an appropriate or useful documentation:

> 4/18/95   Mother in a bad mood and wouldn't participate in teaching.

In the assessment of SCAN in Virginia, *prima facie* evidence of medical neglect can be provided by a physician's statement that if a child does not receive certain care, harm or death may occur. The following statement is an example:

> The trach tube is a critical life support device and it requires constant attention. Someone needs to be present at all times who can manage the trach tube. This requirement exists because there is a constant possibility that the tube will become dislodged or plugged and C would suffocate . . . it is possible that C could die if appropriate attention is not paid to his trach tube care. (Dr. Strope, cited in Mitnick, 1995).

Once suspected abuse or neglect is reported to the appropriate authorities, a Child Protective Service (CPS) worker is engaged. The health care team should collaborate with the CPS worker, providing education addressing the following areas: the child's illness or disability, anticipated impact on the family system, and the prescribed individualized care plan. The health care team should provide ongoing docu-

mentation of both concerns as well as increased family compliance with the plan of care. Health care providers should additionally provide CPS with notification of any changes in the child's plan of care. Persistence on the part of health care providers in following the progress of the investigation is crucial. A focus on the needs of the technology-dependent child for safe and appropriate medical and developmental care is required while pursuing concerns of suspected abuse and neglect.

When neglect or abuse have been documented and reported, the CPS worker will initiate an investigation guided by agency policies regarding timeframes, evidence collection, and assessment. A home evaluation will be conducted, family and health care providers interviewed, and pertinent documentation secured.

Family members should be encouraged to participate in the investigation process and will have the opportunity both to communicate their understanding of the child's needs and how to provide for those needs as well as to detail their own compliance with the child's plan of care. Often, services not otherwise available to the family may be secured as a result of the CPS referral (i.e., financial resources, counseling, child care for siblings, or home adaptations necessary to support the child's care plan).

Collaboration between the CPS agency, the family, and the health care team is necessary to ensure the safety and the appropriate care of the medically fragile child referred for suspected abuse or neglect. Knowledge of minimal care standards, provision of thorough and appropriate documentation, close work with the family, and awareness of both the definitions of abuse and neglect in the state of residence and procedures for reporting suspected abuse and neglect are essential. Persistence in advocating for the child's needs is the professional responsibility of all health care team members.

REFERENCES

Ahmann, E. (1994). Thinking critically about family-centered home care. *Pediatric Nursing, 20*(6), 588–590.

Ahmann, E., & Bond, N.J. (1992). Promoting normal development in school-age children and adolescents who are technology dependent: A family-centered model. *Pediatric Nursing, 18*(4), 399–405.

Hogue, E. (1992). Parental noncompliance in home care. *Pediatric Nursing, 18*(6), 603–606.

Klug, R. (1993). Clarifying roles and expectations in home care. *Pediatric Nursing, 19*(3), 374–376.

Mitnick, D. (1995, April 27). *Suspected child abuse and neglect of the technology-dependent child.* Paper presented at the University of Massachusetts Medical Center conference: Continuing care of the chronically ill and technology-dependent child and family."

Chapter 5

Discharge Planning for the High-risk Infant

Revised by Margaret Cox, RN, BSN, A-CCC

Effective and efficient discharge planning continues to gain importance in the management of health care services. The concept and principles of continuity of care are especially important when a child has multiple and/or complex medical, nursing, and developmental needs. To achieve the goal of a smooth transition for the infant or young child from the hospital to another environment requires skill and collaboration (both multidisciplinary collaboration and collaboration with families). This is especially true as hospital stays are shortened and more support services are needed for the transition to home (Hamilton & Vessey, 1992). However, the rewards of careful attention to discharge planning can be seen in optimum family functioning, optimum health, and efficient use of financial resources.

Simmons (1992) describes the discharge planning process as "a systematic, coordinated program that is designed to bring about a timely discharge of a patient from a hospital to the next appropriate level of care or return to their normal living situation." Discharge planning is a process that should begin even before a patient is admitted to the hospital. Generally, the preferred discharge plan involves what would be a person's normal living situation—at home with family, for example. When this is not a viable possibility, other alternatives are explored. (See Special Issue, "Alternatives to Home Care for Medically Fragile Children.") However, discharge management is broader than simply determining the location for the patient after the acute hospitalization. It includes planning and preparing for all the needs of the patient and family. It is an ongoing process that includes continual refinement and monitoring as the most suitable

plans are developed to meet the patients' postdischarge needs (Simmons, 1992).

RATIONALE

The rationale for discharge planning is both continuity of care and cost-effectiveness. Fiscal restraints have been increased by federal legislation, and cost-containment measures have been implemented by third-party payers. Capitation of payment by state Medicaid programs has increased as well. Lengths of stay require clear documentation of medical necessity and evidence of discharge planning throughout. The Joint Commission of Accreditation of Health Care Organizations (Joint Commission) has integrated discharge planning as part of several review areas.

Critical pathways have been designed to assist in providing optimal care while limiting length of stay and costs. These pathways are defined as "the collaborative guidelines which time and sequence the major interventions of nurses, physicians, and other key departments for a particular case-type . . . sub-set . . . , or condition . . ." (Center for Nursing Case Management, Inc., 1989, pp. 1–2). Discharge planning interventions are an integral part of all critical pathways.

PHILOSOPHY

Every infant has the right to discharge planning. Some infants will require relatively simple preparation for discharge, with a focus on well-baby care and routine medical follow up. A higher level of planning is required for those with more complex care needs. Both the family and each discipline involved in the infant's care should contribute to the processes of assessment and planning. Keeping lines of communication open between the various parties can increase the exchange of ideas and assist in both clarification of needs and identification of optimal solutions. As the discharge planning process evolves, each team member should be considered responsible for documenting discussions, needs, and decisions. (Appendixes 5–A, 5–B, and 5–C provide sample documents.)

The family should be an integral part of the planning team. Including the family will improve the appropriateness of the assessment and the likelihood that the plan is realistic and can be implemented effectively. Parents need accurate, unbiased information to make informed decisions. While information often comes to the family from multiple team members, there should always be a designated person who family members can approach to clarify their concerns, to answer questions, or to whom they can vent in times of particular difficulty. The family may pick a member of the health care team to be its main support. This team member should be identified to others and should be kept informed of any changes affecting the discharge plan.

DISCHARGE PLANNING PROCESS

The discharge planning process is based on a thorough assessment of the needs of the child and family, followed by planning, implementation, and evaluation. Although there is a logical progression of these components, two or more may be operational at the same time. In fact, as indicated in Figure 5–1, there may be constant movement between the components. Movement between planning, implementation, and evaluation can be seen particularly clearly as health care providers attempt to be proactive in setting up home services in order to prevent any discharge delays. For example, it may occur that arrangements are made for home oxygen and oxygen is delivered to the home, only to have it discontinued the day of discharge when the condition of the infant improves, and oxygen is no longer needed. While it is better to have planned for the worst-case scenario, there is a price in time, effort, and sometimes product when services are cancelled at the last minute. Some of this price may not be reimbursable. Explaining to parents the rationale for advance planning and including the family in decisions is especially important so they will understand any last-minute changes.

ASSESSMENT

In the hospital nursery, the assessment phase of discharge planning begins with the admissions interview. At this time,

Figure 5–1 Discharge Planning Process

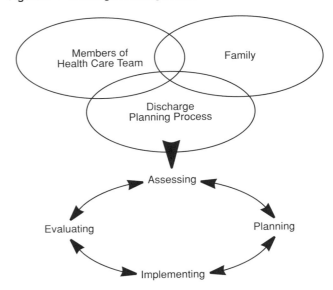

Source: Courtesy of Sally McCarthy, MSN, RN.

the nurse assesses the infant and meets with the family to obtain information for a nursing database. Information about both the infant and the family should be considered in discharge planning. A comprehensive assessment is essential in order to provide direction for effective discharge planning. Additional information obtained during the hospital stay should be documented and considered as discharge planning progresses. The nurse or social worker can work with a family in assessing their own strengths, an important foundation for a home care plan. Another consideration is family member willingness and ability to learn all the skills needed to care for the infant at home. As the technology, health care, and developmental needs of the infant become more clear, a clinical evaluation of the appropriateness of providing the care in the home should also be made. The family should participate with health care providers in these critical discussions.

Use of an assessment tool helps to make the discharge planning assessment process more objective. A tool that is helpful in predicting the need for pediatric home care services is provided in Appendix 5–B. During a long hospital stay, periodic reassessment of the need for home care services may be required as the infant's status or family preparedness change.

PLANNING

The second phase of the discharge planning process is a planning phase. It begins with the formulation of the plan of care or with the use of a critical pathway. The plan of care is based on the initial and ongoing assessments of the needs and strengths of the infant and family. Placement on a critical pathway is dependent on clinical or diagnostic grouping. Either approach to documentation should include documentation of the discharge planning process. Each allows for ongoing adjustments in discharge planning as the child's health status changes.

There are many forums for discharge planning. Whether the forum(s) for discharge planning include rounds, meetings or conferences, family members should be invited to participate in the discussions. Daily physician and nursing rounds frequently provide an opportunity for discussion of discharge planning. Additionally, most hospitals have weekly discharge planning meetings on each unit. As hospital lengths of stay decrease, many pediatric units have begun to use nursing and physician rounds for brief planning periods, supplemented with care conferences for the more complex patients. Another planning model involves the use of a clinical case manager, often a nurse, whose role is to coordinate the care of a group of patients, including both their inpatient and subsequent home care services (Zander, 1994).

Planning for hospital discharge should incorporate information from multiple disciplines. In more complex cases, this is best achieved by the use of a care conference. Parents, primary caregivers, and consultants from various disciplines involved in patient care should attend this conference. For example, those attending care conferences in the hospital nursery might include the family; physicians; nurses; social workers; physical, occupational, speech, or respiratory therapists; dietitians; an insurance representative; a utilization management representative; and (after a company is identified) home care representatives from appropriate community agencies or vendors (see Exhibit 5–1). When family members and representatives of various pertinent disciplines are present, everyone benefits from the information exchange, and everyone hears the same information.

An effective conference is set up well ahead of time so that the largest number of people can schedule the time. Each attendee should know both the identified goal of the conference and what information they will be responsible to present. Exhibit 5–1 gives examples of the role of various disciplines in a discharge planning case conference.

It is ideal if the family already has met most of the staff working with the child prior to a care conference. Family members will be able to contribute more if they are comfortable with the team members. Family members can be invited to have a parent advocate present at a care conference to assist them if they feel it would be helpful. Family members should be given an opportunity to discuss their concerns regarding home care and to participate in the problem-solving process.

For example, sometimes the idea of home care can seem overwhelming to a family. The family and other team members can address this concern, perhaps by adjusting the plan in some way to make it possible for the family to provide the care that is needed. Examples of adjustments include an

Exhibit 5–1 Patient Care Conference Participants and Expected Contributions

Discipline	Contribution
Family	Identifies strengths, resources, needs, and concerns of family unit; Determines own role in home care and discharge planning process; Functions as decision makers
Clinical nurse specialist	Identifies teaching needs & special concerns
Dietitian	Makes nutrition assessment; Sets intake goals for growth and development
Insurance representative	Gathers information & identifies payer support expected
Nurse	Describes expected care routines including medications and treatments
Physician(s)	Determines medical history, status, and prognosis; Identifies postdischarge medical management plans
Respiratory therapist	Describes current respiratory support; Determines frequency of treatments or adjustments
Social worker	Provides family support; Assesses emotional readiness for discharge; Makes suggestions for financial or emotional support postdischarge
Speech, occupational, physical therapist(s)	Assesses need for home program vs. therapist visits; Identifies adaptive equipment needs
Utilization management representative	Predicts expected length of service coverage by payer
Home equipment provider	Assesses for teaching & equipment needs & availability of equipment for home use
Home infusion provider	Assesses teaching & equipment needs
Home health agency representative	Assesses for amount of nursing needed
Discharge planner	Serves as facilitator*; Predicts expected payer support for postdischarge services if insurance representative not present

*Conference facilitator role can be performed by any of the planning team members.

additional amount of in-home nursing support or a change in the scheduling of medications and treatments. On the other hand, the family should be supported in finding an alternative to home care if they do not feel they have the resources to manage caring for their child at home. (See Special Issue, "Alternatives to Home Care for Medically Fragile Children.")

When families participate in discharge planning conferences, the family and health professionals can mutually establish the goals for the discharge plan and assess readiness for discharge. This involvement also enables parents to begin establishing the advocacy role they must later assume for their child. The family's involvement in the decision-making process ensures their commitment to the plan, develops their confidence, and increases the likelihood of a successful discharge plan.

Readiness for discharge is assessed at a care conference, and potential community resources for assisting the family in providing continuity of care are identified. It is important that as discharge planning needs are identified, specific disciplines or individuals who are accountable for making plans that address these needs also be identified. Documentation of the conferences, the outcomes, and identified responsible team members increases accountability and facilitates implementation of the discharge plan.

The timeliness of individual predischarge conferences is an important factor. They must be held early enough in the hospitalization to allow for comfortable planning and implementation rather than crisis intervention. For infants and children with complex care needs, several conferences over time may be necessary for a complete and effective discharge planning process.

IMPLEMENTATION

Implementation of the discharge plan includes discharge teaching, ordering home equipment, arranging for follow-up appointments, and making appropriate referrals to community agencies, home health agencies, and/or vendors.

Discharge Teaching

Home care of the high-risk premature infant may be very complex. Thorough teaching, emphasizing the details of each aspect of routine and potential emergency care, is essential. Teaching methods should include discussion, the provision of instructional materials, and demonstration by the nurse, with a return demonstration by each caregiver. The nurse should also observe for evidence of the caregivers' confidence and competence, as indicated through routine performance. Those who are doing the teaching should assist the family in continually evaluating their ability to learn the required care. Teaching or training methods should be adapted, when necessary, to promote increased

learning ability. For example, the family with an acutely ill child may feel very stressed and, as a result, may have difficulty retaining what is taught. If the teaching plan is adapted for them to ensure introducing only small increments of information at a time, then small successes in learning can encourage them in going forward to each next step. Teaching should progress from more simple care needs, such as bathing and feeding, to the more complex skills, such as medication administration; medical or nursing procedures; and eventually competent, safe use of the child's medical equipment.

Teaching about medical equipment to be used in the home is increasingly done by the company providing the equipment. This teaching is usually done very close to the discharge day. If a family has a high level of anxiety or has demonstrated that its members learn more slowly, special arrangements should be made with the company providing the equipment to give instruction over a longer period of time. The use of complex equipment, such as tracheal continuous positive airway pressure (C-PAP) and ventilators, should be taught at least several days before discharge. Optimally, the same equipment that will be used in the home should be used in the hospital for a minimum of 24 to 48 hours prior to discharge to ensure safe, reliable operation by family members. Because of the differences between equipment used in the hospital and that available for home use, this 24- to 48-hour period is very important.

For infants with complex care needs, it is helpful for the family members to provide total care in the hospital setting for 8 to 24 hours as a prerequisite for discharge. This arrangement ensures that the family has professional nurses available for any problems but has the chance to demonstrate to themselves and hospital staff their ability to provide competent care. Families have often commented that this "trial run" gave them confidence that they would be able to handle the care requirements at home. Some hospitals have special home-like rooms available for this purpose.

An essential component of the discharge teaching plan is the identification and training of at least one secondary or "back-up" caregiver. These back-up caregivers must comprise a reliable support system that is readily available to the primary caregiver. Even when two parents are trained in the care, one may not be readily available for providing care to the infant; for example, the father may work very long hours or be employed in two jobs. In such cases, a relative or neighbor can then be trained as a secondary caregiver. Single parents may also need assistance in identifying a second person to provide care for the child.

Documentation of discharge teaching should include both what teaching has occurred and what degree of understanding and skill the family is able to verbalize or demonstrate. Standardized teaching criteria and discharge teaching checklists facilitate measurement and documentation of the skills and knowledge acquired by the family. A brief overall view of discharge teaching is reflected in a checklist; a more detailed view of the progress is reflected in the nursing progress notes accumulated by all staff participating in the teaching. An example of a discharge teaching checklist for a specific condition (tracheostomy) is provided in Appendix 5–C. Ideally, the checklist should be shared with the home health nurse to enable confirmation and enhancement of discharge teaching in the home setting.

Written discharge instructions are an important part of teaching and should be given to families and caregivers whenever possible. These should address well-baby care as well as pertinent medical/nursing care issues. Providing families with information on well-baby care will be an invaluable aid in helping them to focus on the "normal" aspects of their infant's care, which is often difficult after the infant has spent several weeks in a hospital nursery. Written instructions documenting the infant's special care needs are an important reference for the family once at home.

Preprinted instruction sheets for certain disease conditions or medications can also be devised to assist the caregiver and to streamline the teaching process. (See Appendix 5–D for an example: gastroesophageal reflux.) These must be individualized, however. Written instructions do not substitute for individualized teaching but serve as a source of reference. For maximum benefit, instruction sheets should be given to the family prior to discharge, allowing them time to read and formulate questions while health care team members are available for clarification.

Equipment and Home Health Referrals

Early identification of equipment and nursing support needed for home care is important in order to avoid obstacles in obtaining reimbursement and resulting delays in discharge. Individual state Medicaid programs as well as commercial insurances and health plans have varied limitations regarding how equipment and nursing support are reimbursed. Letters of medical necessity as well as copies of particular tests and confirmation of diagnosis may be required prior to authorization of coverage.

The home health agencies or vendors used should be a matter of the family's choice within the constraints of their insurance company's list of preferred providers. While a family may technically be allowed to use an "out of network" provider, to do so generally results in an increase in the family's copay. On occasion, a dilemma will arise if the agencies on the preferred provider list cannot offer appropriate care. The discharging hospital has a responsibility to discharge the patient to agencies that can provide appropriate care. If the preferred providers are not appropriate, then the insurance company should be given factual information about the concern, and an agreement should be reached that will be safe for the patient.

Families should be given an idea of criteria to use in choosing an agency or vendor. Agencies that have Joint

Exhibit 5–2 Criteria To Consider in the Selection of a Home Care Agency or Vendor

- pediatric experience
- 24-hour availability
- appropriate range of equipment and supplies available for ordering and reordering
- provision of preventive maintenance on equipment
- provision of written instructions for operation and maintenance of equipment
- availability of copy of teaching checklist on request
- provision of timely response to telephone calls regarding problems
- professional, licensed staff
- appropriate state license.

Commission accreditation have demonstrated that they meet high quality standards. Some criteria to consider are listed in Exhibit 5–2.

Many times, insurance companies will assign a case manager to make better use of the health care dollars. The case manager can be a very good advocate for services for the family. The more complete the information they are given, the better they can assist the infant and family. There are times when using some community services can save on the insurance payer dollars. This is most true of therapy services if they are available. Another example is the use of a volunteer group in the community to provide transportation or respite care. Many states have Medicaid waiver programs that will cover major expenses, such as hourly nursing.

The amount of home nursing support requested for an individual child is determined by the assessment information reviewed at the patient care conference. Families of infants who have a large number of medications, enteral feedings, and oxygen and monitor needs, as an example, can often benefit from hourly nursing support. If an infant's care is less complex or if a family prefers no hourly nursing in the home, intermittent nursing visits (i.e., visits that last $\frac{1}{2}$ to 1 hour) can be supportive and provide a professional assessment as frequently as every day or as infrequently as once every 1 to 2 weeks.

Whether services are to be hourly or intermittent, the home health agency and the home health nurse will have an advantage if a complete referral is made at least a few days prior to discharge. Hourly nursing requires more time to schedule and coordinate. Along with demographic data, such as address, names of parents, emergency contact, insurance, and diagnosis, the referral should include the name of the attending physician who will be responsible for ordering home health services, a summary of the hospital stay, the plan or goal for home services, scheduled appointments, and copies of completed discharge teaching checklists.

Prior to hospital discharge, nursing staff should explain to parents what they may expect of the home health nurses. Several major roles can be described (K. Huddleston, personal communication, May 1995):

- assessment of the infant
- direct care provision for the infant
- instruction for the parents
- case-management, advocacy, referral source.

Parents should be informed that the role of the nurse is to assist them in caring for the infant and not to judge them as parents or a family.

Follow-up Appointments

Arranging for appropriate medical follow up with specialty clinics (e.g., for pulmonary or neurologic problems) is also an essential component of the discharge plan. Prior to discharge, the family should be asked about preferences regarding return appointment times. Using these preferences, the family should have the appointments scheduled for them and be given a list of the specific dates and times.

The number of appointments the infant may need for follow up can be overwhelming to the family. Scheduling several appointments on the same day may be most convenient for a family who has to travel a distance to the hospital. Providing the home health nurse with the schedule will enable some reinforcement of the importance of the follow up. Families should also be assisted in developing plans for safely transporting the child to and from the hospital.

Families should be assisted as necessary in identifying a source of primary pediatric care prior to discharge. Care should be taken that any insurance company preferred provider limitations are noted in choice of a primary care provider. The primary care provider should be given a complete history of the neonatal course, a summary of the infant's current status (including immunization status), information about home care services that will be provided, and a list of specialty care providers who will be following the child.

Plans should also be made for follow-up developmental assessment and intervention as may be appropriate. (See Part VI on developmental and sensory concerns.) Many services can be obtained free under Part H of Individuals with Disabilities Education Act (IDEA). See Special Issue titled "Early Intervention Services for the High-risk Infant."

Transportation Plans

No infant can be sent home without an appropriate car seat. Special arrangements may be needed for very small infants and infants with certain disabilities as the standard infant car seats may not provide adequate safety restraint (Bull, Stout, Stroup, & Rust, 1991; Bull, Weber, & Stroup, 1988; Everly et al., 1993; Stroup, Everly, Weber, & Doll, 1994). Special arrangements may also be necessary for sup-

Exhibit 5–3 Sample Consumer Satisfaction Survey

Please rate your satisfaction with the discharge planning process for your child as follows:

	Excellent	Very Good	Good	Fair	Poor
1. Parent involvement in planning discharge					
2. Parent instruction in preparation for discharge					
3. Coordination of care between the hospital and home care providers					
4. Equipment and service provided by home care company					
5. Satisfaction with home nursing services					

Comments: _____
_____
_____

plies, equipment, and ready attention in case of emergency during transportation of the infant with special needs. (Various chapters of this book provide condition- and equipment-specific transportation guidance.)

EVALUATION

Evaluation of discharge planning is essential in order to make home care a safe and successful experience for infants and families. Discharge planners and all health professionals are responsible for evaluating the adequacy of home health agencies, equipment companies, and any community agency providing services or support at home.

Through a consumer survey, families can be helpful in providing feedback about experiences such as the reliability of equipment companies or the readability and usefulness of parent teaching materials. They may also provide valuable information regarding what additional assistance might have helped them in the transition to home care. Consumer surveys are often mailed to a family after hospital discharge. Exhibit 5–3 provides a simple example of the questions that might be used in a consumer survey about the discharge planning process.

A separate survey can be sent to the agencies accepting a referral for home services. The feedback on this survey, in conjunction with the family survey, can identify opportunities for improvement in the discharge planning process. Changes made in response to the survey data should lead to an improved process for the hospital, community agencies, child, and family. The goal is improved continuity of care.

REFERENCES

Bull, M.J., Stout, J., Stroup, K.B., & Rust, J. (1991). Safe transportation home for infants with severe hydrocephalus. *Journal of Neuroscience Nursing, 23*(6), 369–373.

Bull, M.J., Weber, K., & Stroup, K.B. (1988). Automotive restraint systems for premature infants. *Journal of Pediatrics, 112*(3), 385–388.

Center for Nursing Case Management, Inc. (1989). Second generation critical paths. *Definition, 4*(4), 1–2.

Everly, J.S., Bull, M.J., Stroup, K.B., Goldsmith, J.J., Doll J.P., & Russell, R. (1993). A Survey of Transportation Services for Children with Disabilities. *American Journal of Occupational Therapy, 47*(9), 804–810.

Hamilton, B., & Vessey, J. (1992). Pediatric discharge planning. *Pediatric Nursing, 18*(5), 475–478.

Simmons, J. (1992, September). *Risks, rights and realities of discharge planning.* Paper presented at the meeting of the American Association of Continuity of Care, Las Vegas, NV.

Stroup, K.B., Everly, J.S., Weber, K., & Doll, J.P. (1994). Child safety seat use for infants with Pierre Robin syndrome. *Archives of Pediatric and Adolescent Medicine, 148*(3), 301–305.

Zander, K. (1994, October). *Case management: Coming of age.* Paper presented at the Case management: A commitment to advocacy meeting of the Association for the Care of Children's Health, Baltimore, MD.

ADDITIONAL RESOURCES

Ahmann, E. (1994). Family-centered care: Shifting orientation. *Pediatric Nursing, 20*(2), 113–118.

Ahmann, E., & Bond, N.J. (1992). Promoting normal development in school-age children and adolescents who are technology-dependent: A family-centered model. *Pediatric Nursing, 18*(4), 399.

Baginski, Y. (1994). Roadblocks to home care. *Continuing Care Magazine, 12*(4), 16–29.

Birmingham, J. (1992). *Discharge planning: A practitioner's guide to policies, procedures and protocols.* Los Angeles, CA: Academy Medical Systems, Inc.

Bond, N., Philips, P., & Rollins, J.A. (1994). Family centered care at home for families with children who are technology-dependent. *Pediatric Nursing, 20*(2), 123–132.

Center for Nursing Case Management, Inc. (1992). Physicians, caremaps, and collaboration. *Definition, 7*(1), 1–2.

Fenerty, N.J. (1993). Interdisciplinary discharge planning. *Cancer Practice, 1*(2), 147–152.

Howard-Glenn, L. (1992). Transition to home: Discharge planning for the oxygen-dependent infant with bronchopulmonary dysplasia. *Journal of Perinatal and Neonatal Nursing, 6*(2), 85–94.

Lewis, C., Alford-Winston, A., Billy-Kornsas, M., McCaustland, M., & Tachman, C.P. (1992). Care management for children who are medically fragile/technology-dependent. *Issues in Comprehensive Pediatric Nursing, 15,* 73–91.

Ondeck, D.A., & Gingerich, B.S. (1993). Discharge planning: An act of caring. *Journal of Home Health Care Practice, 5*(4), 41–48.

Pray, D., & Hoff, J. (1992). Implementing a multidisciplinary approach to discharge planning. *Nursing Management, 23*(10), 52–56.

Richardson, M., Student, E., O'Boyle, D., Smith, M., & Wheeler, T.W. (1992). Establishment of a state-supported, specialized home care program for children with complex health care needs. *Issues in Comprehensive Pediatric Nursing, 15,* 93–122.

Sheikh, L., O'Brien, M., & McClusky-Fawcett, K. (1993). Parent preparation for the NICU to home transition: Staff and parent perceptions. *Children's Health Care, 22*(3), 227–239.

Society for Social Work Administrators in Health Care of the American Hospital Administration. (1994). Evolution of discharge planning in rehabilitation: A perspective. *Discharge Planning Update, 14*(3), 1–6.

Thompson, D.G. (1994, January-February). Critical pathways in the neonatal intensive care and intermediate care nurseries. *Maternal & Child Nursing, 19,* 29–32.

Wells, P., Watherson, P., DeBoard-Burns, M.B., Cook, R.C., & Mitchell, J. (1994). Growing up in the hospital, Part II: Nurturing the philosophy of family-centered care. *Journal of Pediatric Nursing, 9*(3), 141–149.

Appendix 5-A

Neonatal Intensive Care Unit (NICU) Discharge Planning Checklist

Patient Name:

Primary Nurses:

Caregiver #1

Caregiver #2

WELL BABY CARE	TAUGHT #1	#2	CARDIOVASCULAR	TAUGHT #1	#2	FEEDING TECHNIQUE	TAUGHT #1	#2	EQUIPMENT/LIST
Bathing			CPR			GT Feeding			
Diapering			Film			chg dressing/site care			
Cord Care			Demonstration			replacing GT			REFERRALS
Perineal Care			Redemonstration			feeding technique			Written
S/S Illness			S/S CHF			NEUROLOGICAL			Faxed
Temperature Taking			S/S Hypoxia/Blue Spells			S/S Seizures			PKU
Use/Bulb Syringe			SBE Prophylaxis			S/S Shunt Failure			Admit
Crying/Sleep Patterns			GENITOURINARY			RESPIRATORY			D/C
Safety Education			Clean Intermittent catheterization			S/S Respiratory Distress			TESTS
Growth & Development			NUTRITION/GI			Home Apnea Monitor			Sleep
Ped MD's Name & Phone No.			PO feeding technique			demonstration			Eye Exam
Emergency Phone #s			Breastfeeding			redemonstration			BAER/hrng
Immunizations			Formula Prep			O₂/Nasal Cannula Use & Safety Precautions			FOLLOW-UP APPTS/SCHED-LIST
MEDICATIONS			S/S feeding intolerance			CPT			
Purpose/Side Effects			S/S intestinal obstruction			Suctioning Technique			
Adm Techniques & time schedule			Reflux precautions			NP with catheter			
Immunizations			NG Feeding			trach			
Prescriptions			placing tube			Trach Care			
Drawing up med from filled Rx			checking placement			Aerosol treatment			

Note: S/S = signs & symptoms, Adm = administration, CPR = cardiopulmonary resuscitation, CHF = congestive heart failure, CPT = chest physiotherapy, GT = gastrostomy, D/C = discharge, NG = nasogastric, NP = nasopharyngeal, PKU = phenylketonuria, SBE = subacute bacterial endocarditis.

Source: Courtesy of Children's National Medical Center, the Department of Nursing Education, Washington, DC.

Risk Factors Indicating a Need for Home Care Intervention

Circle appropriate points in each area

HOME CARE INTERVENTION (any of the following is an automatic home care referral)					
4	IV	4	TPN / ENTERAL	4	Trach
4	Monitor	4	Oxygen	4	Vent
4	Injection	3	DME	4	Broviac
3	RT	3	OT / SPEECH / PT	3	Hospice
3	SW	4	Private Duty	3	Skilled Nurse

ADMISSION STATUS					
4	Followed by a Home Care Agency prior to admission	2	Unplanned readmission within 2 weeks of discharge	4	Unplanned readmission within 72 hours or less
2	Unplanned admission following an OP treatment procedure	4	Unplanned visits to ER within 24 hours of prior visit/within 48 hours of discharge	4	Admitted to PICU
2	Admitted through ER	4	Admitted to NICU	1	AMSAC

DIAGNOSIS					
2	AIDS	1	Diabetes	3	Obstruction
4	Apnea/bradycardia	1	Diarrhea, dehydration	3	Osteomyelitis
2	Asthma	2	Failure to thrive	4	Ostomy
3	BPD	1	Feeding Disorder	3	Pulmonary _____
2	Bronchiolitis	2	Fever, R/O sepsis	3	Pneumonia
	Burns % _____	2	Fracture	3	Prematurity
4	Cancer _____	3	GE Reflux	3	RDS, hyaline membrane
3	Cardiac anomaly	3	Hemiparesis	2	Renal _____
3	Cellulitis	1	HIV infection	2	Seizure disorder
3	Central line infection	3	Hydrocephaly	2	Spina bifida
1	Cerebral palsy	2	Meningitis	4	Tracheostomy
2	Congenital anomaly	1	Mental retardation	3	Trauma _____
1	Cystic fibrosis	3	Microcephaly		Other
1	Developmentally delayed	1	NEC		

LIVING ARRANGEMENT					
3	Teen Parent	2	Unemployed family/lower SES	2	Rural area
3	Single Parent	3	Living in shelter	4	Disabled/MR
2	First time, anxious parents	4	Homeless	4	Home environment
2	No family support	2	Unstable/overcrowded living conditions	2	Foster family

(Continued on next page)

PSYCHOSOCIAL ISSUES

4	Suspected abuse/neglect	2	Evidence of bonding problems	3	Possible
3	History of noncompliance	3	Language barrier	2	Behavioral problems
2	Ineffective family coping patterns	4	Previous fetal/infant death	4	Minimal/no history
3	Frequent hospitalization, same diagnosis	4	Coping with life-threatening diagnosis	3	Long acute
3	Caregiver learning barriers	4	Coping with trauma	2	Cultural differences

LEARNING NEEDS

4	Management of new chronic diagnosis	2	Life style adjustment change	1	Diet change
2	Change in medications	1	Medication (inhalation)	1	Change in activity
4	Medication (IV, IM, SC)	3	Equipment	3	Procedures
3	Tests	4	Complex oral medications	3	Follow-up care

PROGNOSIS

1	Good to excellent	3	Fair rehab. potential	3	Poor
3	Terminal				

FINANCIAL

4	No insurance	2	Case managed insurance	3	Financial aid
2	Managed Care (HMO)	4	Self-pay	4	Medicaid pending
4	Medicaid Waiver	1	Co-pay		

OUTCOME INTERVENTION (fill in score and check appropriate interventions)

TOTAL SCORE	High risk for Home Care intervention, referral process begun _____
Referred to credit office: _____	High risk for SW intervention, referred to _____ on _____

RISK FACTOR
High Risk Factor > 25 points
Mod. Risk Factor > 15 to 24 points
Low Risk Factor < 14 points

KEY
Auto. Home Care referral
Monitor further for risk validation
No intervention needed/send to CR

POINT WEIGHT
1 point   Possible concern; chronic condition.
3 points High risk indicator on its own.
2 points On its own it raises a possible concern, however, in combination with other factors it becomes high risk.
4 points High risk, life threatening if not provided.

OUTCOME INTERVENTION
1. If the first seven categories equal 14 points or less, there is no apparent need for Home Care and the screening may stop here.
2. If the first seven categories total 15 or more points, continue the screen.
3. If category 3 and 4 are greater than 25% of the screening score, an automatic referral to the hospital's social service department is made, regardless of need for Home Care intervention.
4. If the Financial section indicates no insurance, self-pay, Medicaid pending or financial planning needed, a referral to the credit office is indicated.
5. Score of 15 to 24 indicates a moderate risk for Home Care intervention, these children will be further monitored before a home care referral is generated.

Appendix 5–C

Discharge Checklist: Tracheostomy Home Care

Nurse's Name   Initials

_____ _____

_____ _____

_____ _____

_____ _____

Caretaker _____

(Indiv. checklist for each caretaker)

Caretaker's level of
Performance
   V—Verbalized
   D—Demonstrated
   RP—Routinely Performs

	Disch. Std.	NURSING ACTIVITIES			CARETAKER ACTIVITIES			COMMENTS
		Disc. Date/Intl.	Demon. Date/Intl.	Reinf. Date/Intl.	V Date/Intl.	D Date/Intl.	RP Date/Intl.	
"Home Care of Your Child with a Tracheostomy" booklet given to caretaker.	V							
Anatomy and physiology of the upper airway system explained and how it is related to a tracheostomy.	V							
Purpose of tracheostomy for this child explained.	V							
Identified general symptoms of respiratory distress.	V							
Identified appropriate steps in handling respiratory difficulty.	V							
Identified the difference between moist and dry breath sounds.	V							
Identified significance of changes in color, nature and amount of secretions.	V							
Demonstrated use of mist collar.	RP							
Instilled normal saline into child's tracheostomy tube.	RP							
Demonstrated correct technique for suctioning.	RP							
Verbalized understanding of purpose and use of resuscitation bag.	V							
Demonstrated use of resuscitation bag.	RP							

B-114/Disk11

    [Explanation of abbreviations on checklist:

    Disch. std. =   Discharge Standard (level of performance)

    Disc.   =   Discussed

    Demon.   =   Demonstrated

    Reinf.   =   Reinforced

    Intl.   =   Initial (of nurse)]

Source: Courtesy of Children's Hospital National Medical Center, Division of Nursing, Washington, D.C.

(Continued on next page)

	Disch. Std.	NURSING ACTIVITIES			CARETAKER ACTIVITIES			COMMENTS
		Disc. Date/Intl.	Demon. Date/Intl.	Reinf. Date/Intl.	V Date/Intl.	D Date/Intl.	RP Date/Intl.	
Demonstrated chest physical therapy.	RP							
Provided skin care around the tracheostomy area and explained how to assess for skin breakdowns.	RP							
Prepared and changed child's tracheostomy ties.	RP							
Explained and demonstrated correct technique in changing child's tracheostomy tube: with assistance without assistance	RP							
Described correct procedure to follow when tracheostomy tube is difficult to insert.	D							
Verbalized and demonstrated on a doll what to do if child accidentally decannulated himself/herself.	D							
Identified appropriate steps in handling plugging of tracheostomy tube.	D							
Demonstrated correct CPR procedure for a child of this age with a tracheostomy.	D							
Provided total care for 24 hours or more.	RP							
Travel kit assembled and given to caretaker with purpose and contents explained.	D							
Home Care supplies: ordered: delivered and demonstrated by vendor Caretaker has demonstrated competence in troubleshooting problems with equipment.	V V D							
Caretaker describes arrangement of supplies/equipment at home.	V							
Parents instructed to post emergency phone #'s by telephone.	V							
Parents instructed to post CPR guidelines by child's bed.	V							
Community Support and Resources	Completed Date/Initials							
Nursing referral written and sent Name of Agency _____								

(Continued on next page)

COMPLETED
DATE/INITIALS

COMMENTS

	Completed Date/Initial	COMMENTS
Local Hospital Emergency Room: Name Phone # Notified in writing of child's need for services Emergency Squad: Name Phone # Notified in writing of child's need for services		
Telephone Company Written notification sent re: child's need for priority service. Instructions given caretaker re: procedure to follow if service is interrupted.		
Electric Company Written notification sent re: child's need for priority service Instructions given caretaker re: procedure to follow if service is interrupted.		

B-114/Disk11

TO ORDER COPIES, CONTACT: Director of Nursing Education and Research
Division of Nursing
Children's Hospital National Medical Center
111 Michigan Ave., NW
Washington, DC 20010

Discharge Instruction Sheet:
Gastroesophageal Reflux (GER) Precautions

WHAT IS GER

Gastroesophageal Reflux (GER) is the movement of stomach contents back up into the throat after they have been swallowed.

GER may be associated with apneic episodes. An infant who has had unexplained vomiting or regurgitation with feeding (GER) will be placed on reflux precautions.

GER PRECAUTIONS

Reflux Precautions consist of the following:

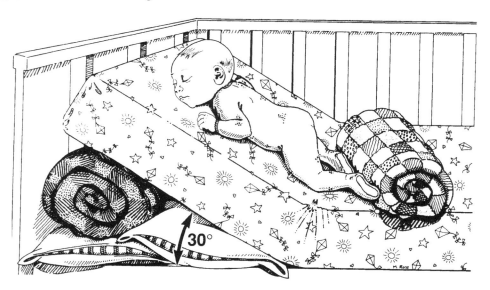

- Place infant on stomach with mattress at a 30–40 angle. (The head should be higher than the feet.) To keep your child from sliding down the mattress, put a blanket roll at his feet. If you wish, you may order a special harness designed to keep your child in the proper position on the mattress.
- Add _____ of rice cereal to each ounce of formula.
- Feed your child slowly and hold him in an upright position.
- Burp after every _____ ounce(s).
- Don't overfeed.

Chapter 6

The Nursing Intake Process
and the Plan of Care

Revised by Elizabeth Ahmann, ScD, RN,
and Christina Floyd, RN, BSN

The role of the home care nurse depends on many factors. These include the following: whether the nurse is providing skilled intermittent visits or shift nursing care in the home; whether a designated case manager is assigned to the client; the complexity of the child's care requirements; the family's level of involvement; the degree of involvement of other disciplines in the child's care; and the policies of the individual home care agency employing the nurse. Although the role of the home care nurse cannot be given one definition fitting all circumstances, this chapter addresses the following generic issues: the nursing intake process, principles of health interviewing, the assessment process, development of a dynamic plan of care, documentation, and case management/care coordination. This chapter should be read in conjunction with the chapter on family-centered care (Chapter 4), which discusses parent–professional collaboration and the parent–nurse relationship.

NURSING INTAKE PROCESS

The first home visit is important for several reasons. First, it is the beginning of the relationship between the community or home health nurse and the family. This visit will in all likelihood set the tone of the relationship and thus influence subsequent visits. Second, in most agencies, the first home visit requires the most documentation (permission forms, insurance information, intake history, and so forth). As a third factor, the first home visit must include an immediate assessment of the child's status and safety at home.

Fourth, nursing interventions including teaching and direct care may be required on the first home visit.

Relationship between Nurse and Family

When family members open their door for the first time to the home care nurse, they may feel that they are opening up their lives for review. Some families may be concerned that the nurse is there to "spy" on them or to evaluate and judge them. Some families feel that the hospital personnel prescribe home care because they view the family as incapable of caring for the child. It is essential for the nurse to dispel these concerns. The nurse should assure the family that the role of the nurse is to assist the family in whatever ways they may identify to ensure optimal health for the child and the greatest possible comfort and well-being for the family as they care for the child.

Most families will know that they have been referred for home care follow up. Ideally, family members will have participated in a discharge planning conference and will have elected to have home care services. Nonetheless, families may be uncertain as to just what services home care personnel will provide. A key aspect of the first home visit is for the nurse to explain to the family the purpose of home visits by nurses and any other personnel who will be part of the team of services the child and family receive.

For example, the home care nursing role can be explained as including the following: assessing the infant's health status, reviewing care procedures with the family and assisting them to determine any learning needs they may have, providing information and training as necessary, providing referrals to primary health care and other community resources as appropriate, and assisting the family with care coordination (case-management) tasks until such time as they can assume these tasks independently. The collaborative nature of home care service provision should be emphasized.

Documentation Concerns

Because of the necessary assessment and documentation requirements, the first visit may tend to be lengthy. It should generally be limited, however, to 1½ to 2 hours; longer periods may seem overwhelming and invasive to a family. In this regard, parents should be informed before the visit of the expected amount of time the nurse will need. They should also be reassured that not all visits will be as lengthy. The first home visit should be planned at a time when parents will be relatively free from interruptions (e.g., older children at school and baby napping). However, patience is necessary if interruptions do occur; the home environment is quite different from the hospital or clinic.

To ensure an acceptable time period for the first home visit, the nurse may need to assign priorities among necessary intake activities. Of course, certain permission forms will need to be signed and insurance information verified.

Although it is often thought that obtaining a complete health history is the first step in providing health care services, the first visit need not be devoted to obtaining a complete history. Prior to the first visit, the nurse can obtain data for the health history from the discharging institution. This health history can be augmented as necessary on the first and subsequent home visits. (Appendix 6–A includes a form for documenting a complete health history.)

Assessment

On the first home visit, the infant's condition must be assessed; equipment must be checked for proper functioning; the presence of all needed supplies must be determined; and a preliminary assessment must be made of the parents' preparation for providing appropriate routine and emergency care. The exact format and content for the assessment will be determined by the child's diagnoses, current condition, and equipment and care requirements (see Chapters 9–25).

Intervention

Most children and families have many care needs that cannot be addressed on the first visit. The nurse and family will have to use their talents to sort through and prioritize pressing concerns. While, ideally, discharge teaching has prepared the family for all aspects of home care, the nurse

and family should review care requirements and implement additional teaching as necessary. Priority must be given to those care needs that are basic to the survival of the child over the next day or two until the nurse can return to continue assessment and teaching. Priority should also be given to areas of concern that parents voice.

For example, if a child has a tracheostomy, maintaining an open airway is critical. To ensure the maintenance of an open airway, two conditions must be met: (1) the caregiver must be able to suction the trach tube properly (this can be ensured by explaining, demonstrating, and eliciting a return demonstration), and (2) a "ready-to-go" replacement trach tube must be available (see Chapter 15). Addressing speech and language concerns can be postponed to a later visit when caregivers are knowledgeable and competent in the direct and emergency care requirements for the child.

As another example, for any infant or child on medication, a review of medication schedules, dosages, concentrations, storage, and administration techniques is essential on the first visit. Medication errors are widespread and can be hazardous in the young child. Key concerns are concentration (as some pharmacies are not familiar with pediatric concentrations of certain medications) and measurement (e.g., 2 mL and 0.2 mL must be distinguished as must a measuring teaspoon and a kitchen spoon).

PRINCIPLES OF HEALTH INTERVIEWING

The health history, including a review of systems, with a physical assessment of the child and an interview with the family, provides the data on which the family and nurse will base both the initial care plan and ongoing nursing interventions. The history-taking process not only provides facts but allows the nurse and family to identify key concerns, care priorities, and learning needs.

The elements of a complete health history are listed in Exhibit 6–1, and a sample form for documenting a complete history is included in Appendix 6–A. Many aspects of a complete health history may not be critical in developing the plan of care. As a result, many home health nurses and agencies have elected to use a focused approach to obtaining a health history. Key components of any pediatric health history include the following:

- primary caregivers
- primary health care provider
- diagnoses (from medical record or referral forms)
- parental description of the health history and current health status of the child
- any previous hospitalizations
- immunization records
- birth history and gestational age at birth
- nutritional history and current diet

Exhibit 6–1 Elements of a Complete Health History for the High-risk Infant*

- Home and family data
- Family health history
- Prenatal history
- Birth history
- Newborn history
- General health history—immunizations, allergies, accidents, illnesses, previous hospitalizations.
- Parent–child interaction
- Daily patterns—feeding, sleeping, urinary and bowel habits
- Nutrition†
- Development
- Special care needs—equipment, treatment, diet, medications
- Review of body systems.‡

*See also Appendix 6–A.
†See Appendix 9–A for nutritional assessment.
‡See Appendix 6–B.

Exhibit 6–2 Considerations Regarding a Family's Right to Privacy and Confidentiality

1. The family may reveal private information that will enhance treatment; in return, the nurse must keep the information confidential.
2. Families have the right to access personal health records and to obtain a copy of records.
3. The nurse must maintain health records in a secure, controlled manner.
4. The nurse only reveals information with the family's permission or when required by law.

Source: Reprinted from *Pediatric Nursing,* Vol. 20, No. 2, March–April, p. 124, with permission of Jannetti Publications, Inc., Pitman, New Jersey, © 1994.

- complete systems review (see Appendix 6–B), including developmental status
- key support persons and organizations for the family (e.g., relatives, friends, neighborhood or church groups).

Parents of children with multiple and complex problems are repeatedly interviewed by numerous health professionals. This can be a frustrating and burdensome experience. When possible, the nurse can streamline some aspects of data gathering by obtaining information from other records and simply verifying it with parents. Explaining the reasons for other questions is considerate.

Families should be assured that any information they provide the nurse will be held in confidence. They should also be told why any questions are asked, how the information will be used, and who will have access to it (Bond, Phillips, & Rollins, 1994). A family's right to privacy and confidentiality must be respected (see Exhibit 6–2). Additionally, a family member's right to withhold information he or she considers too personal should be respected.

When either the initial history or interim histories are obtained, attentiveness and a nonjudgmental attitude are important both for establishing rapport and for creating an environment in which the parent feels free to discuss any concerns openly. In most cases, health interviewing and history taking will be most productive when open-ended questions are used (e.g., "Can you tell me about your infant's health?") rather than a series of direct questions (e.g., "When did you first know the diagnosis?" "How stable has the infant's course been?"). When open-ended questioning is used, the parent (or patient, if old enough to be questioned) should rarely be interrupted. If pauses occur, they can be used for the interviewer to indicate interest or to ask for clarification. Open-ended questions usually generate sig-

nificant health information and reveal parental perceptions and concerns and family dynamics.

If specific details needed for a complete history or assessment are not addressed by the parent in response to open-ended questions, some direct questions may be necessary. The following principles, suggested by Bernstein, Bernstein, and Dana (1974) outline the most appropriate way to use direct questions: "a) The sequence of questions should progress from the general to the specific; b) The questions should progress from the less personal to the more personal; c) The questions should be worded to elicit answers of a sentence or more and to avoid "yes" or "no" responses; d) The questions should be worded to avoid bias" (p. 103).

In any health interview, it is important to use language comprehensible to the persons being interviewed. Although language that is too elementary may be insulting, medical jargon is often not understood, and some parents may be hesitant to ask for an explanation. In addition, some questions that seem important to health care providers may seem unnecessarily prying to parents, who then become reluctant to reply openly. This problem can often be avoided by explaining to the parents what will be asked and why, for example, "Now I am going to ask about the health of the family members. It is important to know if there are any hereditary or contagious diseases." A child at home is part of the family, and that child's problems and care occur in the family context, both affected by and affecting each family member and the family as a whole. For this reason, the reaction of family members to any problem the child has, whether chronic or acute, is important and should be an aspect of both the initial history and subsequent interviews. It is particularly important to explore the parent's main concern or worry at each visit and the reason for this concern. If these concerns are not addressed, the level of parental frustration will be high, and interventions will be less effective and useful.

ASSESSMENT PROCESS

The thoroughness of the discharge planning process, the degree of collaboration between hospital and home care personnel during the child's transition to home, and the family's comfort with the plans for home care will inform the direction and comprehensiveness of the initial assessment provided by the home care nurse. Certain aspects of assessment, such as the physical assessment of the child, are not affected, however.

Part of the purpose of the nursing intake process is to conduct an assessment that will inform the development of an individualized plan of care. Obtaining the health history, including a review of systems, lays the foundation for the nurse's physical assessment of the child. In addition to the physical assessment, the nurse works with the family members as they assess their own strengths, needs, and goals. Multidisciplinary evaluation, as appropriate, is another part of the assessment process.

While an assessment is essential at the onset of providing home care services, in reality, assessment is an ongoing process, extending over the entire period of working with a family (Ahmann & Bond, 1992). Care plans developed as a result of the assessment process must be flexible enough to respond to the child's changing health and developmental needs, multidisciplinary input, and the family's changing priorities.

Physical Assessment of the Child

The physical assessment of the child can be performed using any of a number of methodologies, including a systems approach or a "head to toe" approach. Vessey (1995) has outlined developmentally appropriate approaches to the pediatric physical assessment. Table 6–1 includes some pointers applicable to the infant, toddler, and preschooler. In general, the nurse should be creative and flexible in con-

Table 6–1 Age-specific Approaches to Physical Assessment

Age	Developmental indicators	Positioning	Sequence	Preparation
Infant (0–1)	Stranger anxiety begins at 7 mo; peaks at 9 mo. Resists being restrained Responds to simple commands by age 9 mo. Separation anxiety peaks at 13 mo.	Supine or prone, before 4 to 6 months: can place on examining table After 6 mo. sits alone: use this position whenever possible in parent's lap If on table, place with parent in full view	If quiet, auscultate heart, lungs, abdomen Palpate and percuss same areas Proceed in usual head–toe direction Perform traumatic procedure last (eyes, ears, mouth, [while crying], rectal temperature [if taken]) Elicit reflexes as body part examined, elicit generalized primitive reflexes last	Completely undress if room temperature permits Leave diaper in place Gain cooperation with distraction, bright objects, rattles, talking Smile at infant: use soft, high-pitched voice Pacify with pacifier or sugar water or feeding Enlist parent's aid for restraining to examine ears, mouth Avoid abrupt, jerky movements
Toddler (1–3)	Autonomy important Egocentric Stranger anxiety decreases at 18 mo. Speech begins Negativism present Knows several external body parts Separation anxiety decreases at 2 yr.	Sitting on or standing by parent Prone or supine in parent's lap	Inspect body areas through play: "count fingers," "tickle toes" Minimize physical contact initially Introduce equipment slowly Auscultate, percuss, palpate whenever quiet Perform traumatic procedures last (same as for infant)	Have parent remove outer clothing Remove underwear as body part examined Allow to inspect equipment; demonstrating use of equipment usually ineffective If uncooperative, perform procedures quickly Use restraint when appropriate; request parent's assistance Talk about examination if cooperative; use short phrases Praise for cooperative behavior
Preschool child (3–5)	Likes to "help" More cooperative, follows simple instructions Knows most external body parts, 3–5 internal parts Fears bodily harm	Prefer standing or sitting Usually cooperative Prefer parent's closeness	If cooperative, proceed in head to toe direction If uncooperative, proceed as with toddler	Request self-undressing Allow to wear underpants if shy Offer equipment for inspection, briefly demonstrate use Make up "story" about procedures Use paper doll technique Give choices when possible Expect cooperation; use positive statements

Source: Adapted from *Nursing Care of Infants and Children,* 5th ed., by D. Wong with permission of Mosby-Year Book, © 1995.

ducting the physical assessment. The nurse should start the assessment with the least invasive procedures, such as observing for facial symmetry, and conclude with the most traumatic, including examining the eyes, ears, and mouth.

The home care nurse must be an expert in physical assessment, for his or her judgment of the child's status in the home is often relied upon by the physician to determine the child's health status and medical stability. Findings on physical assessment should also be shared with parents. A sample form for documentation of the physical assessment is provided in Appendix 6–C.

Collaborative Process

Collaboration in the assessment process, as in service provision, has two realms: (1) collaboration between the family and the nurse or other professionals (parent–professional collaboration) and (2) collaboration between the many disciplines that may be involved in the care of the child and family (multidisciplinary collaboration).

Parent–Professional Collaboration

To best meet the needs of the child and family, the plan of care must reflect the family's values, goals, and priorities. To accomplish this, a central aspect of the assessment process is for the family to identify both needs or problems and strengths or resources.

Involving families in the assessment process may be new to many nurses. The process can be facilitated in several ways. First, the nurse can state to the family members that their observations, goals, and priorities are central to developing the plan of care. A number of written surveys are available that can assist families in identifying their concerns, priorities, and resources (see Table 4–1). Additionally, the nurse can ask open-ended questions (e.g., "Tell me about . . ." or "What are your goals for your child?") and can request clarification as necessary. Examples of questions that can be used to encourage the family's participation in assessing its own needs are included in Exhibit 6–3.

The nurse brings a special experience and expertise to the collaborative effort. This expertise can be shared with the family in a way that can further collaboration. Results of physical assessments, referral assessments, and observations should be shared with the family. The nurse can share observations, comments, and knowledge with the family in a neutral manner, without value judgment and without subverting the family's central decision-making role (Bond et al., 1994).

Multidisciplinary Collaboration

An essential part of the assessment process is assisting the family in determining whether the child and/or family may need additional services and disciplines not originally prescribed as part of the plan of care. Such services might include those of a social worker; a physical, occupational, or speech therapist; or a registered dietitian. Each home care agency should have preestablished criteria that can guide the nurse in deciding when such referrals are appropriate for more in-depth assessment or intervention.

As the team extends beyond the physician, nurse, and family, multidisciplinary collaboration becomes crucial. Jointly defining initial goals for the patient followed by providing consistent communication among disciplines will benefit the family and staff in several ways. Close collaboration will result both in a more rapid attainment of goals and in a higher level of desired patient outcomes. Joint visits and team conferencing are two ways multidisciplinary collaboration can be facilitated.

DEVELOPING A DYNAMIC PLAN OF CARE

The overall purpose of the assessment process is to determine priorities, goals, and intervention strategies that will constitute the plan of care or will continue to give direction to the home care plan as collaboratively developed during the discharge planning process. Active participation of the family members in developing the plan of care ensures a plan that meets their needs.

Areas addressed in the plan of care can include medical, nursing, psychosocial, emotional, parenting, financial, educational, nutritional, developmental, and environmental concerns. Identification of specific needs is based on information obtained in the initial history, the review of systems, the physical assessment, assessments by other professionals, and discussions between the nurse and family.

The plan of care may consist of several components. It may include, for example, further data collection, therapeutic interventions, education, and coordination. The care plan should address the identified needs while building on the strengths of the child and family. It should be developed jointly by the nurse and family and should reflect the specific needs and concerns of the individual child and family. The plan may include not only nursing services but also services such as social work, therapy, and/or home health aides. (Sample care plans are provided in the Appendixes of Chapters 8 through 17 and 24.) In developing individual care plans, the nurse and family should think in terms of realistic and achievable outcomes.

Generally, nurses and families agree on the goals of care to be addressed in the plan of care. On occasion, however, the nurse and family may not agree on the goals of care. A family-centered approach requires respecting the family's choices (Bond et al., 1994). Exhibit 6–4 suggests some steps that can be followed when the nurse and family disagree on priorities.

The care plan should in all cases be documented in writing, and a copy should be made available to the family. Sharing a copy of the plan of care with other professionals

Exhibit 6–3 A Sampling of Questions from the Family Profile

Family Structure/Roles

Do you want to care for your child at home?

Are you aware of any alternatives to home care?

Who are your child's primary caregivers?

Who are the other members of your household?

Can you identify another person to act as back up caregiver for your child?

Are there others (friends/family members) who can assist you with your child with special needs, your other children, or with your family obligations?

Medical Management

Have you completed the hospital training in your child's care? If no, what is left to learn?

Has your child's back up caregiver completed training? If no, what is left to learn?

Do you or your back up caregiver need refresher training for anything?

Do you have transportation to medical appointments?

Do you need help in selecting a nursing provider?

Do you need help in selecting a vendor?

Nutrition

How is your child fed?

If formula, will you need help to buy/locate the formula?

Have you applied for WIC?

Does your child have a need for diapers that is greater than the norm?

Education

Will your child be going out to school?

Do you know which school your child will attend?

Has your child been referred for the Infant and Toddler program?

Do you have an IFSP for your child? An IEP?

Do you have a contact person in the school program?

Will your child need adaptive equipment at home?

Parenting/Child Care

What hours/shifts do you think that you will need nursing for your child?

In the event you need to leave home quickly or if you become incapacitated, who will watch your child with special needs? Your other children?

What is your plan for child care in the event of the nurse's absence?

Will you need help in finding day care for your other children?

Do you work outside the home? Any plans for the future?

Do you go to school? Any plans for the future?

Financial Resources

Does your child have medical insurance? Are your other children covered under a family insurance plan?

Do you need more information about or referrals to WIC, SSI, AFDC, Food Stamps, Housing, Respite Care?

Do you need help in obtaining everyday supplies for your child?

Do you need a referral for help in obtaining other items for your child, such as furniture, clothing, toys?

Do you need help with budgeting?

Community Resources

Are you involved with any other helping agencies or persons, especially those you would like to include in this planning process?

Do you or other family members belong to a church? Social groups? Clubs? Associations?

Would you like to talk to another parent who has a child with special needs?

Would you like a referral to a support group?

Do you want a referral for counselling? Individual? Marital? Family? Child? Sibling?

Family Life

Do you see your child's homecoming as making a significant change in your lifestyle, and if so, how?

Do you have concerns about your other children?

Can you describe how you will see your child in a few months? What are your short term goals for your child?

Can you describe how you will see your child in a few years? What are your long term goals for your child?

How would you describe your family strengths?

What are your family's needs at this time?

Source: Reprinted from *Family Profile* by B. McCord with permission of the Coordinating Center for Home and Community Care, Millersville, Maryland, © 1993.

involved in the child's care will assist in coordination of services.

The nurse should have a plan for each home visit that addresses one or more aspects of the overall plan of care. Throughout each home visit, the information elicited from parents and other caregivers, with the nurse's skilled observation and assessment, will provide the basis upon which the nurse, other disciplines, and the family update the plan of care. Regular evaluation and refinement of the care plan are essential from one visit to the next. Periodically, a more formal review of the entire plan of care, including reassessment of the goals, is advised. This process should include the nurse, family, and other key providers.

DOCUMENTATION

Standard Plans of Care

The thrust in health care is toward streamlining documentation and standardizing patterns of care with a combined purpose of reducing costs and coordinating and improving care practices. Most agencies have standardized plans of care for homogenous patient types that can be individualized for each patient. (Examples are provided in the Appendixes to many chapters of this text.) Standard care plans will act as a guide for the nurse and parents for assessment, teaching, and intervention needs after the initial home visit.

Exhibit 6–4 Guidelines for Resolving Parent–Professional Disagreement about Goals and Priorities in the Home Care Plan

---

If nurses disagree with family goals/priorities or see them as unrealistic, several approaches can be taken simultaneously or over time. Each approach maintains respect for the family's right to determine the priorities of care.

OPTION 1: Work with the family's priorities and reevaluate over time.

OPTION 2: Share the nursing perspective and explain the nurse's choice of priorities.

OPTION 3: Explain the risks or drawbacks, if any, if the priorities the family recommends are implemented.

OPTION 4: Suggest adding an additional priority goal, addressing the nurse's concern, if the family agrees.

OPTION 5: In the unusual event that the nurse has a liability concern resulting from implementing a family's priority (or not implementing the nurse's priority), communicate this concern respectfully to the family, and document the conversation.

Source: Reprinted from *Pediatric Nursing,* Vol. 18, No. 4, p. 402, with permission of Jannetti Publications, Inc., Pitman, New Jersey, © 1992.

Standard plans of care can have several formats: traditional care plans with medical or nursing diagnoses, critical pathways, and Care Maps (Care Maps are a registered trademark of the Center for Case Management, 6 Pleasant Street, South Natick, MA 01760). In fact, there is increasing interest in developing Care Maps or critical pathways for pediatric home care services, particularly for the care of children with respiratory disorders (Zander, 1994).

Care Maps and Critical Pathways

The Center for Case Management (1992) defines a Care Map as "a cause and effect grid which identifies expected patient/family and staff behaviors against a timeline for a case type or otherwise defined homogenous population." Its components include a timeline, an index of problems with intermediate and outcome criteria, a critical path, and a record of variance from the path and timeline. A critical pathway is distinguished from a Care Map in that it does not list outcome criteria (Zander, 1994).

While a Care Map or critical pathway might be a useful tool for the home care nurse, it is most likely that the population of high-risk infants would be difficult to fit onto a specific pathway because of the complex and interacting nature of their problems. In fact, most of the infants in this population are likely to account for the variance in outcomes of mapped care in the tertiary care setting. When care maps are developed for the home care setting, specific aspects of care in the home could be mapped (e.g., seizure care, bronchopulmonary dysplasia), and the nurse might then combine

several pathways for documentation. In the meantime, standard care plans and assessment lists (included in the appendixes of many chapters of this book) can be individualized and used as suggested in each specific chapter to plan, deliver, monitor, and evaluate home care for the high-risk infant.

Documentation of Home Visits

Thorough documentation of each home nursing visit is important. Several formats can be used for this purpose. Previously common narrative nursing notes and charting using the SOAP (Subjective Data, Objective Data, Assessment, Plan) format are increasingly being replaced by the use of "PIG" notes (Plan, Implementation, Goal) and flowsheets, such as that provided in Appendix 6–D. These more streamlined methods of documentation will provide a greater consistency in the quality of documentation from nurse to nurse and, as a result, will assist nurses, individually and as a team, in more effectively achieving the goals outlined in the plan of care.

CASE MANAGEMENT OR CARE COORDINATION

Traditional definitions of case management generally focus on controlling cost, attaining desired clinical outcomes, and monitoring and evaluating care provided. Perrin, Shayne, and Bloom (1993) submit that "benefits management," which is focused on cost control (the role of insurance case managers), is distinct from care coordination that is focused on the needs of the child and family. For optimum home care of the child who is technology dependent, case management—or care coordination—should be viewed quite broadly.

Care coordination should have several purposes. It should have as a primary goal ensuring continuity for the child and family across various care settings: hospital, home, educational, therapeutic, and so forth. Care plans and care provision should be coordinated among multiple providers to reduce the complexity of care for the child, reduce fragmentation of care, and reduce the burden of care for the family. For the child with multiple and complex care needs, care coordination is also important in order to ensure that health maintenance needs, including developmental and behavioral support, immunizations, dental care, and the like, are not overlooked. Family support, education, and empowerment should be a priority of the case manager as well. Exhibit 6–5 lists many tasks and responsibilities involved in care coordination.

Any model of care coordination should address, at a minimum, the following areas of care (much of the following is from Lobosco et al., 1991, p. 77, and from Perrin et al., 1993, p. 12):

Exhibit 6–5 Aspects of Care Coordination

Assess needs.
  Assess medical, nursing, and other needs of child.
  Assess resources and needs of family.
  Assess home environment.
  Assess resources of community.

Plan for comprehensive care.
  Develop overall integrated plan of care.
  Combine plans of various disciplines.
  Highlight family goals.
  Assure health maintenance needs are addressed.

Link client(s) with service provider.
  Provide information about available services.
  Initiate referrals to desired services.
  Arrange appointments.
  Assist with transportation arrangements.

Coordinate services.
  Specify responsibilities of family and service providers.
  Obtain agreements.
  Help avoid service duplication.
  Arrange conferences as necessary.
  Assist in trouble shooting and problem solving between family and service providers.

Monitor and evaluate service provision.
  Maintain regular contact with family and providers.
  Review care plan on a regular basis.
  Supervise quality of care.
  Assess safety in provision of care.
  Assess family satisfaction with care provided.

Advocate for appropriate services.
  Address problem areas in home care services.
  Encourage educational opportunities.
  Negotiate insurance coverage.
  Lobby for needed services and benefits.

Provide administrative support.
  Inventory equipment and supplies.
  Assist in financial planning.
  Complete paperwork for insurance, other agencies.
  Oversee scheduling of provider visits and appointments.

Source: Copyright © 1996, Elizabeth Ahmann, ScD, RN.

- medical and nursing needs of the child
  1. competent home care nursing
  2. education and training of family and other care providers
  3. reliable vendor
  4. physical preparation of the home
- financial concerns
  1. cost of equipment and services
  2. insurance restrictions
  3. multiple application procedures

- psychosocial concerns
  1. disruptions of family life
  2. availability of support groups
  3. availability of respite services
- developmental and educational issues
  1. barriers to in-center medical/nursing support
  2. interruptions of developmental programming or education secondary to repeat hospitalizations
  3. inflexibility of many educational programs
- educational and support needs of the family
  1. information about the child's condition
  2. how best to care for the child
  3. how to manage the service systems
  4. where to find support.

Care coordination will be most effective if a single person works with the family to accomplish the many tasks and responsibilities involved.

To be effective in the case management role, the American Nurses Association (ANA; 1988) recommends that a nurse case manager should have a minimum of a bacclaureate degree in nursing and 3 years of experience. Skills in active listening, diplomacy, and other excellent communication skills are important. The nurse also should be knowledgeable about available community resources, including the following (Davis & Steele, 1991):

- primary, secondary, and tertiary health care services
- early intervention services
- speech/hearing/language/vision resources
- respite services
- financial assistance programs
- parent groups
- advocacy groups
- local, state, and federal public officials
- transportation services
- private-sector individuals with an interest in children with disabilities. (p. 16)

While professionals must always see part of their role as ensuring that integrated, coordinated care is provided, care coordination should promote the family's role as primary decision maker and enhance the family's capacity to meet the special needs of the child and family unit (Johnson, Jeppson, & Redburn, 1992; McGonigel, Kaufman, & Johnson, 1991). Families may choose to be involved to varying degrees in the tasks involved in coordination of their child's care. Many parents will take on increasing responsibility for care coordination as time goes on; they should be encouraged and supported in this role.

REFERENCES

Ahmann, E., & Bond, N. (1992). Promoting normal development in school-age children and adolescents who are technology-dependent: A family-centered model. *Pediatric Nursing, 18*(4), 399–405.

American Nurses Association. (1988). *Nursing case management.* Kansas City, MO: American Nurses Publishing.

Bernstein, L., Bernstein, R.S., & Dana, R.H. (1974). *Interviewing: A guide for health professionals* (2nd ed.). New York, NY: Appleton-Century-Crofts.

Bond, N., Phillips, P., & Rollins, J.A. (1994). Family-centered care at home for families with children who are technology-dependent. *Pediatric Nursing, 20*(2), 123–130.

Center for Case Management. (1992). *Definitions* (photocopy). South Natick, MA: Author.

Davis, B.D., & Steele, S. (1991). Case management for young children with special care needs. *Pediatric Nursing, 17,* 15–19.

Johnson, B.H., Jeppson, E.S., & Redburn, L. (1992). *Caring for children and families: Guidelines for hospitals.* Bethesda, MD: Association for the Care of Children's Health.

Lobosco, A.F., Eron, N.B., Bobo, T., Kril, L., & Chalanick, K. (1991). Local coalitions for coordinating services to children dependent on technology and their families. *Children's Health Care, 20*(2), 75–86.

McGonigel, M., Kaufman, R., & Johnson, B. (Eds.). (1991). *Guidelines and recommended practices for the individualized family service plan* (2nd ed.). Bethesda, MD: Association for the Care of Children's Health.

Perrin, J.M., Shayne, M.W., & Bloom, S.R. (1993). *Home and community care for chronically ill children.* New York, NY: Oxford University Press.

Vessey, J.A. (1995). Developmental approaches to examining young children. *Pediatric Nursing, 21*(1), 53–56.

Zander, K. (1994, October 21). *Case management: Coming of age.* Paper presented at the ACCH Midatlantic Affiliate Fall Program: Case management: A commitment to advocacy, Baltimore, MD.

Nursing Intake History

Name _____ DOB _____

Address _____ Phone _____

Mother's name _____ Work Phone _____

Father's name_____ Work Phone _____

DIAGNOSES _____

_____

_____

Doctors _____ Phone _____

_____ Phone _____

_____ Phone _____

_____ Phone _____

_____ Phone _____

_____ Phone _____

HOME & FAMILY

Description of home and community (Observation for safety, location of equipment, availability of telephone, transportation) _____

_____

_____

_____

_____

Family constellation (List names and ages of family members) _____

_____

_____

_____

Family dynamics (Parental confidence, parental interaction, sibling roles, parent–child interactions) _____

_____

_____

_____

FAMILY HEALTH HISTORY

Source of information _____
(Note if positive for asthma/allergies, diabetes, hypertension, anemia, sickle cell, cancer, alcoholism, drug abuse, hearing/vision loss, mental retardation, deaths)

(Continued on next page)

Mother _____

Father _____

Siblings _____

_____

Maternal grandmother _____ Paternal grandmother _____

Maternal grandfather _____ Paternal grandfather _____

PRENATAL HISTORY

Age of mother _____ # of pregnancies _____ # of births _____

# of miscarriages _____ # of abortions _____

Prenatal care (frequency, source) _____

Complications of pregnancy (infections, bleeding, etc.) _____

_____

Alcohol _____ Smoking _____ X-rays _____ Weight gain _____

Caffeine _____ Medications _____

BIRTH HISTORY

Hospital_____

Gestational age _____ Type of Delivery _____

Length of labor _____ Apgars(blue?) _____

Birth weight _____ Length_____ Head circumference _____

Comments_____

_____

_____

NEWBORN PERIOD

Respiratory difficulties (describe) _____

_____

Jaundice _____ Seizures_____ Anemia _____

Feeding problems (describe) _____

_____

Infections (describe) _____

_____

Physical abnormalities (describe)_____

_____

ICU _____ Length of stay _____

Length of initial hospitalization _____

Comments _____

_____

_____

IMMUNIZATIONS

DT or DPT (circle), CPV, (I) _____ (II) _____ (III) _____ MMR _____

· reactions _____

(Continued on next page)

ALLERGIES

Foods _____   Medications _____

Other_____

ACCIDENTS

_____

_____

_____

ILLNESSES

measles _____	chickenpox_____	scarlet fever _____
meningitis _____	pneumonia_____	tuberculosis _____
febrile convulsions _____	rubella _____	mumps _____
strep throat _____	hepatitis_____	otitis _____
abscesses _____	other _____	

PREVIOUS HOSPITALIZATIONS

_____

_____

_____

_____

Brief history of most recent hospitalization _____

_____

_____

_____

_____

THE CHILD

Source of information _____

Parental description of child _____

_____

How do you know when your child is upset? _____

_____

How do you quiet your child?

_____

_____

Do you recognize different cries?_____

_____

_____

DAILY PATTERNS

Caretakers _____

_____

(Continued on next page)

Feeding (see nutritional assessment)

Appetite _____ schedule _____

Problems _____

Sleeping schedule (including naps) _____

Where child sleeps _____

Bedtime routine_____

Problems _____

Urinary habits (freq/amount/odor)_____

Bowel habit (freq/type/color)_____

Problems _____

Bathing (freq/method) _____

Discipline _____

_____

Activity/play/toys _____

_____

Peer relationships_____

_____

School (performance/reactions) _____

_____

Self-care: feeding _____   bathing _____

             dressing _____   toileting _____

             _____

Do you have any problems managing your child in the home? _____

_____

_____

_____

DEVELOPMENT

Source of information _____

Development milestones (List age acquired)

hold up head _____   responds to name _____   smile responsively _____   cruise _____

roll prone to supine _____   walk_____   roll supine to prone _____   babble _____

voluntary grasp-release toys ___   first word_____   sit alone _____   finger feed _____

4-point crawl _____   cup drink_____   pull to stand _____   spoon feed_____

Parent summary of child's development (compared to normal child) _____

_____

Summary of developmental screening: (DDST & Milani under 1 yr.*; DDST, 1–3 yrs.) _____

_____

*Denver Developmental Screening Test (DDST)
Milani-Comparetti Motor Development Screening Test

(Continued on next page)

SPECIAL CARE NEEDS

Source of information _____

Parental description of child's medical problems _____

_____

_____

EQUIPMENT (type, location, arrangement, and prescribed settings)

_____

_____

_____

Supplier(s) _____   Phone _____

             _____   Phone _____

             _____   Phone _____

TREATMENTS (frequency, schedule)

_____

_____

_____

DIET PRESCRIPTION

_____

_____

_____

_____

MEDICATIONS

_____

_____

_____

_____

Nursing completing intake _____ Date _____

Source: Courtesy of Children's Hospital National Medical Center, Home Health Care Services, Washington, D.C.

Review of Systems

LIST AREAS OF CONCERN
OR AREAS WNL

Review of Systems (Circle if Present)

1. SKIN: Itching, dryness, rashes, acne, bruises easily, hypersensitivity to tactile input, hyperpigmented spots, nodules.

2. EYES: Glasses _____ Last Eye Exam _____
   Itch, water, tire easily, redness, stands close to TV, clumsy, sensitive to light, cross, rubs eyes, squints, slanted downward, upward, epicanthal folds, wide spacing. Other _____
   Risk factors from history _____

3. EARS: Earaches, hearing loss, infections, sensitive to noise, drainage, ringing, fears strangers, wakens from sleep when called, low set, malformed. Other _____
   Risk factors from history _____

4. NOSE: Frequent colds, itching, discharge, infections, paroxysmal sneezing, nose bleeds, broad flat bridge.
   Other _____

5. MOUTH-THROAT: Dental cavities, toothache, bleeding gums, sore throat, strep, hoarseness, swollen glands, loss of color of teeth, pitted teeth, thin upper lip.
   Other _____

6. CARDIO-RESPIRATORY: Coughing, wheezing, shortness of breath, cyanosis, tires easily with running, hyperventilates.
   Other _____

7. GASTRO-INTESTINAL: Diarrhea, constipation, bleeding, abdominal pain, vomiting. Other _____

8. GENITO-URINARY: Strong stream, dribbling, dysuria, burning, frequency, odor, color, undescended testicles. Other _____

9. MUSCULO-SKELETAL: Pain, swelling, leg pains, redness in joints, limited range of motion in joints, back pains, fractures easily or multifractures, lax joints, nails malformed, webbing of digits, hyper or hypomuscle tone.

10. NEUROLOGICAL: Headaches, dizziness, twiches, blackout spells, tremors, fainting spells, reflexes appropriate for age.

11. ENDOCRINE: Deviation in growth pattern, hyper or hypo activity, excessive thirst, frequent voiding, coarse hair texture, hair pattern whorls, excessive body/facial hair.

12. GENETIC: Family history of delays, seizures, mental retardation, still births, diagnosed genetic or congenital defect, failure to thrive. Other _____

Source: Reprinted from *FAT: The Family Assessment Tool for School Nurses and Other Professionals* by Sandra Holt and Thelma Robinson, revision authors, Thelma Robinson (school-aged) and Melissa Van Wey (infant/preschool) with permission of Family Assessment Tools, © 1979, 1985.

Appendix 6–C

Sample Form for Documentation of the Physical Assessment

1. Patient Name		2. Date of Birth	3. Medical Record No.

4. Diagnosis	5. Measurements HT _____% _____ WT _____% _____	HC _____% _____ WT/HT % _____	6. Vital Signs T _____ R _____ P _____ BP _____

7. General Survey (*Sex, race, overall health, activity, personal hygiene, etc.*)

NO PROBLEM		ABNORMAL	NOTES (Describe abnormality in detail) Enter item # before each comment.
	8. HEAD & FACE fontanel (size) _____		
[ ]	fontanel soft, flat/closed	[ ]	
[ ]	symmetry of all movements	[ ]	
	9. NECK & MOUTH		
[ ]	no masses	[ ]	
[ ]	full ROM	[ ]	
[ ]	mucous membranes pink, moist, no lesions	[ ]	
	10. EYES, EARS & NOSE		
[ ]	PERRLA	[ ]	
[ ]	EOMs	[ ]	
[ ]	moist, no discharge or inflammation	[ ]	
[ ]	normal placement	[ ]	
[ ]	Tm(s) pearly gray	[ ]	
[ ]	patent	[ ]	
[ ]	no discharge	[ ]	
	11. CHEST		
[ ]	symmetry	[ ]	
[ ]	clear equal lung sounds	[ ]	
[ ]	brisk cap. refill	[ ]	
[ ]	peripheral pulses equal, present	[ ]	
	12. ABDOMEN		
[ ]	audible bowel sound all four quadrants	[ ]	
[ ]	no masses, hernia	[ ]	
[ ]	no tenderness	[ ]	
	13. GENITALIA		
[ ]	testes present, descended	[ ]	
[ ]	placement of urethral opening	[ ]	
[ ]	uncircumcised, foreskin retractable or circumcision	[ ]	
[ ]	no vaginal discharge	[ ]	
	14. NEUROLOGICAL		
[ ]	age appropriate DDST	[ ]	
[ ]	reflexes present, symmetrical	[ ]	
[ ]	good muscle tone	[ ]	
	15. MUSCULOSKELETAL		
[ ]	equal muscle mass, movement and alignment full ROM of all extremities	[ ]	
	16. SKIN		
[ ]	normal racial tone	[ ]	
[ ]	no lesions, scars, bruising	[ ]	
[ ]	smooth texture, turgor, elastic & mobile	[ ]	

17. *Nurse's Signature:* _____	18. *Date of Exam* _____

Source: Courtesy of Children's Hospital National Medical Center, Home Health Care Services, Washington, DC.

Sample Visit Report Summary

The following were assessed (specify): (*Items not checked are not applicable)

☐ VITAL SIGNS

Temp_____ B/P _____
HR _____ Rhythm_____
RR _____ Quality _____

☐ CARDIO-PULMONARY

☐ RESPIRATORY ONLY

Retraction	☐ Yes	☐ No
Cough	☐ Yes	☐ No
Productive	☐ Yes	☐ No

Chest P.T. _____ Suction _____
Activity _____
Lung Sounds:
    Rt. Clear ☐ Yes ☐ No
    Lt: Clear ☐ Yes ☐ No
Oxygen: Flow Rate _____
☐ APNEA MONITOR/SETTINGS
High HR: _____ Low HR: _____
Apnea Delay: _____
Alarms: Loose Lead ☐
☐ Apnea # ____ ☐ Bradycardia # ___
Action Taken/Infant Response:

☐ CARDIAC ONLY
Color _____
Peripheral Pulses: Equal/Strong
                    ☐ Yes ☐ No

Capillary Refill: Brisk
                    ☐ Yes ☐ No
Edema _____ Abd. Girth _____

☐ GROWTH PARAMETERS

                    Next Assessment
Weight: _____ _____
Length: _____ _____
Head
Circumference: _____
Fontanelle: Closed ☐
Flat ☐ Bulging ☐ Depressed ☐

☐ NUTRITION

☐ INTAKE
Diet (Cal/oz-Formula)_____

☐ P.O. Frequency: _____
    Amount: _____
☐ Enteral Tube Type/Size: _____
Tube Change: _____
    Gravity/Pump
    Schedule/Rate: _____
    Correct Tube Placement
                    ☐ Yes ☐ No
Vomiting: _____
☐ TPN: (See Hyperalimentation
    Flow Sheet)

☐ GI

Oral Mucosa: Clear/Intact
                    ☐ Yes ☐ No

BM: Number _____
Color _____
Consistency _____

☐ GU

Urine: Color/Frequency_____

☐ NEUROLOGIC

Asleep	☐	Irritable	☐
Quiet	☐	Lethargic	☐
Alert	☐	Fussy	☐
Playful	☐	Overactive	☐
Pupils			
S/S ICP	☐	Seizure Activity	☐

☐ SKIN INTEGRITY

Hygiene: _____
Turgor: _____

Diaphoresis	☐ Yes	☐ No
Discoloration	☐ Yes	☐ No
Incision	☐ Yes	☐ No
Break in Skin	☐ Yes	☐ No
Rash	☐ Yes	☐ No
Sensation	☐ Yes	☐ No
Edema	☐ Yes	☐ No

Location: _____
Size: _____
Drainage: _____
Tx/Dressing Change: _____
_____

☐ MEDICATIONS

☐ ORAL/NG/GT/SQ/PR
Patient/Caregiver Independent:
    ☐ Yes ☐ No _____

☐ PARENTERAL
☐ Central Line ☐ Peripheral Line
Type of Catheter: _____
Location of Catheter: _____
Site Status:

Patent	☐ Yes	☐ No
Phlebitis	☐ Yes	☐ No
Drainage	☐ Yes	☐ No

☐ Dressing changed on: _____
☐ Cap changed on: _____
☐ PIV changed on:_____
☐ Medication administered by:_____

Saline/Heparin Flush
    (Dose & Frequency):_____

☐ Medication Reactions (if any):

☐ Labs Drawn (list): _____

☐ OTHER ASSESSMENT TOOLS USED

☐ Safety Assessment
☐ DDST II
☐ Growth Chart
☐ Tracheostomy Flow Sheet
☐ Diabetic Flow Sheet
☐ Hyperalimentation Flow Page 2
☐ Infusion Flow Sheet Page 2
☐ Burn Diagram
☐ Pain Assessment
☐ Other: _____

☐ OTHER ASSESSMENTS

1. _____
_____
_____
_____
_____

2. _____
_____
_____
_____
_____

3. _____
_____
_____
_____
_____

4. _____
_____
_____
_____
_____

Summary of Significant Findings Noted Above: _____
_____
_____

Teaching/Reinforcement Provided:_____
_____
_____

Patient/Caregiver Response to Teaching and Interventions: _____
_____
_____

Plan: _____
_____
_____

Date of Next Nursing Visit: _____ Date of Physician(s) Follow-up: _____
Diet/Frequency/Medication Change: ☐ No ☐ Yes (See Change Order/Home Instruction Sheet)
Plan of Care Modifications: ☐ Not Required — Reflects Current Needs ☐ Required — See Modified Care Plan

Signature: _____ Date:_____

Source: Courtesy of Children's Hospital National Medical Center, Home Health Care Services, Washington, DC.

Chapter 7

Community Resources for the Family

Revised by Ann Scher, ACSW, and Elizabeth Ahmann, ScD, RN

For the high-risk infant or chronically ill child, the transition from the hospital to the home must be well planned to ensure continuity of care (see Chapter 5). An essential component of the planning process is the identification of community resources that are available to assist the family in providing care at home.

The availability and quality of resources in any given community is influenced by many factors, including economics, politics, and societal attitudes. As a result, available health care services, social services, and other community resources often vary greatly among different communities. Even federal programs, such as Medicaid, have eligibility requirements and home care coverage provisions that vary from state to state. The home care professional must become aware of the range of available community services and resources that can benefit families caring for the high-risk infant at home. Financial, therapeutic, family support, and informational resources are identified and discussed in this chapter.

FINANCIAL RESOURCES

Financial concerns are often a major stressor for families providing home care for the high-risk infant. These families not only have the basic living expenses faced by any family but have the following additional expenses:

- special supplies and equipment
- medications

- special formulas or foods
- transportation to frequent medical appointments
- increased utility bills related to use of medical equipment
- insurance copays and sometimes even hospital and outpatient bills.

Even if a family has insurance coverage, is a member of a health maintenance organization (HMO), or has Medicaid, many of these increased expenses will not be covered. The home care professional and the family may need to work together to develop a creative package of programs and funding resources in order to meet the many needs of the child and family while maintaining the family's financial viability. Sources of funding that may assist the family to provide home care include the following:

- private insurance
- HMOs
- Medicaid
- Supplemental Security Income (SSI)
- Women, Infants, and Children (WIC) programs
- food stamps
- state Crippled Children's services (may also be known by other names)
- Part H of the Individuals with Disabilities Education Act (IDEA) (see Special Issue, "Early Intervention Services for the High-risk Infant")

- state and local social service agencies
- community organizations
- disease-specific organizations
- religious organizations
- state and local public health departments
- state and local departments of education
- private contributions.

Families may find the following resource useful as they consider how to finance their child's care: Rosenfeld, L. (1994) *Your Child and Health Care: A "Dollars and Sense" Guide for Families with Special Needs*. Baltimore, MD: Paul H. Brookes Publishing. The rest of this section discusses some considerations in identifying and choosing appropriate funding sources.

Insurance or HMO

If a family has insurance coverage, is a member of a preferred provider plan or an HMO, several points are important. First, it is essential to know whether the policy includes a lifetime limit for reimbursement. Families with infants who have been hospitalized for extended periods may have depleted a substantial portion of their available coverage. Second, to avoid sudden, unexpected costs, it is essential to query the company in detail about its home care coverage. Coverage may vary by service provided, and the family can request monthly or quarterly reviews detailing both services used and coverage remaining for each service (e.g., occupational therapy, physical therapy). Similarly, it is important to track prescription expenses, as many insurance policies have prescription caps. Some companies can be convinced to provide coverage for home care if their representatives are provided with figures that demonstrate the cost-effectiveness of this approach for an individual. This may also be true in regard to the costs of durable medical equipment. On a case-by-case basis, some insurers are also willing to "barter" coverage, for example, trade in 30 days of coverage in a long-term care facility for an equal number of hours of home care per year (Stepanek, personal communication, September 1995).

Medicaid

If a family's insurance limit is reached, or if a family does not have insurance, the Medicaid program may provide coverage for medical and related expenses. Although specific criteria related to Medicaid eligibility vary from state to state, one of the three following factors must apply:

1. Family income is below the state-determined poverty level.

2. Child's medical expenses are high in relation to family income.
3. Child is blind or disabled, and family is living on a limited income.

The local agency of the U.S. Department of Health and Human Services and the local Social Security office can supply eligibility criteria and application materials to interested families or professionals. The following materials are generally required when applying for Medicaid: birth certificate(s), identification, verification of income, medical bills or statements, and verification of residency.

Some states are also participating in the Medicaid Home and Community Based Waiver Program. This program extends Medicaid coverage to some persons who, on the basis of diagnostic criteria, would otherwise not be eligible for Medicaid coverage. Services covered by the waiver program vary from state to state, but may include a variety of services generally not covered by Medicaid, such as case management, respite care, and even home repair.

The SSI Program

The SSI program is a federal income-maintenance program for the aged, blind, and disabled. Disabled children meeting eligibility criteria can receive monthly SSI payments, the amount of which is based on family income. In addition, if SSI eligibility criteria are met, the child automatically qualifies for Medicaid, regardless of the family's income. However, eligibility for other assistance programs, such as Aid to Families with Dependent Children (AFDC), may be adversely affected by receipt of SSI payments. For this reason, the family applying for such assistance should determine which programs offer the most advantages. Further information about the SSI program and application materials can be obtained at any Social Security office. The following materials are generally required when applying for SSI: Social Security number, proof of age, verification of income, medical records, and verification of residency.

The WIC Program

The WIC supplemental food program provides eligible low-income persons with both specific nutritious supplemental foods and nutrition education at no cost. Pregnant women, those who have just given birth, and breastfeeding women, as well as infants and children up to their fifth birthday are eligible if they meet income standards and if they are determined to be at nutritional risk. Additional information and application materials are available through the local health department.

Food Stamps

The food stamps program provides monthly benefits that help low-income persons buy food needed to maintain good health. Eligibility is based on the family's gross income. For the family with a disabled child, eligibility is based on meeting income guidelines after deductions. Further information and application materials can be obtained at the local Department of Human Services or Social Security office.

Other Financial Resources

Each state has a Crippled Children's program. (Although the name or title of the program may vary from state to state, asking the local health department about the Crippled Children's program is generally a useful way to track it down.) In some states, a portion of the funds for this program may be used to assist families in the purchase of equipment, supplies, or services needed by disabled children.

Assistance in purchasing durable medical equipment or special supplies is also sometimes available from community organizations or disease-specific associations (such as the American Lung Association) if a special request is made. Church organizations and philanthropic contributions are yet another possible source of financial assistance.

THERAPEUTIC RESOURCES

Home care of the high-risk infant may require any of a wide variety of therapeutic services, including the following:

- infant stimulation
- educational programs
- occupational therapy
- physical therapy
- speech therapy
- respiratory therapy
- nutritional consultations
- audiologic evaluation and follow-up
- pharmacy services
- home nursing services
- durable medical equipment and supply services
- transportation
- emergency services
- primary and specialty medical care
- parent support
- respite care.

Effective case management can assist families in locating the needed services, coordinating schedules and care, and arranging for payment. When any service is needed, payment mechanisms should be explored. Some agencies may provide a service only to self-pay families; others may accept reimbursement from third-party payers or Medicaid; still other agencies may provide services on a sliding scale or even free of charge if a family's resources are limited. (Obviously, this will be true for only certain types of services.) Certain evaluations and services are provided free through federally mandated programs (Education, 1991). Payment options will influence the family's choice of service provider.

Infant stimulation and education programs can generally be located through the local school system, health department, or Child Find Program. As a result of federally mandated entitlement programs, including PL 94-142 and its subsequent amendments 98-199, 99-457, and 101-476 (IDEA), early intervention, special education, and related services including occupational, physical, and speech therapy, audiologic evaluation and follow-up, must be made available to children with special needs and some others from birth to age 21. (See Special Issue, "Early Intervention Services for the High-risk Infant" and the NICHCY News Digest, Volume 1, No. 1, 1991, which focused on the topic The Education of Children and Youth with Special Needs: What Do the Laws Say? NICHCY, P.O. Box 1492, Washington, DC 20013.)

Early intervention programs may be home or center based. Center-based programs may or may not be prepared to provide services to children with a tracheostomy or to those on oxygen. However, some program personnel may be willing to provide services to such children if special training can be arranged through the hospital or home health agency.

If nutrition or occupational, physical, or speech therapy services are indicated, a physician's referral may be necessary (though not for services and evaluations provided through Part H of PL 99-457). A hospital rehabilitation department or the school system may be able to provide referrals to therapists with a pediatric background, an important criterion in the choice of provider. Only certain providers work with the federal entitlement programs.

Some infants with respiratory compromise may need medications that are not readily available in local pharmacies. If a family has difficulty obtaining specific medications, a hospital pharmacy is a possible resource. Alternatively, if a willing community pharmacist can be identified, special orders may be arranged, or the hospital pharmacist can instruct the community pharmacist in any unusual medication "recipes."

Several transportation issues may affect the family of a high-risk infant: cost, convenience, and special needs. If a family has Medicaid coverage, some states may provide transportation assistance to medical appointments. Transportation to certain appointments can be arranged as part of the services provided under IDEA. Handicap tags or stickers for privately owned vehicles may assist the family in parking convenience. If an ambulance or van is needed to transport a ventilator-dependent child to medical appointments, the Medicaid program, Red Cross, or the local ambulance or rescue squad may be of assistance. Other therapeutic services are discussed in Chapters 2 and 4.

FAMILY SUPPORT RESOURCES

When the high-risk infant first comes home from the hospital, the family is most likely to need concrete instrumental support. For example, assistance in arranging transportation to and from the clinic, in finding a pharmacy that can supply the needed medications, and in arranging daily schedules to accommodate the child's care may be most welcome initially.

With time, most families caring for a child with chronic illness or disability will identify a need for respite care. (See Special Issue, "Alternatives to Home Care for Medically Fragile Children.") Because of the complexity of care and the relative instability of some high-risk infants, an appropriate source of back-up or respite care may be home nursing services. Unless insurance or Medicaid covers the cost of home nursing, this arrangement may not be financially feasible for a family. As an alternative, a family may try to locate a babysitter willing to be trained to care for the infant. (Such training, however, must be as complete as that for the primary caregiver.) Some communities have respite care programs that may serve as a source of relief for parents. In most cases, however, these programs are targeted to care for the mentally retarded and developmentally disabled populations, and the respite providers do not have the training to care for a child with medical impairments. Nevertheless, it may be possible to make special arrangements for training of program personnel if no other source of relief is available to a family. United Cerebral Palsy offers a "Respitality" program in many locations; information about the program can be obtained by calling 1-800-872-5827.

In addition to some source of respite care, an important resource for parents of the high-risk infant can be sharing both information and support with other parents. Support groups, arranged by hospitals, social service agencies, Infant and Toddler programs of Part H of PL 99-456, or parents themselves, provide a useful forum for promoting coping; problem solving; exchanging experiences, challenges, and ideas; encouraging advocacy; and reducing isolation (Worthington, 1992). If no such appropriate support groups are available, or if a parent is unable to attend meetings, telephone contacts with one or two other parents may be a helpful alternative. However, a family's desire for privacy should always be respected. Some of the organizations listed in Appendix 7–A provide peer support as well as information for parents. The Association for the Care of Children's Health publishes a parent-resource directory.

Psychosocial counseling intervention is a service some families may want to use. Although the cost of this service often is not reimbursable by third-party payers, the importance of social work, psychotherapeutic, and psychologic support services should not be overlooked. This service may be covered under IDEA.

When the infant has been at home for some time, the family's needs may change; the home care professional must be sensitive to cues signaling such changes. A variety of community resources are available to provide needed support to families caring for the high-risk infant at home:

- back-up caregivers
- babysitting services
- respite caregivers
- parent groups
- sibling groups
- neighborhood organizations
- church groups
- psychosocial support services
- national disease-specific organizations.

INFORMATION RESOURCES

Family members and other caregivers may be interested in obtaining information about the infant's condition, prognosis, available treatments or services, and other topics. The physician, community health nurse, and other professionals involved in the infant's care may be helpful in this regard. Individual parents and parent groups may also be an important information resource.

In addition, books, articles, pamphlets, and newsletters are available to augment discussions with both professionals and other parents. (See Appendix 7–A for some suggestions.) National organizations that provide information, publications including newsletters, peer support, and contacts with local affiliates are listed in Appendix 7–B.

REFERENCES

NICHCY (1991). The education of children and youth with special needs: What do the laws say? *The NICHCY News Digest, 1*(1). NICHCY, P.O. Box 1492, Washington, DC 20013, telephone 800-999-5599.

Worthington, R.C. (1992). Family support networks: Help for families of children with special needs. *Family Medicine, 24*(1), 41–44.

Publications for Parents, Children, and Professionals

Lyn Ingersoll, MLS

Family Librarian, Children's Hospital National Medical Center, Washington, DC

This resource list for parents, children, and professionals covers the following topics:

- General Bibliographies
- Acquired Immune Deficiency Syndrome (AIDS) and human immunodeficiency virus (HIV)
- Breastfeeding
- Coping
- Death: preparation for and coping with (including sudden infant death syndrome [SIDS] and infant death)
- Development
- Disabilities: General and Specific

- Parenting and Child Care
- Parent–Professional Collaboration
- Premature Infants
- Safety
- Sensory Deficits
- Siblings of Children with Illness and Disability.

Many of the suggestions in this list are drawn from the Health Resource Collection of the Family Library at Children's National Medical Center, Washington, DC, the largest such library collection in the United States.

GENERAL BIBLIOGRAPHIES

Cuddigan, M., & Hanson, M.B. (1988). *Growing pains: Helping children deal with everyday problems through reading.* Chicago, IL: American Library Association.

Dreyer, S.S. (1992). *The best of bookfinder: A guide to children's literature about interests and concerns of youth aged 2–18.* Circle Pines, MN: American Guidance Service.

Moore, C. (1990). *A reader's guide: For parents of children with mental, physical or emotional disabilities.* Bethesda, MD: Woodbine House.

Rudman, M.K., Gagne, K.D., & Bernstein, J.E. (1993). *Books to help children cope with separation and loss.* New Providence, N.J.: R.R. Bowker.

AIDS AND HIV

Aiello, B., & Shulman, J. (1991). *Friends for life.* New York, NY: Twenty-First Century Books (The Kids on the Block Book Series).

Baker, L.S. (1991). *You and HIV . . . a day at a time.* Philadelphia, PA: W.B. Saunders.

Girard, L.W. (1991). *Alex, the kid with AIDS.* Morton Grove, IL: Albert Whitman & Company.

Hausherr, R. (1989). *Children and the AIDS virus: A book for children, parents & teachers.* New York, NY: Clarion Books.

Madaras, L. (1988). *Lynda Madaras talks to teens about AIDS: An essential guide for parents, teachers and young people.* New York, NY: Newmarket Press.

Quakenbush, M., & Villarcal, S. (1988). *"Does AIDS hurt?" Educating young children about AIDS.* Santa Cruz, CA: ETR Associates.

BREASTFEEDING

Gotsch, G. (1994). Breastfeeding pure and simple. Schaumburg, IL.: La Leche League.

Huggins, K. (1995). *The nursing mother's companion.* Boston, MA: The Harvard Common Press.

La Leche League International. (1991). *The womanly art of breastfeeding.* New York, NY: New American Library-Dutton.

Pryor, K. (1991). *Nursing your baby.* New York, NY: Pocket Books.

Walker, M. (1989). *Breastfeeding your premature or special care baby: A practical guide for nursing the tiny baby.* Weston, MA: Lactation Associates.

COPING

Association for the Care of Children's Health. (1989). *Your child with special needs at home and in the community* [Pamphlet]. Bethesda, MD: Author.

Buck, P.S. (1992). *The child who never grew.* Bethesda, MD: Woodbine House.

Callanan, C.R. (1990). *Since Owen: A parent-to-parent guide for care of the disabled child.* Baltimore, MD: The Johns Hopkins University Press.

Canfield, J. (1993). *Chicken soup for the soul.* Deerfield Beach, FL: Health Communications.

Featherstone, H. (1990). *A difference in the family: Life with a disabled child.* New York, NY: Penguin Viking.

Goldfarb, L.A. (1986). *Meeting the challenge of disability or chronic illness: A family guide.* Baltimore, MD: Paul H. Brookes Publishing.

Kersey, K. (1986). *Helping your child handle stress.* Berkeley, CA: Berkeley Publishers.

Marshall, R.E. (1982). *Coping with caring for sick newborns.* Philadelphia, PA: W.B. Saunders.

McAnaney, K.D. (1992). *I wish . . . Dreams and realities of parenting a special needs child.* Sacramento, CA: United Cerebral Palsy Association of California.

McCollum, A.T. (1981). *The chronically ill child: A guide for parents and professionals.* New Haven, CT: Yale University Press.

Miller, N.B. (1993). *Nobody's perfect: Living and growing with children who have special needs.* Baltimore, MD: Paul H. Brookes Publishing.

Routburg, M. (1987). *On becoming a special parent: A mini-support group in a book.* Chicago, IL: Parent/Professional Publications.

Russell, L.M. (1993). *Planning for the future: Providing a meaningful life for a child with a disability after your death.* Evanston, IL: American Publishing Company.

Segal, M. (1988). *In time and with love: Caring for the special needs baby.* New York, NY: Newmarket Press.

Simons, R. (1987). *After the tears: Parents talk about raising a child with a disability.* San Diego, CA: Harcourt Brace.

Thompson, C.E. (1986). *Raising a handicapped child: A helpful guide for parents of the physically disabled.* New York, NY: Ballantine.

Weinhouse, D., & Weinhouse, M. (1994). *Little children, big needs: Parents discuss raising young children with exceptional needs.* Niwot, CO: University Press of Colorado.

DEATH: PREPARATION FOR AND COPING WITH, SIDS, INFANT DEATH

Adult resources:

Davis, D.L. (1991). *Empty cradle broken heart: Surviving the death of your baby.* Golden, CO: Fulcrum Publishing.

DeFrain, J., et al. (1986). *Stillborn: The invisible death.* Lexington, MA: Free Press.

DeFrain, J., et al. (1991). *Sudden infant death: Enduring the loss.* Lexington, MA: Free Press.

Donnelly, K.F. (1994). *Recovering from the loss of a child.* Berkeley, CA: Berkeley Publishers.

Donnelley, N.H. (1987). *I never know what to say: How to help your family and friends cope with tragedy.* New York, NY: Ballantine Books.

Fitzgerald, H. (1992). *The grieving child: A parent's guide.* New York, NY: Simon & Schuster.

Gilbert, K.R., & Smart, L.S. (1992). *Coping with infant or fetal loss: The couple's healing process.* New York, NY: Brunner/Mazel.

Goldman, L. (1994). *Life and loss: A guide to help grieving children.* Muncie, IN: Accelerated Development.

Ilse, S. (1990). *Empty arms: Coping after miscarriage, stillbirth and infant death.* Maple Plain, MN: Wintergreen Press.

Kohn, I. (1992). *A silent sorrow: Pregnancy loss.* New York, NY: Dell Publishing.

Schiff, H.S. (1984). *The bereaved parent.* New York, NY: Penguin Books.

Schiff, H.S. (1987). *Living through mourning: Finding comfort and hope when a loved one has died.* New York, NY: Viking.

Toder, F.A. (1986). *When your child is gone: Learning to live again.* Sacramento, CA: Capital Publishing.

Children's resources:

Fox, M. (1994). *Tough Boris.* San Diego, CA: Harcourt Brace.

Greenlee, S. (1992). *When someone dies.* Atlanta, GA: Peachtree Publishers.

Mellonie, B. (1983). *Lifetimes: The beautiful way to explain death to children.* New York, NY: Bantam Books.

Viorst, J., & Ingren, R. (1987). *The tenth good thing about Barney.* New York, NY: Simon and Schuster.

DEVELOPMENT

Ames, Louise Bates. (Various dates). *Your One Year Old/Your Two Year Old/Your Three Year Old/Your Four Year Old/Your Five Year Old/Your Six Year Old/Your Seven Year Old/Your Eight Year Old/Your Nine Year Old/Your Ten to Fourteen Year Old.* New York, NY: Delta. (Gesell Institute of Human Development).

Brazelton, T. B. (1994). *Touchpoints: Your child's emotional and behavioral development, The essential reference.* Redding, MA: Addison-Wesley Publishing.

Caplan, F. (Ed.). (1984). *The first twelve months of life: Your baby's growth month by month.* New York, NY: Bantam. (The Princeton Center for Infancy and Early Childhood).

Caplan, Theresa (Ed.). (1984). *The early childhood years: The 2 to 6 year old.* New York, NY: Bantam. (The Princeton Center for Infancy and Early Childhood).

Eisenberg, A. (1994). *What to expect the first year.* New York, NY: Workman Publishing.

Eisenberg, A., et al. (1994). *What to expect during the toddler years.* New York, NY: Workman Publishing.

Fraiberg, S.H. (1966). *The magic years: Understanding and handling the problems of early childhood.* New York, NY: Charles Scribner's Sons.

Leach, P. (1989). *Your baby & child: From birth to age five.* New York, NY: Alfred A. Knopf.

DISABILITIES: GENERAL AND SPECIFIC

General

Adult resources:

Batshaw, M.L. (1993). *Your child has a handicap: A practical guide to daily care.* Boston, MA: Little, Brown.

Blackman, J.A. (1990). *Medical aspects of developmental disabilities in children birth to three,* 2nd ed. Rockville, MD: Aspen Publishers.

Pueschel, S.M. (1994). *The special child: A source book for parents of children with developmental disabilities,* 2nd ed. Baltimore, MD: Paul H. Brookes.

Children's resources:

Bergman, T. (1989). *On our terms: Children living with physical disabilities.* Milwaukee, WI: Gareth Stevens Children's Books.

Krementz, J. (1992). *How it feels to live with a physical disability.* New York, NY: Simon & Schuster.

Mills, J.C. (1992). *Little tree: A story for children with serious medical problems.* New York, NY: Magination Press.

Westridge Young Writers Workshop Staff. (1994). *Kids explore the gifts of children with special needs.* Santa Fe, NM: John Muir Publications.

Specific

Geralis, E. (Ed.). (1991). *Children with cerebral palsy: A parents' guide.* Bethesda, MD: Woodbine House.

Hanson, M.J. (1987). *Teaching the infant with Down syndrome: A guide for parents and professionals,* 2nd ed. Austin, TX: Pro-Ed.

Kumin, L. (1993). *Communication skills in children with Down syndrome: A guide for parents.* Bethesda, MD: Woodbine House.

Moller, J.H. (1988). *A parents' guide to heart disorders.* Minneapolis, MN: University of Minnesota Press.

Moller, K.T., et al. (1990). *A parents' guide to cleft lip and palate.* Minneapolis, MN: University of Minnesota Press.

Reisner, H. (Ed.). (1987). *Children with epilepsy: A parents' guide.* Bethesda, MD: Woodbine House.

Schleichkorn, J. (1993). *Coping with cerebral palsy: Answers to questions parents often ask.* Austin, TX: Pro-Ed.

Smith, R. (Ed.). (1993). *Children with mental retardation: A parents' guide.* Bethesda, MD: Woodbine House.

Stray-Gundersen, K. (Ed.). (1995). *Babies with Down syndrome: A new parents' guide.* Bethesda, MD: Woodbine House.

Van Dyke, D.C., et al. (Eds.). (1995). *Medical & surgical care for children with Down syndrome: A guide for parents.* Bethesda, MD: Woodbine House.

PARENTING AND CHILD CARE

Brazelton, T. Berry. (1983). *Infants and mothers: Differences in development.* New York, NY: Dell Publishing.

Evans, J., & Ilfeld, E. (1982). *Good beginnings: Parenting in the early years.* Ypsilanti, MI: High Scope Press.

Finston, P. (1990). *Parenting plus: Raising children with special health needs.* New York, NY: Penguin Books USA.

Kelly, M. (1992). *The mother's almanac revised.* New York, NY: Doubleday.

Marsh, J.D.B. (Ed.). (1995). *From the heart: On being the mother of a child with a disability.* Bethesda, MD: Woodbine House.

Meyer, D.J. (Ed.). (1995). *Uncommon fathers: Reflections on raising a child with a disability.* Bethesda, MD: Woodbine House.

Mrazek, D. (1993). *A to Z guide to your child's behavior.* New York, NY: Putnam Publishing Group.

Segal, M., & Adcock, D. (Various years). *Your Child at Play: Birth to One Year/One to Two Years/Two to Three Years/Three to Five Years.* New York, NY: New Market Press. (4 books).

Shelov, S.P., & American Academy of Pediatrics. (1991). *Caring for your baby and young child: Birth to age 5.* New York, NY: Bantam Books.

PARENT–PROFESSIONAL COLLABORATION

Beckman, P., & Boyers, G.B. (1993). *Deciphering the system: A guide for families of young children with disabilities.* Cambridge, MA: Brookline Books.

Hochstadt, N.J., & Yost, D. (Ed.). (1991). *The medically complex child: The transition to home care.* Newark, NJ: Gordon and Breach Science Publications.

Larson, G. (Ed.). (1986). *Managing the school age child with a chronic health condition.* Wayzata, MN: DCI Publishing.

Leff, P.T., & Walizer, E. (1992). *Building the healing partnership: Parents, professionals and children with chronic illnesses and disabilities.* Cambridge, MA: Brookline Books.

White, B. (Ed.). (1992). *Self-help sourcebook: Finding and forming mutual aid self-help groups.* Denville, NJ: St. Clares-Riverside Medical Center.

PREMATURE INFANTS

Adult resources:

Ballard, R.A. (1988). *Pediatric care of the ICN graduate.* Philadelphia, PA: W.B. Saunders.

Hales, Dianne. (1990). *Intensive caring: New hope for high-risk pregnancy.* New York, NY: Crown Publishers.

Harrison, H., & Kosititsky, A. (1983). *The premature baby book: A parents' guide to coping and caring in the first years.* New York, NY: St. Martin's Press. With an expanded and updated resource section.

Henig, R.M. (1983). *Your premature baby.* New York, NY: Ballantine Books.

Jason, J., & Van der Meer, A. (1989). *Parenting your premature baby.* New York, NY: Henry Holt and Company.

Manginello, F.P., & Di Gesonimo, T.F. (1991). *Your premature baby: Everything you need to know about the childbirth, treatment and parenting of premature infants.* New York, NY: John Wiley & Sons.

Children's resources:

Althea. (1986). *Special care babies.* London, England: Dinosaur Publications (Collins Publishing Group).

Pankow, V. (1987). *No bigger than my teddy bear.* Nashville, TN: Abingdon Press.

SAFETY

Chewning, E.B. (1984). *Emergency first aid for children.* Reading, MA: Addison-Wesley.

Vogel, S.N., & Manhoff, D.H. (1989). *Emergency medical treatment: Children. A handbook of what to do in an emergency to keep a child alive until help arrives.* Wilmette, IL: EMT, Inc.

Vogel, S.N., & Manhoff, D.H. (1989). *Emergency medical treatment: Infants. A handbook of what to do in an emergency to keep an infant alive until help arrives.* Wilmette, IL: EMT, Inc.

SENSORY DEFICITS

Adult resources:

Schwartz, S. (Ed.). (1987). *Choices in deafness: A parent's guide.* Bethesda, MD: Woodbine House.

Scott, E.P., et al. (1994). *Can't your child see? A guide for parents and professionals about young visually impaired children,* 3rd ed. Austin, TX: Pro-Ed.

Future Reflections: The National Federation of the Blind Magazine for Parents of Blind Children (edited by Barbara Cheadle). Baltimore, MD: The National Federation of the Blind.

Children's resources:

Aiello, B., & Schulman, J. (1988). *Business is looking up.* Frederick, MD: Twenty-First Century Books (The Kids on the Block Book Series).

Arnold, C. (1991). *A guide dog puppy grows up.* San Diego, CA: Harcourt Brace Jovanovich.

Barrett, M.B. (1994). *Sing to the stars.* Boston, MA: Little, Brown.

Bove, Linda. (1985). *Sesame Street sign language ABC with Linda Bove.* New York, NY: Random House.

Karim, R. (1994). *Mandy Sue Day.* New York, NY: Clarion Books.

Lakin, Pat. (1994). *Dad and me in the morning.* Morton Grove, IL: Albert Whitman & Company.

Levine, E.S. (1984). *Lisa and her soundless world.* New York, NY: Human Sciences Press.

Litchfield, A.B. (1976). *A button in her ear.* Chicago, IL: Albert Whitman & Company.

SIBLINGS OF CHILDREN WITH ILLNESS AND DISABILITIES

Adult resources:

Klein, S.D., & Schleifer, M.S. (1993). *It isn't fair! Siblings of children with disabilities.* Westport, CN: Bergin & Garvey.

Meyer, Donald J. (1985). *Living with a brother or sister with special needs.* Seattle, WA: University of Washington Press.

Powell, T.H., & Gallagher, P.A. (1992). *Brothers & sisters: A special part of exceptional families,* 2nd ed. Baltimore, MD: Paul H. Brookes.

Children's resources:

Baznik, D. (1981). *Becky's story: A book to share.* Bethesda, MD: Association for the Care of Children's Health.

Brandenberg, F. (1990). *I wish I was sick, too!* New York, NY: Greenwillow Books.

Peterkin, A. (1992). *What about me? When brothers and sisters get sick.* New York, NY: Magination Press.

Thompson, M. (1992). *My brother, Matthew.* Bethesda, MD: Woodbine House.

Resource Organizations for Parents and Professionals

Access to Respite Care Help (ARCH)
800 Easttowne Drive
Chapel Hill, NC 27514
800-473-1727

American Heart Association
7320 Greenville Avenue
Dallas, TX 74231
800-242-8721

American Lung Association
1740 Broadway
New York, NY 10019
800-586-4872

Association for the Care of Children's
Health
7910 Woodmont Avenue, Suite 300
Bethesda, MD 20814
301-654-6549
1-800-808-2224

Clearinghouse on Infant Feeding and
Nutrition
American Public Health Association
1015 15th Street, N.W.
Washington, DC 20005

Cystic Fibrosis Foundation
6931 Arlington Road
Bethesda, MD 20814
301-951-4422
800-344-4823

Epilepsy Foundation of America
4351 Garden City Drive
Landover, MD 20785
301-459-3700
800-332-1000

Exceptional Parent Magazine
1170 Commonwealth Avenue, Third
Floor
Boston, MA 02134-4646
617-730-5800

Family Voices
P.O. Box 769
Algodone, NM 87001
505-867-2368

National Coalition of Hispanic
Health & Human Services
Organizations (COSSMHO)
1501 16th Street, N.W.
Washington, DC 20036-1401
202-387-5000

National Hydrocephalus Foundation
22427 S. River Road
Joliet, IL 60436
815-467-6548

National Information Center for
Children and Youth with
Disabilities
P.O. Box 1492
Washington, DC 20013
800-999-5599

National Information Center for
Infants with Disabilities and Life-
Threatening Conditions
Association for the Care of Children's
Health
7910 Woodmont Avenue, Suite 300
Bethesda, MD 20814
800-922-9234

National Information Center on
Deafness
Gallaudet University
800 Florida Avenue, N.E.
Washington, DC 20002-3625
202-651-5051

National Institute on Deafness and
Other Communication Disorders
Clearinghouse
P.O. Box 3777
Washington, DC 20013-3777
301-565-4020
800-241-1044

National Maternal and Child Health
Clearinghouse
38th and R Streets, N.W.
Washington, DC 20057
202-625-8410

National Organization for Rare
Diseases (NORD)
P.O. Box 8923
New Fairfield, CT 06812
203-746-6518

National Parent Network on
Disabilities
1600 Prince Street, Suite 115
Alexandria, VA 22314
703-684-6763

National Self Help Clearinghouse
CUNY Graduate School and
University Center
25 W. 43rd Street, Room 620
New York, NY 10036
212-354-8525

Olney Foundation
(parenteral/enteral feeding)
124 Hun Memorial A-23
Albany Medical Center
Albany, NY 12208
518-262-5079

Respitality Program
c/o United Cerebral Palsy Association
1660 L Street, N.W., Suite 700
Washington, DC 20036
800-872-5827

Sibling Information Network
1776 Ellington Road
South Windsor, CT 06074
203-648-1205

SKIP [Sick Kids Need Involved
People]
8360 Route 3
Millersville, MD 21108
301-621-7830

United Cerebral Palsy Association,
Inc.
1660 L Street, N.W., Suite 700
Washington, DC 20036
800-872-5827

Promoting Health Maintenance for the High-risk Premature Infant

Elizabeth Ahmann, ScD, RN

Health maintenance for the infant with chronic illness and technology dependence poses special challenges for the family and for health care providers. For example, some families may have difficulty finding a source of pediatric care; immunizations may be significantly off schedule; and managing minor illnesses can be complicated. Although this chapter is not meant to provide a complete guide for primary care, it will assist the community health or home care nurse in knowing when referrals, parent guidance, or case management efforts may be useful in promoting appropriate health maintenance for the high-risk infant.

The topics addressed in this chapter include primary pediatric care, immunizations, minor illnesses, dental care, nutrition, growth, developmental intervention, parenting, activities of daily living, safety, and family adjustment and use of community resources. An overview of primary care concerns is provided in Table 8–1. A sample plan of care for promoting health maintenance is provided in Appendix 8–A.

PRIMARY PEDIATRIC CARE

Families should be assisted in arranging for pediatric primary care either prior to or shortly after the infant's arrival home from the hospital. Pediatricians and nurse practitioners can provide primary care to the high-risk preterm infant. If a family previously has worked with a certain provider, this may be the best source of primary care for the infant. A pediatrician or nurse practitioner may be more confident in the provision of care to the infant with multiple and complex

medical and developmental needs if this care is a collaborative effort. The opportunity for regular telephone consultations with the hospital neonatologist or other specialist, preferably one who has followed the child's early course, will assist the primary care provider in gaining a complete understanding of the child's medical course, status, prognosis, and needs. The primary care provider should also be informed where the developmental assessment and intervention are being provided, that a nurse will be making regular home visits, and what other disciplines and specialties are involved in the child's care.

IMMUNIZATIONS

Increasingly, intensive care nurseries routinely start immunizations at 2 months chronological age for infants who are clinically stable; however, the oral polio vaccine (OPV) is not given inpatient. Immunizations received in the ICN should be documented in the discharge summary (Miller, 1993). Nonetheless, immunizations may be significantly off schedule owing to prolonged hospitalization or repeated minor illnesses.

Parents may be relieved to know that immunizations can be given on an altered schedule. They may have questions related particularly to the immunizations for pertussis, measles, Haemophilus influenza type B (Hib) and influenza (flu) vaccines. Review articles on childhood immunization include that by Osguthorpe and Morgan (1995) and Yoon (1992). Parents should discuss risks and benefits of various

Table 8–1 Overview of Primary Care Concerns for the Intensive Care Nursery (ICN) Graduate (Table developed by Nancy Miller, RN, FNP)

	1 Month after D/C from ICN	3 Months corrected age	6 Months corrected age	12 Months corrected age	18–24 Months corrected age
I. Growth parameters	*Head circumference*—There is dramatic catch-up growth in the first 3 months corrected age that continues until 6–8 months. A positive neurological history such as an intraventricular hemorrhage (IVH) and an HC above 95% would warrant a cranial ultrasound or CT scan.[1] *Weight and length*—A period of rapid weight gain occurs slightly before a gain in length.[2]	Continued catch-up growth in HC, but reevaluation should be considered if the HC is growing more than 1.75cm/week.[2]	Referral or reevaluation needed if the HC levels off at 5–6 months of age.[2]	Many premies who were SGA never catch up like the AGA does.	The premie should be almost caught up to his or her chronological age size.
II. Nutrition	*Formula*—What type of formula is used and what is the calorie content? How much is taken at each feeding, how often, and how long does it take to finish? *Breastfeeding*—If there are questions or concerns refer to a lactation consultant.	Healthy premies require 110–130 kcal/kg/day, but chronically ill premies may need 200 kcal/kg/day.[3] Feeding difficulties and gastroesophageal reflux are common and can compromise adequate nutrition.[4]	*Solids*—The corrected age should be used to determine when solids should be started and they can be started now. Supplements of polycose or oils may be added for BPD premies who need more calories.[3]	*Formula*—Using the corrected age, this is the time to switch from formula to whole milk.	*Formula*—Children with BPD who still need nutritional supplements can now used Pediasure.[3]
III. Screenings	*Vision*—Most premies have one or more eye exams in the ICN. What were the results of the exams? Does the baby need followup with a pediatric opthalmologist as in retinopathy of prematurity (ROP)? *Hearing*—Many premies have had a Brainstem Auditory Evoked Response (BAER) test done in the ICN. An abnormal BAER is usually repeated in 6 months. *Development*—In most large hospitals there is a Premature Follow-up Program. Will the baby be followed in a premie follow-up program and will they send written reports? Inform parents regarding Part H services.	*Vision*—Continue opthalmology followup for any positive findings since premies have an increased incidence of myopia and strabismus.[1] *Hearing*—If the baby didn't have a BAER done in the ICN and was VLBW, they should have a BAER done now.[3] *Development*—A baseline developmental screening should be done at 3–4 months.	*Hearing*—If the BAER was abnormal in the ICN, it should be repeated now. *Development*—Premies often present with transient neuromuscular abnormalities that usually resolve by 18 months.[3]	*Development*—Premies who weighed 1,500 g or less have an overall 25% disability rate and a 7.7% incidence of CP.[7]	*Vision*—Myopia and strabismus can increase up to this age, especially in the lowest birthweights and those with increased severity of ROP.[5] *Hearing and Speech*—A formal speech and hearing evaluation should be considered if the child is delayed in the language area. Premies have an increased risk of a hearing loss and delays in speech.[6] *Development*—Premies have a very high incidence of learning disabilities and should continue screenings.[8]

(continues)

Table 8–1 (continued)

	1 Month after D/C from ICN	3 Months corrected age	6 Months corrected age	12 Months corrected age	18–24 Months corrected age
IV. Medical problems	*Diagnoses*—Does the baby have ROP, anemia, bronchopulmonary dysplasia (BPD), apnea of prematurity, IVH, or hernias? *Medications*—What medications are given, how much and when? Do levels need to be checked? Are there any problems giving the medication or any side effects? *Equipment*—What equipment is being used? Are there any problems with operating them?	*Equipment*—Apnea monitors need the resting heart rate adjusted as the premie grows. Have there been any true apneas?	*Medications*—BPD infants may be weaning from diuretics, bronchodilators or oxygen. Their weight and respiratory status should be monitored closely. Their pulse oximeter should continue to read 95 through all activities of living.[3]	*Diagnoses*—Many premies are hospitalized at least once in their first year for respiratory infections. BPD infants can have a severe problem with RSV infections.[9]	
V. Anticipatory guidance	*Sleep*—Premies have shorter sleep-wake cycles and it is common for them to wake and fuss every 2 hours until 3–4 months corrected age. Some may need to be weaned off all the light and noise they were used to in the ICN using a radio or soft light. Others may need a dark quiet room. *Crying*—The amount and intensity of crying peaks at 3–4 months corrected age.[10]	*Sleep*—It can take up to 6–8 months corrected age before premies sleep 8 hours at night.[10]	*Safety*—It's time to start baby proofing the house with safety latches, plug covers, and gates.	*General*—Emphasizing that the child is normal now and doesn't need to be protected as much, help prevent the parents from labeling their premie as forever vulnerable (the Vulnerable Child Syndrome).[2]	*General*—Cup drinking should be well established and premies should be weaning from the bottle and pacifiers.

Note: D/C = discharge, KN = intensive care nursery, HC = head circumference, CT = computed tomography, VLBW = very low birth weight, CP = cerebral palsy, RSV = respiratory syncytial virus, SGA = small for gestational age, AGA = appropriate for gestational age.

Source: Adapted from Miller, N., Guidelines for Primary Care Follow-Up of Premature Infants, *Nurse Practitioner*, Vol. 18, p. 10, with permission of Springhouse Corporation, © 1993.

Table references:

1. Goldman, D.J. and Goldman S.L. "Prematurity," in Jackson, P.L. and Vessey, J.A., *Primary Care of the Child with a Chronic Condition*, St. Louis, Mosby-Year Book, Inc., 1992, pp. 446–464.
2. Hack, M. and Fanaroff, A.A.: "Growth Patterns in the ICN Graduate,": in Ballard, R.A.: *Pediatric Care of the ICN Graduate*, Philadelphia, W.B. Saunders, 1988, pp. 33–39.
3. Bernbaum, J.C. and Hoffman-Williamson, M.: *Primary Care of The Preterm Infant*, St. Louis, Mosby-Year Book Inc., 1991, pp. 7, 53–74, 87–119, 194, 234.
4. Gardner, S.L. and Hagedorn, M.I.: "Physiologic Sequelae of Prematurity: The Nurse Practitioner's Role. Part V. Feeding Difficulties and Growth Failure," *Journal of Pediatric Health Care*, 1991, 5:3, pp. 122–134.
5. Page, J.M., et al: "Ocular Sequelae in Premature Infants," *Pediatrics*, 1993, 92:6, pp. 787–790.
6. Ryan, J.: "Hearing and Speech Assessment,": in Ballard, R.A.: *Pediatric Care of the ICN Graduate*, Philadelphia, W.B. Saunders Co. 1988, pp. 111–120.
7. Escobar, G.J., et al: "Outcome Among Surviving Very Low Birthweight Infants: A Meta-Analysis," *Archives of Disease in Childhood*, 1991, 66, pp. 204–211.
8. Batshaw, M.L. and Perret, Y.M.: *Children with Disabilities*, Baltimore, Brookes Pub. Co., 1992, p. 104.
9. Chiocca, E.M.: "RSV and the High-Risk Infant," *Pediatric Nursing*, 1994, 20:6, pp. 565–568.
10. Gorski, P.A.: "Fostering Family Development After Preterm Hospitalization,": in Ballard, R.A.: *Pediatric Care of the ICN Graduate*, Philadelphia, W.B. Saunders 1988, pp. 27–32.

vaccines with the primary care provider. Primary care providers can provide parents with information sheets on each vaccine. The information in Exhibit 8–1 while not comprehensive regarding vaccine risks and benefits, addresses specific concerns related to the high-risk preterm infant and may be helpful to share when parents have questions.

MINOR ILLNESSES

Fever, respiratory infections, vomiting, diarrhea, and constipation are minor illnesses discussed in this section. The reader is referred to other resources for a more in-depth discussion of minor illnesses.

Fever

Temperature taking is an important skill for any parent. The nurse can stimulate a discussion on this subject by requesting to use the family's thermometer. Asking caregivers whether they have ever been taught to take temperatures correctly and then observing them using the thermometer during home visits is a nonthreatening way to explore their knowledge. If temperature taking is to be taught, demonstration, parents' return demonstration, and written instructions left in the home can be helpful.

Guidelines for treatment of fevers should be worked out with the child's pediatric care provider. Generally, if the infant has a rectal temperature of 101°F (39.5°C) or more, the pediatrician or nurse practitioner should be notified. Since fever can be associated with shunt malfunction or infection, otitis media, bronchiolitis, pneumonia, or other serious condition, an episode of fever should be thoroughly assessed.

The family should be encouraged to keep acetaminophen drops (e.g., Tylenol or Tempra) available at home for use if needed. Aspirin is not recommended, particularly for varicella infections or respiratory febrile illnesses, because of the association with an increased incidence of Reye's syndrome.

Respiratory Tract Infections

Respiratory viruses are a major cause of morbidity in the preterm infant. Children with bronchopulmonary dysplasia are very susceptible to viral and bacterial respiratory infections, and many will require rehospitalization for respiratory problems during the first year of life. Some clinicians recommend that during the first year, susceptible infants should be in minimal contact with relatives who have symptoms of a cold or flu (Arvin, 1988).

The first signs of infection that the parents or nurse may notice include irritability, lethargy, decreased appetite, fever, or changes from the infant's individual baseline respiratory rate and quality. Respiratory tract infection can be manifest

Exhibit 8–1 Information about Immunizations for Parents of High-risk Preterm Infants

Pertussis (usually administered as diptheria, tetanus, pertussis [DTP] vaccine). If the infant has any history of seizures or other central nervous system (CNS) disorders, a decision about the the pertussis portion of the vaccine is to be made on an individual basis, with consideration given to risks and benefits (American Academy of Pediatrics, 1991). Infants and children with bronchopulmonary dysplasia are at a high risk of serious morbidity with pertussis infection (Conte, 1992). As a result, while pertussis immunization may be deferred in the child with a neurological disorder, if neurological disease is not progressive, the vaccine will usually be given at or before the first birthday (American Academy of Pediatrics, 1991). Postimmunization seizures are rare (occurring less than once for every 1,750 doses). Since they are generally related to fever, antipyretic prophylaxis can be provided. Children with a history of seizures are at an increased risk of seizures after a DTP (Livengood et al, 1989), so emergency care should be reviewed in case a seizure should occur (see Chapter 17).

Diptheria and Tetanus. If the pertussis vaccine will be withheld, the diptheria, tetanus (DT) vaccine can be administered instead of the DTP.

Measles (administered as measles, mumps, rubella [MMR] vaccine). The measles vaccine has been implicated in postvaccine seizures with a higher incidence of these occurring in children with a history of seizures (American Academy of Pediatrics, 1988). According to the American Academy of Pediatrics (1988), these postvaccine seizures are not thought to produce permanent neurologic damage, and the risk of measles morbidity justifies routine immunization. MMR administration is recommended for human immunodeficiency virus (HIV)-infected persons and is not associated with an increased risk of adverse reactions in this population (American Academy of Pediatrics, 1989, 1991).

Poliomyelitis vaccines (live virus [OPV] or inactivated/ killed poliovirus vaccine [IPV]). The OPV is contraindicated in individuals with HIV or acquired immune deficiency syndrome (AIDS) or with immunocompromised family members; the IPV may be administered (Yoon, 1993).

Haemophilus influenza type B (Hib). Children with shunts for hydrocephalus are at an increased risk of Hib infections of the central nervous system, and for this reason should receive the conjugated Hib vaccine (Jackson, 1990).

Influenza. Subviron influenza vaccines are recommended for children over 6 months of age with bronchopulmonary dysplasia and for their caretakers (American Academy of Pediatrics, 1991), as the flu may further compromise the tenuous respiratory status in this population. Persons with HIV, AIDS, or other immunosuppression are also a high-risk target group to receive the vaccine (Osguthorpe & Morgan, 1995).

Note: This exhibit is not a complete listing of indications, contraindications, precautions, adverse reactions, or educational needs related to childhood immunization. For additional information, see Osguthorpe & Morgan (1995) and Yoon (1992, 1993).

as pneumonia, bronchiolitis, increased reactivity in the airways, or apneic episodes (Arvin, 1988; Davis, Sinkin, & Aranda, 1990). Otitis media and sinusitis can also be associated with a respiratory tract infection. Parents should be advised that cough suppressants, antihistamines, and other over-the-counter cold remedies should not be used without the advice of the primary care provider. More frequent use of respiratory support measures, including increased humidity and more frequent chest physical therapy, may be required during the course of an infection (Conte, 1992). Respiratory care is discussed in detail in Chapters 12 through 16.

Vomiting

Management of vomiting in the high-risk infant can be complicated, and parents should contact the infant's primary care provider when vomiting occurs. Although some spitting up may be normal, prompt identification and treatment of certain vomiting problems are important.

Causes

Vomiting may be associated with a number of problems. Some infants with copious secretions may cough and vomit. Other infants receiving theophylline and medicated aerosol treatments may vomit if fed shortly after treatments; vomiting can also signal toxic theophylline levels. If an infant has a history of intraventricular hemorrhage or hydrocephalus, vomiting may be a sign of increased intracranial pressure (see Chapter 18). Gastroenteritis is another possible cause. Vomiting can place the infant at risk of more serious problems by upsetting a tenuous fluid or electrolyte balance. In addition, feeding problems may contribute to vomiting, and vomiting can, conversely, contribute to failure to thrive.

Reflux

Reflux vomiting is an additional area of concern. The term *reflux* refers to the return flow of stomach contents into the esophagus, caused by relaxation at the distal esophagus. Mild reflux is reported for many infants. It presents as regurgitation or vomiting after meals, usually when the infant is laid down after feeding. The majority of infants with functional reflux may become asymptomatic by 18 months of age.

Reflux is more prevalent in premature infants and children with mental retardation and cerebral palsy. It can contribute to the risk of aspiration and aspiration pneumonia, may also be related to the development of recurrent apnea and cyanosis in some infants, and may aggravate existing lung disease. In children with frequent and copious vomiting, reflux can contribute to failure to thrive. (Reflux vomiting is discussed in Chapter 9.)

Assessment of Vomiting

Because of the many possible causes of vomiting and the associated risks, episodes in the high-risk infant should be assessed thoroughly. A thorough assessment of vomiting episodes includes amount; frequency; timing; and related activities, such as positioning, use of aerosol medications, coughing, and general activity. Overestimation of the volume of emesis is a common problem: 15 mL—about a teaspoon—makes a spot 4 inches in diameter on clothing or sheet; 60 mL—2 oz—makes a spot 8 inches in diameter.

Diarrhea

Diarrhea is also a signal for parents to contact the infant's health care provider, since dehydration can occur rapidly in infants. Diarrhea can signal several serious concerns. Formula intolerance (dairy or soy) should be ruled out. Occasionally, acute diarrhea and abdominal pain can signal peritoneal shunt malfunction. The infant with short bowel syndrome may be at particular risk of diarrhea, and intake and output should be closely monitored (see Chapter 11).

Nursing assessment of diarrhea addresses the following: amount, frequency, color, odor, texture, and relationship to feedings. Hydration status should also be assessed. If diarrhea is a recurrent problem for the infant, parents may wish to keep a supply of oral electrolyte solution available in the home for use in accordance with recommendations by the primary care provider.

Constipation

Constipation (difficulty in passing stools, which typically are hard and rocklike) can become a problem for a variety of reasons. Inadequate dietary fluids, hyper- or hypotonus, limited mobility, and medication side effects are common contributors to constipation in this population.

Both nutritional and nonnutritional interventions for constipation can be considered. As a nutritional intervention, unless fluid restriction is necessary for management of cardiac or pulmonary problems, fluids should be offered frequently. Prune juice, an ounce at a time, can also be given as needed. Karo syrup, 1 tsp in 2 to 3 oz of formula, as needed, can help loosen stools and is often used in infants requiring fluid restriction; however, there may be an associated risk of botulism. If solids have been introduced very early or increased quickly, they can be discontinued until the constipation is relieved. Subsequently, solids should be reintroduced slowly and in small amounts to prevent a recurrence of constipation.

Nonnutritional interventions include rectal stimulation with a thermometer and the use of glycerine suppositories in an acute episode. Only in extreme cases of impaction should an enema be used.

DENTAL CARE

Although a dentist is not needed in the first 2 years of life, there are several important dental issues that warrant discussion with families. First, many parents wait expectantly for the infant's first tooth. It will normally erupt between 4 and 10 months of age. The high-risk infant's schedule should not be any slower, if correction for prematurity is taken into account in determining age.

Good dental hygiene can prevent possible discoloration from the use of oral iron preparations. For young children with oral defensiveness, daily toothbrushing can be made easier by the use of soft toothettes or foam-tipped brushes and with baking soda in place of stronger-tasting toothpaste (Conte, 1992).

As with any baby, concerns about "bottle mouth" should be addressed as a preventive measure before teeth erupt. Bottle mouth is a form of decay of the primary teeth that is associated with frequent and prolonged sucking on a bottle containing carbohydrate liquids, such as milk or juices. Bottle mouth occurs most commonly when the infant is often given a bottle at nap or bed time. Optimally, a bottle should be given only while the infant is being held; however, if parents feel a bottle is necessary at nap or bed time, only water should be used.

NUTRITION

Attention to nutrition is essential in the care of the high-risk infant. Adequate nutrition is necessary to maintain health and resistance to disease, to promote growth, to provide the energy necessary for developmental pursuits, to build and repair tissue, and to promote resolution of health problems (Gardner & Hagedorn, 1991). At the same time, the chronic respiratory, cardiac, neurological, and gastrointestinal complications of prematurity can interfere with achieving optimal nutritional status. It can be challenging to meet simultaneously the high caloric requirements related to prematurity and the increased work of breathing associated with bronchopulmonary dysplasia (BPD) while neither requiring a great deal of energy for consumption, nor creating fluid overload (Conte, 1992). Oral defensiveness, gastric reflux, and short gut can further complicate the picture.

Assessment of both nutrition and feeding status, as well as interventions for the infant with problems of nutrition or feeding, are discussed in Chapter 9. The mother who wishes to breastfeed her infant may need both information and support; breastfeeding is addressed briefly in Chapter 9 and discussed as a Special Issue in the section on nutrition. Enteral and parenteral feeding are discussed in Chapters 10 and 11.

GROWTH

Parents will be curious about growth patterns to expect. While growth is individual and based on a number of factors, data from several research studies can be used to give parents general guidelines.

Most preterm infants born at a size appropriate for gestational age (AGA) follow the same growth pattern as full-term infants, if plotted on the growth charts by corrected rather than chronological age. While "healthy" preterm infants may catch up to the full-term charts by 1 year, smaller or sicker infants may not reach their growth potential until 3 or more years of age (Hack & Fanaroff, 1988). Preterm infants born small for gestational age (SGA), but with a normal head circumference, tend to have normal weights by 33 months (Hack et al., 1984). However, SGA infants who are symmetrically growth retarded (all growth parameters are small for gestational age) do not catch up to children born AGA (Gardner & Hagedorn, 1991). As a group, low birth weight (LBW) and very low birth weight (VLBW) infants may remain smaller than normal children at 3 years of age, even when corrected age is used (Casey et al., 1990). One study found that a group of VLBW infants, smaller than term peers at 1 and 3 years of age, had caught up by 8 years (Ross, Lipper, & Auld, 1990).

DEVELOPMENTAL INTERVENTION

Prematurely born infants are at an increased risk of neurodevelopmental problems that range from mild developmental delay to more profound disorders, such as cerebral palsy or mental retardation. Chapter 19 provides an overview of developmental issues in the care of the preterm infant.

Developmental assessment and intervention are important aspects of health maintenance. Appropriate developmental intervention should be based on the infant's developmental age, developmental strengths and needs, and current health status. Activities can be planned in conjunction with an occupational, physical, or speech therapist if the child needs such services. Chapter 20 explores the nurse's role in developmental assessment and intervention. Premature infants, particularly those with chronic medical problems, are at risk for hearing, vision, and language problems and should receive relevant screening and referral for services (see Chapters 21 through 23 and Special Issue, Early Intervention Services for the High-risk Infant). Recent research suggests the need for assessment in the learning and behavioral realms as the child born prematurely approaches school age (Hack et al., 1994).

Developmental intervention must also address the "normal" needs of the infant or young child. For example, devel-

Exhibit 8–2 Infant Characteristics Found in Disturbed Parent–Infant Interactions

Feeding disorders	Developmental delay
Failure to gain weight	Listlessness or lethargy
Food refusal	Sleep disturbances
Recurrent vomiting	Minimal vocalization
Recurrent diarrhea	Decreased "cuddliness"

Source: Compiled from Green, M., A Developmental Approach to Symptoms Based on Age Groups, *Pediatric Clinics of North America,* Vol. 22, pp. 571–583, W.B. Saunders, © 1975.

Exhibit 8–3 Nursing Interventions To Promote Healthy Parent–Child Interactions

Support
Point out strengths.
Offer praise and reinforcement when appropriate.
Offer parent acceptance and support.
Avoid blame or criticism.
Mother the parent: "And how are you doing?"
Respect different coping mechanisms.
Invite telephone calls from parents.

Empowerment
Use a collaborative model of nursing practice.
Encourage parent to attend to his or her own needs.
Promote family communication.
Assist parents to identify and use personal support systems.
Provide referrals for family-to-family support.

Education
Assist parents in close observation of infant's traits and skills.
Assist parents in understanding infant's cues and needs.
Instruct in age-, condition-, and development-appropriate behaviors and expectations.
Provide information in response to parental requests.

Modeling
Role model appropriate developmental interventions.
Role model responding to the infant's cues.
Role model meeting the infant's needs.

Note: Based on Brazelton (1973), Clark (1976), Clark and Alfonso (1976), Shelton and Stepanek (1994), and Webster-Stratton and Kogan (1980).

opment of trust is a critical developmental task of infancy. The nurse can assist family members in identifying the "normal" developmental tasks and in strategizing to meet their infants' needs in these areas. (See Special Issue, Normalization.)

PARENTING

Increasingly, intensive care nurseries are acknowledging the important role of the parent in the care of the preterm infant. Twenty-four-hour visitation and other family-centered policies make it easier for parents to come to know their infant. Nonetheless, parents may feel quite challenged when transitioning from hospital to home care.

Parenting an infant with multiple and complex medical problems can be anxiety provoking and exhausting. Typical characteristics and behaviors of the high-risk preterm infant are challenging and are among those Green (1975) identified years ago in association with disturbed parent–infant interactions (See Exhibit 8–2).

The nurse can help parents explore both their perceptions of the infant and their awareness of his or her abilities. "How would you describe your baby?" is a useful open-ended lead question. The questions listed both in the Neonatal Perception Inventory and in the Degree of Bother Inventory can also be helpful for assessing the parent–infant interaction (Broussard & Hartner, 1970).

The question, "What do you find most difficult about parenting your infant?" can help the nurse and parent focus effort, information, and support where the parent feels the greatest need. Asking, "What do you find most satisfying in parenting your infant at home?" can help parents focus on the positive aspects of a challenging experience.

Nursing interventions to support the parent and promote healthy parent–child interactions can be undertaken quite easily in the context of the nursing visit and the nurse's therapeutic relationship with the family. Suggestions, presented in Exhibit 8–3, focus on support, empowerment, education, and modeling behaviors.

Social support has been demonstrated repeatedly to influence parent–child interactions. The parent's own support network, parent-to-parent support from other parents of premature infants, and support provided by professionals can all be influential.

In this regard, Lang, Behle, and Ballard (1988) suggest that the community or home health nurse has many opportunities to foster parent–infant attachment and nurture and promote positive parenting and good coping skills. They suggest that asking the parent to "tell me about the last 24 hours" can help focus a discussion. The nurse can then confirm parental observations, thereby validating the parent as historian and accurate observer. The nurse can dispel unnecessary anxieties a parent may have (e.g. skin mottling or a pulsing fontanelle), and can clarify any misconceptions a parent may have about real problems. Furthermore, the nurse can assist the parent to notice strengths the infant has (e.g., visual tracking, a strong grasp) and progress the infant makes. Helping the parent see the child as an individual with skills and strengths can foster a healthy parent–infant relationship and good parenting skills.

ACTIVITIES OF DAILY LIVING

The adjustment home from the hospital can be difficult for baby and family. The medical condition contributes to the challenge; uncertainty about activities of daily living does as well. Many parents of preterm infants have questions about normal activities, such as sleep and bathing (McKim, 1993). The community or home health nurse can provide guidance on sleep, bathing, and crying, and anticipatory guidance on toileting and discipline.

Sleep

Sleep patterns in the premature infant may be irregular for a variety of reasons. Neurologic immaturity and nutritional needs may rouse the premature infant from sleep. Infants transitioning from hospital to home may be used to sleeping in bright, noisy rooms, and they may need help in the transition to "normal" nighttime sleeping patterns at home. The use of a nightlight or radio may ease the transition. Parents can be assisted to arrange medication and treatment schedules to minimize disruption of the nighttime hours for the infant and family. Parents should be able to hear machine and monitor alarms at night, and an intercom or baby monitor can be used to ensure this. However, frequent false alarms should be brought to the attention of the primary care provider; readjustment of alarm limits may lead to less disruption of infant and parent sleep (Conte, 1992). At the same time, parents should be reassured that it is common for "healthy" preterm infants to rouse and fuss every 2 hours until 3 to 4 months corrected age and not settle in to more lengthy sleep periods until 6 to 8 months (Gorski, 1988). The nurse can support parents through this period and encourage mothers to nap when possible.

Bathing

Daily bathing is not necessary. Regularly cleaning the face, hands, and diaper area will generally be sufficient for the first several weeks (Lang & Ballard, 1988). The infant who is upset during bathing may be soothed by wearing a tee shirt during the bath. Depending on the infant's condition, special precautions may apply. For example, an infant must be removed from an apnea monitor during bathing. Special care should be taken when bathing the infant with a tracheostomy. Petroleum-based oils or lotions should not be used on the infant requiring oxygen therapy.

Crying

The parents of the premature infant may see a peak in amount and intensity of crying at 3 to 4 months corrected age, lagging behind the peak for term infants (Gorski, 1988).

Crying can be vexing to parents and can undermine self-confidence in the parenting role. Techniques for quieting a crying baby, listed in Exhibit 8–4, may be shared with parents. Parents should be assured that they will learn to interpret their infant's cries over the first several weeks at home. In the interim, parents can facilitate communication efforts by playing with the infant only when fully awake, feeding promptly when hungry, and allowing undisturbed sleep (Lang & Ballard, 1988).

Some premature infants may seem irritable or hypersensitive to noise, touch, and other stimulation. Responsiveness to the cues of the sensitive infant can promote calming and assist adaptation. For example, removing the infant from the sources of stimulation into a quiet area may be soothing. At the same time, some infants may be temperamentally more irritable or excitable. Parents should be assisted to recognize when this is the case so that they do not feel frustrated when their efforts to calm the infant are ineffective. Exhibit 8–5 lists both books that will help parents care for the preterm infant and books that can assist in understanding and managing temperament.

Toilet Training

Prolonged hospitalization, prematurity, neurodevelopmental delay, and abnormalities of muscle tone can con-

Exhibit 8–4 Techniques for Quieting a Crying Infant

1. Place your hands on the baby's abdomen or hold his or her arms close to the body. Talk in a soothing voice. If the baby is jumpy, slow your movements.
2. Help the infant to bring a hand to the mouth to suck on it.
3. Try a change of the baby's position to the tummy or side.
4. Pick up the baby if he or she is still upset, trying a variety of rhythmic movements.
5. Hold the infant across your lap on his or her tummy, massage the back. Burp the baby again.
6. Check the clothing. The baby may be too hot or too cold.
7. Try swaddling the infant. Try a pacifier.
8. Walk with the infant. Try a Snuggli.
9. Try a wind-up swing, but only if this does not make the baby more jumpy (increase or cause tremors or startles).
10. Try soft music or turn on TV.
11. Turn on a monotonous sound, e.g., a vacuum cleaner or hair dryer.
12. Put the baby back in the crib for 15 minutes, then hold him or her for 15 minutes.
13. Take a ride in the car or walk with the stroller.
14. Try to relax yourself with breathing or other relaxation techniques.
15. In the end, remember that parents may need to "spell" each other, taking turns with the baby.

Source: Reprinted from *Pediatric Care of the ICN Graduate* by R.A. Ballard, p. 42, with permission of W.B. Saunders, © 1988.

Exhibit 8–5 Books for Parents

Topic: Caring for the Preterm Infant

Harrison, H. (1983). *The premature baby book*. New York, NY: St. Martin's Press.

Henig, R.M. (1983). *Your premature baby*. New York, NY: Ballantine Books.

Jason, J., & Van der Meer, A. (1989). *Parenting your premature baby*. New York, NY: Holt.

Lieberman, A., & Sheagren, T. (1984). *The premie parents' handbook*. New York, NY: EP Dutton.

Manginello, F.P. (1991). *Your premature baby—everything you need to know* . . . New York, NY: Wiley.

Topic: Crying

Jones, S. (1983). *Crying baby, sleepless nights*. New York, NY: Warner Books.

Sammons, W.A.H. (1989). *The self-calmed baby*. Boston, MA: Little, Brown.

Sears, W. (1989). *The fussy baby*. Franklin Park, IL: LaLeche League, International.

Topic: Managing Temperament

Kurcinka, M.S. (1991). *Raising your spirited child*. New York, NY: HarperCollins.

Turecki, S. (1989). *The difficult child*. New York, NY: Bantam Books.

Note: See also extensive bibliography in Appendix 7–A.

---

tribute to delayed bowel and bladder control (Conte, 1992; Goldman & Goldman, 1992). The use of diuretics or theophylline increase the frequency of urination and can make bladder control more difficult. Short bowel syndrome is associated with high stool output and may delay toilet readiness. Among preterm infants in general, signs of readiness for toileting are more likely to occur at the corrected developmental age (Goldman & Goldman, 1992). Expectations should be individualized.

Discipline

As the infant who is technology dependent grows and develops, issues of appropriate discipline may arise. Families may discipline their children in a variety of ways, and nurses working in the home should respect familial choices.

At the same time, overly cautious or overly indulgent approaches to discipline may not benefit the child. Three decades ago, Green and Solnit (1964) identified a syndrome of imagined vulnerability among some parents of healthy children who had been medically vulnerable early in life. Early parental anxiety had become more generalized, and the parents perceived the children as fragile, overprotecting them from sports, academic pressures, and peer interactions. The children had also grown to perceive themselves as frag-

ile and vulnerable. The term *vulnerable child syndrome* has been used to describe this syndrome of separation anxiety, infantilization, somatic complaints, and school problems among healthy children with prior medical problems.

Helping the parents of a child with complex medical problems focus on the child's strengths and see the many ways in which the child engages in normal age-appropriate activities from infancy on will encourage parents to guide the child appropriately. Normalizing daily activities, setting limits, and providing consistency in expectations for the child will encourage normal behavior and avoid dependent, demanding, or uncontrolled behaviors in the child.

In general, appropriate discipline is guidance, rather than punishment. An environment attentive to safety will permit normal active, curious toddler behavior while minimizing the opportunity for mistakes and consequences. Behavioral expectations should generally relate to the child's mental and corrected age rather than chronological age. It is important that the nurse working in the home understand parental wishes in regard to discipline and that some consistency is maintained between various caregivers.

SAFETY

Accidents are the leading cause of death among children in the United States; most accidents, however, are preventable. Plans for safe transportation of the infant with special needs are of the utmost priority (Bull et al., 1988). The community health nurse visiting the home is in an ideal position to address safety issues. The nurse can identify safety hazards in the home or neighborhood and educate family members about such hazards. Anticipatory guidance and preventive teaching about age- and development-specific safety issues can also be provided. Appendix 8–B lists important general safety precautions for the home, as well as specific considerations for infants and toddlers. Appendix 8–C includes a safety assessment checklist.

Specific safety concerns relevant to home care equipment, supplies, and procedures should be addressed as well. When young children are playing around medical equipment and supplies, special precautions are necessary. Many chapters of this book review safety issues relevant to individual types of equipment and specific procedures. Some general issues related to medical equipment and child safety in the home are addressed in Exhibit 8–6.

FAMILY ADJUSTMENT AND USE OF COMMUNITY RESOURCES

Care of the child with multiple disabilities or chronic illness can have a profound impact on the entire family. Family patterns and routines must change, and normal social support mechanisms may be unavailable due to economic or

Exhibit 8–6 Examples of Safety Issues in Pediatric Home Care

Safe Conduct of Procedures

Safe conduct of medical and nursing procedures is the clear standard of care. Because of the child's small body size, skill and caution are required in carrying out many procedures. Suctioning and administration of IV fluids are two examples. Suctioning that is too vigorous can dangerously deplete the infant's oxygen supply. IV fluids delivered too rapidly can overwhelm the infant's system.

Equipment Precautions

Curiosity is a natural part of childhood. Control panels, buttons, and dials for the ventilator, IV pumps, oxygen, and the like, should be "off limits" to children. As a further precaution, equipment should be secured as far out of reach as possible, and clear plastic panels, covers, or tape can be placed over buttons and dials so that children are not able to change any of the equipment settings.

Medication/Waste Hazards

Medications, syringes, and contaminated materials should be stored well out of reach of curious hands.

Electrical Hazards

Electric equipment and electric outlets can pose a hazard to young children. Safety covers should be in place when wall outlets are not in use. Any equipment not in use should be unplugged, and any wires (e.g., lead wires for an apnea monitor) should be stored out of reach.

Nighttime Precautions

Nighttime care of the child dependent on technology requires special safety precautions. Coiling and taping extra IV tubing and running tubing and apnea monitor wires out the bottoms of pajamas will help prevent accidental strangulation during sleep. An inexpensive intercom or baby monitor will assist parents in hearing machine alarms during the night.

Note: Based on Ahmann (1994) and Berry and Joergensen (1988).

---

time restraints, and sometimes due to fear on the part of friends and relatives. Family adjustment is addressed in greater detail in Chapter 2. Siblings may also face adjustment challenges as the family cares for the chronically ill preterm infant (see Chapter 3). Care of the child can stretch family resources in a wide range of areas, including financial, environmental, emotional, interpersonal, and social. Assisting the family to assess their resource needs (Chapter 4) and care coordination (Chapter 6) and providing information about and referrals to available community resources (Chapter 7) are important ways the home care nurse can promote family adjustment.

REFERENCES

Ahmann, E. (1994). An overview of issues in pediatric high-tech home care. In L.A. Gorski (Ed.), *High-tech home care manual.* Gaithersburg, MD: Aspen Publishers.

American Academy of Pediatrics. (1988). *Report of the committee on infectious diseases.* Evanston, IL: Author.

American Academy of Pediatrics. (1989). Measles reassessment of the current immunization policy. *Pediatrics, 84,* 1,110–1,113.

American Academy of Pediatrics. (1991). *Report of the committee on infectious disease.* Evanston, IL: Author.

Arvin, A. (1988). Infectious disease issues in the care of the ICN graduate. In R.A. Ballard (Ed.), *Pediatric care of the ICN graduate.* Philadelphia, PA: W.B. Saunders.

Berry, R.K., & Joergensen, S. (1988). Growing with home parenteral nutrition: Maintaining a safe environment. *Pediatric Nursing, 14,* 155–157.

Brazelton, T.B. (1973). *Neonatal Behavioral Assessment Scale.* In *Clinics in Developmental Medicine Series 50.* Philadelphia, PA: J.B. Lippincott.

Broussard, E.B., & Hartner, M.S.S. (1970). Further considerations regarding maternal perception of the newborn. In J. Hellmuth (Ed.), *Exceptional infants: Studies in abnormalities 2.* New York, NY: Brunner/Mazel.

Bull, M.J., Weber K., & Stroup, K.B. (1988). Automotive restraint system for premature infants. *Journal of Pediatrics, 112*(3), 385–388.

Casey, P.H., Kraemer, H.C., Bernbaum, J., Tyson, J.E., Sells, J.C., Yogman, M.W., & Bauer, C.R. (1990). Growth patterns of low birthweight premature infants: A longitudinal analysis of a large, varied sample. *Journal of Pediatrics, 117,* 298–307.

Chow, M.P., Durand, B.A., Feldman, M.N., et al. (1984). *Handbook of pediatric primary care* (2nd ed.). New York, NY: Wiley.

Clark, A.L. (1976, March/April). Recognizing discord between mother and child and changing it to harmony. *MCN: The American Journal of Maternal-Child Nursing, 1,* 100–106.

Clark, A.L., & Alfonso, D.D. (1976, March/April). Infant behavior and maternal attachment: Two sides to the coin. *MCN: The American Journal of Maternal-Child Nursing, 1,* 93–99.

Conte, V.H. (1992). Bronchopulmonary dysplasia. In P.L. Jackson & J.A. Vessey (Eds.), *Primary care of the child with a chronic condition.* St. Louis, MO: C.V. Mosby.

Davis, J.M., Sinkin, R.A., & Aranda, J. (1990). Drug therapy for bronchopulmonary dysplasia. *Pediatric Pulmonology, 8,* 117–125.

Gardner, S.L., & Hagedorn, M.I. (1991). Physiologic sequelae of prematurity: The nurse practitioner's role. Feeding difficulties and growth failure (pathophysiology, cause and growth failure). *Journal of Pediatric Health Care, 5,* 122–134.

Goldman, D.J., & Goldman, S.L. (1992). Prematurity. In P.L. Jackson & J.A. Vessey (Eds.), *Primary care of the child with a chronic condition.* St. Louis, MO: C.V. Mosby.

Gorski, P. (1988). Fostering family development after preterm hospitalization. In R.A. Ballard (Ed.), *Pediatric care of the ICN graduate.* Philadelphia, PA: W.B. Saunders.

Green, M. (1975). A developmental approach to symptoms based on age groups. *Pediatric Clinics of North America, 22,* 571–583.

Hack, M., & Fanaroff, A. (1988). Growth patterns in the ICN graduate. In R.A. Ballard (Ed.), *Pediatric care of the ICN graduate.* Philadelphia, PA: W.B. Saunders.

Hack, M., Merkatz, I., McGrath, S., et al. (1984). Catch-up growth in very-low-birthweight infants. *American Journal of Diseases of Children, 138,* 370–375.

Hack, M., Taylor, G., Klein, N., Eiben, R., Schatschneider, C., & Mercuri-Minich, N. (1994). School-age outcomes in children with birthweights under 750 g. *New England Journal of Medicine, 331*(12), 753–759.

Jackson, P.L. (1990). Primary care needs of children with hydrocephalus. *Journal of Pediatric Health Care, 4*(2), 59–71.

Lang, M.D., & Ballard, R.A. (1988). Well-baby care of the ICN graduate. In R.A. Ballard (Ed.), *Pediatric care of the ICN graduate.* Philadelphia, PA: W.B. Saunders.

Lang, M.D., Behle, M.B., & Ballard, R.A. (1988). The transition from hospital to home. In R.A. Ballard (Ed.), *Pediatric care of the ICN graduate*. Philadelphia, PA: W.B. Saunders.

Livengood, J.R., Mullen, J.R., White, J.W., Brink, E.W., & Orenstein, W.A. (1989). Family history of convulsions and use of pertussis vaccine. *Journal of Pediatrics, 115*(4), 527–531.

McKim, E.M. (1993). The difficult first week at home with a premature infant. *Public Health Nursing, 10*(2), 89–96.

Miller, N.P. (1993). Guidelines for primary care follow-up of premature infants. *Nurse Practitioner, 18*(10), 45–48.

Osguthorpe, N.C., & Morgan, E.P. (1995). An immunization update for primary health care providers. *Nurse Practitioner, 20*(6), 52–65.

Ross, G., Lipper, E.G., & Auld, P.A.M. (1990). Growth achievement of very low birthweight children at school age. *Journal of Pediatrics, 117*, 307–309.

Shelton, T.L., & Stepanek, J.S. (1994). *Family-centered care for children needing specialized health and developmental services*. Bethesda, MD: Association for the Care of Children's Health.

Webster-Stratton, C., & Kogan, K. (1980, February). Helping parents parent. *American Journal of Nursing, 80*, 240–244.

Yoon, C.Y. (1992). Childhood immunization: Part I. *Journal of Pediatric Health Care, 6*(6), 370–376.

Yoon, C.Y. (1993). Childhood immunization: Part II. *Journal of Pediatric Health Care, 7*(3), 127–133.

Home Care Plan: Health Maintenance

Date _____   Case manager _____

Name _____   Hosp # _____   DOB _____

PROBLEM: **HEALTH MAINTENANCE**

GOALS/OBJECTIVES	METHODS	STAFF/REVIEW
Family will have a source of primary pediatric care and will appropriately utilize same.	Assist family in obtaining and teach appropriate use of pediatric primary care.	
Child will be up-to-date on immunizations as medically indicated.	Discuss alterations in immunization schedule with family, prn; facilitate obtaining appropriate immunizations.	
Family will demonstrate appropriate well child care re: nutrition, growth and development, stimulation, responses to minor illness, dental and safety needs.	Assess/teach provision of well child care as needed in each aspect. Coordinate with primary care provider prn.	
Parents will become confident in parenting role.	Assist parents in understanding parenting role, building on positive perceptions of infant, and managing activities of daily living with chronically ill infant.	
Family will demonstrate a workable adjustment to care of the child and will utilize available community resources as needed.	Assist family in assessing strengths and weaknesses. Provide referrals for counseling and support to facilitate adjustment prn. Educate family and assist in accessing appropriate community resources prn.	
Child will receive coordinated, integrated care.	Assist in coordination of care and facilitate communication between care providers.	

Source: Courtesy of Children's Hospital National Medical Center, Home Health Care Services, Washington, D.C.

Home Safety Precautions

General Precautions

Use only Underwriter's Laboratories (UL)-approved electrical equipment.

Avoid overloading electrical systems.

Store medicines and poisons in childproof containers and out of reach of children.

When giving medications, measure doses carefully; know side effects and toxic effects.

Do not give any medications without prescription.

Store syringes and contaminated equipment/supplies out of reach.

Post emergency telephone numbers near the home telephone.

Learn first aid and cardiopulmonary resuscitation (CPR).

Immunize pets.

If child is on apnea monitor, make sure alarm can be heard from all parts of house; observe other safety precautions.

If child has tracheostomy or is on oxygen or a ventilator, observe all safety recommendations.

Preventing Falls

Keep crib sides up.

Strap child carefully in infant seat or feeding chair; crotch strap is important.

When child uses infant seat, place on floor or in playpen.

Do not leave infant unattended on bed, couch, or changing table.

Place gates at head and foot of stairways.

Put guards on windows; secure screens.

Keep chairs or stools away from windows.

Keep stairs free of clutter.

Avoid walkers, especially near stairs.

Preventing Choking/Strangulation/Suffocation

Do not use cribs with slats more than $2\frac{1}{8}$ inches apart.

Use bumper pads in crib.

Do not tie anything (including pacifier) around infant's neck.

Remove bib at bedtime.

Thread apnea monitor wires through lower end of clothing.

Remove loose or small parts from toys.

Avoid small hard foods (e.g., candy, nuts, raisins).

Keep all small objects out of reach.

Avoid bottle propping.

Burp infant well before putting into crib.

Keep drapery cords tied up high or cut short.

Tie plastic bags in a knot and discard.

Avoid play with balloons.

Use pacifier with one-piece construction and loop handle.

Know emergency procedures for choking.

Preventing Burns

Label flammable liquids, and store away from heat or sparks.

Develop and practice a fire escape plan.

Install smoke detectors.

Keep a small fire extinguisher available.

Check temperature of bath water carefully.

Use flame-resistant clothing, sheets, and blankets.

Avoid holding infant while cooking or handling hot liquids.

Keep pot handles turned in toward stove.

Keep hot drinks and foods away from counter or table edges.

Do not warm formula in microwave—bottle and formula will be different temperatures.

Avoid use of tablecloths with hanging edges.

Place guards around fireplaces, radiators, and heaters.

Keep crib or bed away from radiators or heaters.

Avoid use of heating pad.

Place safety caps on unused electrical outlets.

Keep electric wires out of reach.

Keep kitchen door closed or gated.

Keep vaporizers out of child's reach.

Limit sun exposure; use sunscreen (6 months).

Preventing Drowning

Do not leave child unattended in bath or pool.

Place fences around pools.

Empty tub or sink when not in use.

Keep bathroom door closed.

Preventing Injuries

Keep sharp items, including diaper pins, out of child's reach.

Pad sharp corners of furniture.

Secure small rugs.

Keep fans out of reach.

Avoid toys with sharp or breakable parts.

Teach safe play.

Car Safety

Always use a federally approved car seat, installed correctly.

Never leave children alone in car.

Keep car doors locked.

Avoid litter and loose objects inside car.

Do not place infant in carriage or stroller behind a parked car.

Source: Compiled from *Handbook of Pediatric Primary Care,* 2nd ed., by M.P. Chow et al., John Wiley and Sons, © 1984; *Lippincott Manual of Nursing Practice,* 3rd ed., by L.S. Brunner and D.S. Suddarth eds. Lippincott-Raven, © 1982; and *Nursing Care of Infants and Children,* 5th ed., by D.L. Wong, Mosby-Year Book, © 1995.

Home Safety Assessment

Patient Name: _____ HC#: _____ Date: _____

	GENERAL HOUSEHOLD SAFETY SCREENING TOOL	N/A	Yes	No
F I R E S A F E T Y	1. Number of smoke detectors in the home? _____ Are they battery operated?			
	2. Are fire extinguishers present in appropriate locations for use?			
	3. Can family members state escape routes and meeting place in the event of a fire?			
	4. Can family members state the actions to be taken if a person catches fire?			
	Comments:			
G A S / E L E C T R I C S A F E T Y	1. If a fuse or circuit breaker box is in the home, is it labeled?			
	2. For pts with electrical medical equipment is there a back-up power source in case of power outage?			
	3. Are flashlights/batteries or candles/matches kept for power outages?			
	4. Are electrical outlets 2 or 3 pronged? _____ 2 pronged _____ 3 pronged			
	5. Are electrical outlets accessible to patient care areas?			
	6. Are electrical cords frayed or are wires exposed?			
	7. What is the source of heating/cooking fuel? ( ) electric ( ) gas ( ) oil ( ) other _____			
	8. If gas, does the family know its odor and actions to be taken if a leak is suspected?			
	Comments			
G E N E R A L H O M E S A F E T Y	1. Does the family know emergency phone numbers?			
	2. Is the number for poison control posted on or near the phone?			
	3. Is there a working telephone in the home?			
	4. Are cleansers, drugs and plants out of reach of children or in locked cabinets?			
	5. If indicated, do family members wear allergy or medic alert bracelets?			
	6. Are fireplaces, radiators, and space heaters screened?			
	7. Is the hot water temperature at or below 130 degrees F?			
	8. Are hallways and stairs free of clutter, banister present for stairs, and rugs secured?			
	9. Is the elevator, hallway, building, or neighborhood safe? (well lit, clean, visible)			
	10. Are rodents, roaches, loose plaster, paint chips, or drugs/alcohol in the home?			
	11. Are age specific safety measures, per CHHCS protocols, followed in the home?			
	Comments:			

Case Manager Signature_____

Source: Courtesy of Children's Hospital National Medical Center Home Health Care Services, Washington, D.C.

Part III

Nutrition and Feeding

Breastfeeding the High-risk Premature Infant: Assessment and Management

Barbara L. Marino, PhD, RN, and Virginia L. Combs, BSN

Until recently, infants born prematurely or with chronic diseases were expected to fail at breastfeeding. Basic textbooks perpetuated the belief that breastfeeding was too hard for the sick infant. Now there is ample evidence that former premature infants can successfully breastfeed (Gross & Slagle, 1993). Studies of other groups of high-risk infants are finding that breastfeeding is possible for them as well (Combs & Marino, 1993; Lawrence, 1994). This is encouraging for many mothers who want to breastfeed a high-risk infant.

Although not every chronically ill child will succeed at breastfeeding, breastfeeding is usually possible with extra commitment and support. Common problems for the breastfeeding mother of a high-risk infant include decreased milk supply, inadequate support or knowledge, and maternal anatomical variations that complicate breastfeeding. For the high-risk infant, the most common obstacles to breastfeeding are learned behaviors about feeding and hyper- or hypotonicity affecting suck, swallow, or positioning.

ASSESSMENT OF BREASTFEEDING

Assessment includes an interview and an observation of an entire feeding. The purpose of the interview is to determine the following:

- the strength of the mother's commitment to breastfeeding
- the mother's previous experience and knowledge of breastfeeding
- the feelings of her partner and other important people in her life (e.g., mother, mother-in-law, pediatrician, sister) about her breastfeeding and their level of support for breastfeeding
- any aspect of her lifestyle that places the infant at risk.

Determining the strength of the mother's commitment to breastfeeding provides information about what she wants and, more importantly, empowers the mother to decide if, for how long, and why she wants to breastfeed. All teaching and professional support should revolve around the mother's definition of successful breastfeeding. Asking her about her experience and the opinions of those around her provides information about knowledge deficits or obstacles that can be addressed. Asking about her lifestyle should elicit information about her use of any substance that may affect the infant. Mothers who are human immunodeficiency virus (HIV)-positive and those who use illegal drugs or certain prescription drugs should not breastfeed.

Observation of the feeding should include the entire process: positioning, latching on, sucking and swallowing, and mother's interpretations of infant feeding behavior. A description of the process can be found in most basic breastfeeding manuals (e.g., Huggins, 1990). Ideally, one feeding each day should be observed until the infant is gaining $\frac{1}{2}$ oz to 1 oz per day, and the mother is confident in her ability to nurse. When daily visits are not possible, a telephone contact is necessary to ensure that the infant is adequately nourished. To ensure accuracy in infant weights, weigh the nude infant before the feeding. Pre- and postfeeding weights may be useful as a rough measure of intake, if electronic scales are being used (Meier, Lysakowski, Engstrom, Kavanaugh, & Mangurten, 1990).

MANAGEMENT OF COMMON MATERNAL PROBLEMS

The following lists recommendations for management of common maternal problems:

- Decreased milk supply
  1. Prevent decreased supply by having the mother pump during the infant's hospitalization.
  2. Ensure adequate rest and oral intake so the mother can produce increasing quantities of milk.
  3. Pump between feedings to rebuild supply once child is nursing.
  4. Plan weaning from bottle to breast on the supply/demand principle.
  5. Use relactation devices if necessary (see section on community resources, below).
- Inadequate support or knowledge
  1. Provide a good basic manual for breastfeeding (e.g., Huggins, 1990, *The Nursing Mother's Companion*).
  2. Empower mother to decide how long/if to continue breastfeeding.
  3. Problem solve with her about demands on her time.
  4. Build supports by including her partner or other important people in education.
  5. Advocate for mother with physicians if they are not supportive of breastfeeding.
- Breast anatomy
  1. Utilize basic breastfeeding manual to address problems such as cracked or sore nipples, flat or inverted nipples, large nipples.

MANAGEMENT OF COMMON INFANT PROBLEMS

The following lists recommendations for management of common infant problems:

- Learned behaviors about feeding
  1. Teach mother that infant has associated bottle with satiation, not that he or she prefers it over breast.
  2. Teach that learned behavior can be unlearned.
  3. Feed infant when he or she is hungry and in quiet alert state, not screaming or sleepy.
  4. Teach mother to recognize infant cues for hunger and satiation.
  5. Express milk onto nipple so infant can smell and taste it.
  6. Help mother to relax.
  7. Feed on demand.
  8. Use relactation device if supply is very low so infant associates breast with satiation.
- Hyper- or hypotonicity
  1. Utilize strategies described in *Breast Feeding: A Guide for the Medical Profession* (Lawrence, 1994).

2. Consult with physical therapy (PT)/occupational therapy (OT) for assistance as needed.

COMMUNITY RESOURCES

Lactation consultants who have been certified by the International Board of Lactation Consultants are ideal resources for both nurses and mothers. The accreditation process includes intensive education and demonstrated competency in management of breastfeeding. Local maternity hospitals may have a list of lactation consultants in the region. Lactation consultants can also be located by contacting International Lactation Consultants Association at 1–708–260–8874.

Relactation devices consist of a container for formula and a tube through which the formula runs. The end of the tube is attached to the mother's nipple. As the infant nurses, the flow of milk from the relactation device supplements the breast milk. By sucking at the breast, the infant stimulates the mother's milk production and learns to associate nursing with satiation. Relactation devices are available through Medela at 1–800–435–8316.

WHEN IT ISN'T WORKING . . .

Inevitably, there will be mothers and infants who are unable to breastfeed or should stop because the infant is being jeopardized (e.g., the HIV-positive mother). Two approaches can be helpful. First, empower the mother to review her options. This step may include her partner if she wishes. Help them think through the consequences of each option for themselves and for the infant. Second, help them plan how to transition the infant to a bottle.

The home care nurse is often crucial in assisting the mother and infant in the transition to successful breastfeeding. The nurse may be an advocate with providers, insurers, or even family members. The nurse can help mothers make decisions about infant feeding that are based on the mother's preferences and the needs and ability of the infant. Not all couples will succeed in breastfeeding, but some will. With the assistance of the community health or home care nurse, each mother and infant can have the opportunity to try.

REFERENCES

Combs, V.L., & Marino, B.L. (1993). A comparison of growth patterns in breast and bottle fed infants with congenital heart disease. *Pediatric Nursing, 19*(2), 175–179.

Gross, S.J., & Slagle, T.A. (1993). Feeding the low birth weight infant. *Clinics in Perinatology, 20*(1), 193–209.

Huggins, K. (1990). *The nursing mother's companion.* Boston, MA: Harvard Common Press.

Lawrence, R.A. (1994). *Breast feeding: A guide for the medical profession* (4th ed). Toronto, Ontario, Canada: C.V. Mosby.

Meier, P.P., Lysakowski, T.Y., Engstrom, J.L., Kavanaugh, K.L., & Mangurten, H.H. (1990). The accuracy of test weighing for preterm infants. *Journal of Pediatric Gastroenterology and Nutrition, 10*, 62–65.

Failure To Thrive

Connie Lierman, RN, MSN

Meeting the nutritional needs of the high-risk premature infant can sometimes pose a challenge to parents and health care providers. A thorough assessment of growth, intake, and feeding skills and behavior is necessary to both ensure that the infant's nutritional needs are met and to pinpoint problem areas (see Chapter 9). Many problems, identified early, are amenable to fairly straightforward interventions. Other difficulties may require the assistance of specialists in feeding skills or behavior—occupational therapists, speech therapists, or child psychologists.

Some infants will not only have feeding difficulties, but may also be diagnosed with "failure to thrive" (FTT). A diagnosis of FTT is made based on one of the following criteria:

- weight below 80% of the median for age
- weight less than the third percentile on the National Center for Health Statistics (NCHS) growth charts
- growth curve that has dropped 2 or more percentile ranks on the NCHS charts (Peterson, Washington, & Rathburn, 1984).

Once the diagnosis of FTT is made, the Waterlow and Gomez classifications (see Tables SI1 & SI2) are used to determine the degree of malnutrition. The degree of malnutrition will often dictate the timing and type of interventions considered appropriate.

CAUSES OF FTT

The causes of FTT can be organic, nonorganic, or mixed (Bithoney, Dubowitz, & Egan, 1992; O'Brien, Repp, Williams, & Christopherson, 1991).

Organic FTT

Organic FTT (OFTT) results from a physical anomaly or a condition affecting a major body system (e.g., gastrointestinal, renal, cardiac, or pulmonary). Examples include cystic fibrosis, celiac disease, Hirshsprung's disease, congenital heart failure, or bronchopulmonary dysplasia.

Nonorganic FTT

Nonorganic FTT (NOFTT) is generally defined by the exclusion of any obvious organic cause for the growth failure. However, a recent study by Ramsay, Gisel, and Boutry (1993) found that review of the early feeding history of infants diagnosed with NOFTT revealed abnormal feeding-related symptoms that were present at birth or shortly thereafter and persisted until later referral for FTT. The authors postulated that impaired oral function may be an unrecognized organic cause of what has generally been called NOFTT. The infant's impaired function would also affect the caregiver–infant interaction (Bithoney & Newberger, 1987).

Some studies have suggested an association between NOFTT and disturbed or different mother–infant interactions. One study documented less visual attention, less demonstration of affection, and more physical punishment in the mother–infant interaction (O'Brien et al., 1991). NOFTT also has been associated with children who have been abused or neglected. The results of the Ramsey group (1993) study raise questions about cause and effect of disturbed parent–infant interactions in NOFTT.

Mixed FTT

A third category, mixed FTT (MFTT), also has been suggested and describes the child with both organic and nonorganic causes of growth failure (Powell, Low, & Speers, 1987). For example, an infant with severe reflux (OFTT) and esophagitis may associate feeding with pain and develop food refusal behaviors (NOFTT). An infant with cardiac or respiratory disease may eventually learn to manipulate parental attention by abnormal feeding behaviors. In these infants, growth failure is secondary to both

Table SI 1 Waterlow Classification for Assessment of Malnutrition

Grade of malnutrition	Weight/height % of standard	Height/age % of standard
0	>90	>95
1	81–90	90–95
2	70–80	85–89
3	<70	<85

organic and nonorganic problems. Mixed FTT may also be a more appropriate diagnosis in many infants previously diagnosed with NOFTT.

NURSING INTERVENTIONS

Interventions for FTT will depend on both the degree of malnutrition and the cause(s).

Nutritional Interventions

In children diagnosed with FTT, hospitalization is often necessary to complete diagnostic tests, to observe for weight gain outside the home, and to offer nutritional intervention in an acute situation. Strategies to improve caloric intake will be implemented (see Chapter 9). These may include concentrated formulas and/or supplements. If malnutrition is severe or oral intake is not adequately effective in improving the child's growth parameters, enteral or occasionally parenteral feeding may be necessary (see Chapters 10 & 11). When appropriate, plans also will be developed to address problems of feeding skills and behaviors (see Chapter 9).

If FTT is found to have a nonorganic component, nutritional recommendations must be augmented by intervention with the parent–infant dyad to improve the feeding interaction. Such intervention begins in the hospital but must be continued at home. Nursing interventions for NOFTT include several strategies, described below.

Nurturing Relationship

The nurse should begin intervention for FTT by establishing a caring and nurturing relationship with the parents that will encourage them to develop trust and begin to improve self-esteem when necessary. Being judgmental and

Table SI 2 Gomez Criteria for Assessment of Malnutrition

Degree of malnutrition	% of standard weight/age
1°	75–85
2°	64–74
3°	<64

authoritarian are inappropriate for the nurse, whereas being concerned and understanding are very important.

Since building self-esteem in the parent is a goal in treating the parent–infant dyad, the nurse should help the parent set small, achievable goals at each home visit so that there is much opportunity for praise and no opportunity for the parent to fail. Offering positive reinforcement whenever the parent exhibits nurturing behavior toward the infant is critical. In addition, describing and praising strengths of the parent and positive interactions with the infant can be helpful.

Experiences and Stressors

The nurse should assist parents in exploring past events, current life stresses, and the parents' experiences with feeding and nurturing. A detailed history of early feeding should be obtained by direct or indirect questions, such as the following: What was it like to feed your baby in the first month? How frequent were feedings, and how long did they take? This information can offer important clues in understanding the feeding and interactional problems. Feelings about the infant, particularly about any physical deformities, chronic illness, or mental retardation, should also be explored.

Any positive or negative feelings expressed should be accepted. Suggestions can be offered about solutions to current problems but should be offered in a collaborative, caring manner rather than authoritatively. In this regard, problems should be framed in terms of how to meet the child's needs rather than how to improve the parents' behavior.

Role Modeling

Role modeling appropriate care of the child is another aspect of nursing intervention for NOFTT. The feeding observation discussed in Chapter 9 describes observing for clarity of the infant's cues and caregiver response to the infant as well as caregiver and infant responses to each other. These areas are of prime importance in intervention. The nurse can assist the parents to identify feeding cues in their infant and can role model appropriate responses. It is especially helpful to role model during feeding and to provide support to the parents when they are feeding the infant. Behavioral interventions discussed in Chapter 9 also may be helpful in improving parent–child interactions.

Referrals

In addition to parent support, role modeling, and behavioral intervention, referral to agencies providing augmentative services may be helpful. Referrals may be made for more in-depth counseling or behavioral management, parent discussion groups, parenting classes, respite care, day care, or infant stimulation. Crisis intervention lines are also available and provide telephone numbers parents can call at any time.

REFERENCES

Bithoney, W.G., Dubowitz, H., & Egan, H. (1992). Failure to thrive/growth deficiency. *Pediatrics in Review, 13*(12), 453.

Bithoney, W.G., & Newberger, E.H. (1987). Child and family attributes of failure to thrive. *Developmental and Behavioral Pediatrics, 8*(1), 32–36.

O'Brien, S., Repp, A., Williams, G., & Christopherson, E. (1991). Pediatric feeding disorders. *Behavior Modification, 15*(3), 394–418.

Peterson, K.E., Washington, J., & Rathburn, J.M. (1984). Team management of failure to thrive. *Perspectives in Practice, 84*(7), 810–815.

Powell, G.F., Low, J.F., & Speers, M.A. (1987). Behavior as a diagnostic aid in failure-to-thrive. *Developmental and Behavioral Pediatrics, 8,* 18–24.

Ramsay, M., Gisel, E.G., & Boutry, M. (1993). Non-organic failure-to-thrive: Growth failure secondary to feeding skills disorder. *Developmental Medicine and Child Neurology, 35,* 285–297.

Chapter 9

Nutrition and Feeding of the Chronically Ill Infant

Connie Lierman, RN, MSN

Providing adequate nutrition for the chronically ill infant poses a challenge to parents and health care providers. Medical and developmental problems may interfere with attaining optimal nutrition (see Exhibit 9–1). Yet, the first 2 years of life are a period of rapid growth, and malnutrition during this time may have long-range effects.

The community health nurse plays an important role in promoting adequate nutrition and feeding of the chronically ill infant. The nurse's role in this regard has several aspects. First, the nurse will need a sound knowledge of the normal progression of feeding behaviors (see Appendix 9–A). Second, the nurse must be able to offer a comprehensive assessment if feeding or nutritional problems are suspected. Third, the nurse must have a knowledge of interventions appropriate to the more common nutrition and feeding problems. Fourth, since nutritional and feeding problems are often multifaceted, the nurse must recognize when consultations with other disciplines are warranted. If nutritional problems are not responsive to the more common interventions, consultation with a pediatric dietitian or a physician may be necessary. Occupational, physical, speech, or behavioral therapists may also be important team members. In cases involving several disciplines, a team approach may be the optimal management strategy.

The first part of this chapter addresses the assessment of feeding and nutrition. The next part addresses common nutritional and feeding interventions that the nurse and parents can utilize. The third part discusses disorders of feeding skills and behavior for which referral to a specialist may be necessary. Two additional issues, Breastfeeding the High-

risk Infant and Failure To Thrive, are discussed in Special Issues.

ASSESSMENT OF NUTRITION

The nurse must complete a thorough assessment of feeding and nutrition in order to determine the most appropriate interventions and to decide if referrals to other specialties are needed. (See Appendix 9–B.) The assessment should include the following areas:

- obtaining and plotting serial measurements of growth parameters
- obtaining a thorough nutrition and feeding history, including a diet record
- obtaining a medical history
- conducting a developmental assessment
- conducting a feeding observation, with attention to both skills and behavior, the feeding environment, and the psychosocial context of feeding.

Paramount in the assessment process is the inclusion of the caregivers. The parents or other caregivers will be the infant's primary feeders, and their cooperation and commitment are essential for any treatment program to be successful. Their concerns, questions, and goals should receive attention in the assessment process.

Exhibit 9–1 Factors Placing an Infant at Risk of Feeding and Nutritional Problems

- congenital abnormalities of the oral motor area
- central nervous system damage
- immature neurologic development secondary to prematurity
- developmental delay
- chronic illness (e.g., bronchopulmonary dysplasia [BPD]) with increased caloric demands and easy fatiguability
- gastrointestinal problems with inadequate/altered absorption
- loss of nutrients secondary to vomiting or diarrhea
- genetic disorders
- oral hypersensitivity secondary to lack of oral experiences or aversive oral experiences (e.g., prolonged intubation)
- delayed onset of oral feedings secondary to need for hyperalimentation or gavage feeding with prolonged NPO
- interactional disturbances

Growth Parameters

The first year of life is often considered the single most important period of growth (Pinyerd, 1992). In a healthy full-term infant during the first year, birth weight triples, length doubles, and head circumference increases by one third. As indicated in Table 9–1, infants normally gain 25 to 35 g per day during the first 3 months of life, 15 to 21 g per day in the second 3 months, and 10 to 13 g per day in the second 6 months. Growth patterns for the chronically ill preterm infant may deviate from accepted norms.

Serial Measurements

Growth refers to proportionate changes in size, and it is assessed by obtaining accurate serial measurements of a

Table 9–1 Growth Velocity in Normal Infants and Children

Age	Weight (g/day)	Length (cm/month)	Head circumference (cm/week)
0 to 3 months	25 to 35	2.6 to 3.5	0.5
3 to 6 months	15 to 21	1.6 to 2.5	0.5
6 to 12 months	10 to 13	1.2 to 1.7	0.5
1 to 3 years	4 to 10	0.7 to 1.1	
4 to 6 years	5 to 8	0.5 to 0.8	
7 to 10 years	5 to 12	0.4 to 0.6	

Note. Sex-specific reference data on gains in weight and length in the first 24 months can be found in Guo et al. (1991).

Source: Adapted from Fomon S.J., et al., Body Composition of Reference Children from Birth to Age 10 Years. *American Journal of Clinical Nutrition,* Vol. 35, p. 1, 169, with permission of the American Society for Clinical Nutrition, © 1982.

child's length (height), weight, and head circumference. Serial measurements should include the measurements taken at birth. These serial data are plotted on a National Center for Health Statistics (NCHS) growth chart or, if appropriate, a Down's syndrome growth chart. (NCHS growth charts are available from Ross Laboratories, Columbus, Ohio and Mead Johnson Nutritionals, Evansville, Indiana.) When assessing and plotting growth for a premature infant, the corrected age should be used.

Corrected Age

To calculate the corrected age for an infant born prematurely, the following simple formula is used:

$$\text{chronological age} - \text{weeks premature}$$

That is, subtract the number of weeks the infant was born prematurely from the infant's chronological age. For example, if the infant was born 6 weeks prematurely and is now 8 weeks old, the corrected age is 2 weeks (8 weeks minus 6 weeks). If necessary, the number of weeks the infant was born prematurely can be obtained by subtracting the gestational age (GA) at birth from 40 weeks (full term). The corrected age is used for the first year and may be used until the infant is 2 or 3 years of age. It is no longer used when the weeks of prematurity become a small fraction of the total age (Groh-Wargo, 1990).

Weight

Weight should be obtained on a balance-beam scale. Spring scales will lose accuracy over time, particularly if they are often carried in a car. For purposes of accurate assessment, the scale should be set to zero before each use, and the infant should be weighed nude. Decreases either in weight or in the percentile for age on the NCHS growth curve indicate an acute nutritional insult.

Length

Length should also be measured. Length is the supine measurement. Length is generally used as the measurement for the first 3 years, after which height, the standing measurement, is used. Length is important in determining the ideal weight and, thus, the calorie needs for the infant. To measure length at home, the infant can be placed supine on an even surface, such as the floor or a table. One person holds the measuring tape even with the top of the infant's head. Another person stretches the tape alongside the infant and straightens the infant's hips and knees to get an accurate measurement. The distance from the base of the heel to the top of the head is the length. Cessation of growth in length or a decrease in the percentile for age on the NCHS growth curve indicates a chronic nutritional insult.

Weight for Length

Weight for length is also an important growth parameter for the infant. To obtain this parameter, weight should be plotted as a function of length on the appropriate portion of the NCHS growth chart. Serial measures should be plotted to obtain a curve. An upward sloping curve suggests that the infant is growing optimally. A downward sloping curve, or a weight for length less than the 5th percentile, would indicate a referral for a more in-depth assessment is needed.

"Ideal" Weight for Length

The "ideal" weight for length is the weight in kilograms (kg) at the 50th percentile for the infant's length on the NCHS growth charts. The Recommended Daily Allowances (RDAs) will allow for normal growth, but additional calories must be provided above the RDA to achieve catch-up growth. The ideal weight for length can be used to calculate the energy and protein needs for catch-up growth (see Exhibit 9–2).

Head Circumference

Head circumference is an index of brain growth. It is also assessed as an indicator of hydrocephalus. Head circumference is measured with a nonstretchable tape placed around the widest part of the head from the maximal occipital prominence to the area over the supraorbital ridges. It should be plotted serially on the growth chart. Head circumference is the last anthropometric parameter to be affected by nutritional status.

Nutritional History

Feeding problems can be very anxiety-producing for caregivers. To facilitate obtaining as much information as possible about the infant's nutrition and feeding, a nonjudgmental approach to interviewing is important. The family's key role in assessment and treatment should also be recognized and acknowledged. The interview should begin with a focus on the family's concerns. Questions that can be used to elicit concerns include the following: What do parents see as a problem? What has been tried to resolve the problem? How did that treatment work? What are parental goals for treatment?

Aspects of the History

In addition to assessing areas pertaining to the family's concerns, a thorough assessment should include the following:

- infant's overall health status, including underlying medical problems and medication regime
- feeding history, including the use of total parenteral nutrition (TPN), a nasogastric (NG) tube, or a gastros-

Exhibit 9–2 Estimating Energy and Protein Needs for Catch-up Growth

Energy

$$\text{kcal/kg} = \frac{\text{ideal weight for height} \times \text{RDA kcal/kg weight age}^{a,b}}{\text{Actual weight}}$$

Protein

$$\text{g Pro/kg}^c = \frac{\text{ideal weight for height} \times \text{RDA g Pro/kg weight age}^{a,b}}{\text{Actual weight}}$$

[a]Some practitioners use the RDA for height age to calculate catch-up requirements. [b]Age at which present weight or height = 50th percentile. [c]Protein: % of calories from protein and grams of protein/kg should not exceed recommended range for age unless medically indicated

Source: Reprinted from Peterson, K.E., Washington, J., and Rathbun, J.M., Team Management of Failure to Thrive, *Journal of the American Dietetic Association*, Vol. 84, No. 7, p. 815, with permission of the American Dietetic Association, © 1984.

tomy (G) tube, age at introduction of oral feedings, any transitions from breast to bottle or to baby or table foods, and past feeding problems (reflux, choking, formula intolerance, or any aversive oral experiences)
- current feeding patterns including breast or formula, how formula is prepared, amount fed, frequency, length of a feeding, other foods offered, normal family/infant feeding routine, self-feeding skills
- current feeding problems (e.g., reflux, choking, formula intolerance, oral refusal).

Diet Record

A diet record should also be obtained; a record is more accurate than mere recall. A record requires parents to record information on feeding practices as feeding occurs, thereby ensuring optimal reliability of the data. Depending on the child's nutritional status and the parent's ability to keep data, a record of from 3 to 7 days is recommended for assessment of intake and feeding patterns. A thorough diet record will yield valuable information about total intake (both calories and nutrients), frequency and amounts of feedings, and the appropriateness of the foods offered. The record should include the following information: time, the food or liquid given, type of preparation, and exact amount in ounces or tablespoons. Any episodes of vomiting or diarrhea should also be noted, including both the time and amount.

To assist in the calculation of calories based on the diet record, the guide in Table 9–2 can be used. The diet record can be given to a dietitian for a more complete assessment of the caloric and nutrient intake.

Medical History

Obtaining the child's health history is important to determine if there are any physical problems affecting growth or

Table 9–2 Guide to Calculation of Caloric Intake

Food	Caloric content
Standard commercial formula	20 cal/oz
Baby rice cereal	15 cal/tbsp
Baby fruits and vegetables	5–10 cal/tbsp
Baby meat	15–18 cal/tbsp

Note. 4 tbsp = ¼ cup = ½ small jar of baby food.

Source: Data from *Bowes & Church's Food Value of Portions Commonly Used, 16th ed.* by J. Pennington, pp. 177–199, Lippincott-Raven, © 1994.

feeding. In some cases, such as frequent episodes of vomiting or recurrent illnesses, the child may need to be referred for further medical evaluations. As part of the health history, it is also important to obtain a list of the child's current medications. Certain medications (see Table 9–3) that may be used in the management of the high-risk infant can affect nutritional status. When necessary, the physician can be consulted to see if laboratory tests are needed or medication changes are possible.

Developmental Status

A developmental assessment should also be completed (see Chapter 20). Feeding skills proceed in a developmental sequence. In defining realistic expectations for the infant's feeding behaviors, the parents and nurse must consider whether an infant's developmental level is congruent with his or her chronological age. (See also Appendix 9–A.)

FEEDING OBSERVATION

Often the nurse, through careful observation, first becomes aware of feeding problems in the high-risk infant. Observation of one or more feedings can provide a wealth of information that will contribute to the overall assessment of an infant's feeding or nutritional problems. Observation should include an assessment of feeding skills and behaviors, assessment of the parental ability to use appropriate positions and techniques in order to feed the infant in a reasonable length of time, the environment in which feeding occurs, and an assessment of the psychosocial context of the feeding.

Feeding Skills and Behaviors

Adequate nutritional intake by the infant can be hindered by delayed or abnormal acquisition of feeding skills and by behavior disorders. Normal development of feeding skills is reviewed briefly in Appendix 9–B. A knowledge of the normal patterns, coupled with an awareness of potential disorders, listed in Table 9–4, provide the basis for a thorough nursing assessment.

Common Problems

Among high-risk premature infants the most common problems of feeding skills and feeding-related behavior include the following:

- ineffective sucking
- poor coordination of breathing with suck-swallow

Table 9–3 Medications Affecting Nutritional Status

Medication	Effect on Nutritional Status	Intervention
Diuretics	Alter fluid and electrolyte balance	Sodium and potassium supplements may be needed. Monitor for fluid overload or dehydration. Fluid restriction may be necessary.
Phenobarbital	Decreases effectiveness of vitamin D and can alter the calcium and phosphorus metabolism	Monitor serum phosphatase levels every 3–6 months. Vitamin D supplements may be needed.
Dilantin	Alters vitamin D, calcium, and phosphorus metabolism and absorption. Can lead to loss of taste and gum irritation	Monitor serum phosphatase levels every 3–6 months. Good oral hygiene is essential; gum massage may relieve irritation.
Iron	May cause constipation	More fluids in formula may be needed.
Steroids	Increase appetite	Restriction of infant's intake may be needed.
Theophylline	Increases risk of reflux	Assess for signs of reflux.

Table 9–4 Common Feeding Disorders in the High-risk Infant

Disorder	Effects on Feeding
Suck-swallow uncoordination	Risk for aspiration Decreased efficiency and increased energy output Prolonged feeding time Frustration
Poor lip seal	Loss of liquid Prolonged feeding time

Abnormal oral development
  Tongue thrust
  Tongue retraction
  Poor tongue control
  Lip immobility
  Lip retraction
  Limited movement of oral musculature
  Structural abnormalities
	Interference with progression of feeding and oral motor skills
	Prolonged feeding time
	Frustration
	Disturbed infant–parent relationship
	Need for tube feeding

Vomiting or reflux	Frustration Need for tube feeding Need for increased frequency of feedings Need for special positions during feeding
Food refusal	Disturbed infant–parent relationship Weight loss Need for tube feeding
Respiratory compromise	Interference with rhythm of suck-swallow-breathe Tiring during feeding Need for prolonged intubation or TPN Tube feeding
Lethargy or agitation	Prolonged feeding time Parental frustration Need for tube feeding
Lack of oral experience	Interference with progression of feeding and oral motor skills Food refusal Need for tube feeding

Source: Developed by E. Ahmann, MS, RN, M. Wilson, OTR, and C. Berg, OTR, and revised by Alicia Ward, MA, CCC-SLP, with permission of Children's National Medical Center, Washington, D.C.

- neck hyperextension
- tactile defensiveness
- lethargy or agitation
- food refusal
- difficulty in transitions (liquid to pureed, pureed to textured)
- poor positioning.

Specific neurologic and neuromotor problems can also contribute to feeding problems.

Sucking Skills

The nurse should observe the infant for sucking skills: the ability to initiate and maintain an effective seal on the nipple with minimal leakage of formula, to initiate and maintain a rhythmic suck, and to coordinate a smooth and rhythmic suck-swallow pattern. In addition, the nurse should observe for coordination of breathing with suck-swallow in a rhythmic pattern. Incoordination can lead to physiologic changes with color, heart rate, and respiratory rate fluctuations.

Hyperextension

A related problem, hyperextension of the neck, is frequently noted in infants with respiratory compromise, a tracheostomy, or certain types of cerebral palsy. Hyperextension during feeding will interfere with both suck and swallow. In addition, it may interfere with the timely development of hand-to-mouth motor skills and oral experiences.

Tactile Defensiveness

Oral tactile defensiveness, seen as an aversive reaction to touch, can develop in the infant who has been without oral intake (maintained with TPN or tube-fed) for long periods or who has had aversive oral experiences. Use of a pacifier for nonnutritive sucking and other means of oral stimulation can help prevent the problem. However, once tactile defensiveness develops, the infant may resist any texture in or around the mouth, and oral motor development and oral feeding are hindered. When tactile defensiveness is present, the infant or child should be referred to a pediatric occupational therapist, speech therapist, and/or to a pediatric feeding disorders clinic.

Lethargy or Agitation

Lethargy and agitation are feeding behaviors that can be observed among many chronically ill premature infants as well as malnourished infants. Lethargy may result from poor bonding and attachment, causing lack of interest, or, more commonly, from exhaustion related to the work required to coordinate breathing with eating. The nurse will observe that the infant seems to tire easily during a feeding and shows little interest in maintaining a suck. Prolonged feeding times may also be noted. In some infants, an agitated state of arousal may be elicited during attempts at feeding. An infant may be easily hyperstimulated by touch, positioning, and the incoordination of the suck-swallow-breathing triad.

Food Refusal

Food refusal is perhaps the most frustrating feeding disorder. It may evolve because of early oral deprivation, resulting from lengthy illness and hospitalization. Forced oral feeding can also contribute to the development of food refusal. Food refusal may manifest similarly to tactile defensiveness: the infant may turn or back away from food stimuli or, in some cases, vomit.

Transitions

Difficulty in transitions usually occurs when the infant is advancing from liquid to pureed foods or pureed to textured foods. The infant may eagerly take formula, but refuse any attempts at pureed foods. Some infants take pureed foods, but if the food has any lumps in it, they will spit them out or refuse any further solid foods. In some cases, these infants may have had prior episodes of choking or gagging with solids and, therefore, refuse these foods in the future.

Environmental Assessment

The nurse should observe the environment in which feeding occurs. Important considerations include the physical location for feeding; environmental characteristics that neither distract the child nor the feeder; the structure of mealtime as a pleasant time; and, if the child is older, the presence of models who are demonstrating appropriate behavior (Wolff & Lierman, 1994). It is most important to observe the environment in which the primary caregiver feeds the infant. However, it may also be helpful to observe the infant being fed by others in a different setting, such as in a babysitter's home or in the day care setting. The nurse may want to feed the infant herself to see if the infant responds differently to others or to try out any techniques she feels may facilitate feeding.

Psychosocial Context of Feeding

A feeding observation should include an assessment of the psychosocial context of feeding. Feeding is a reciprocal process that depends on the abilities and experiences of both the caregiver and the infant (Satter, 1992). The chronically ill premature infant is particularly vulnerable to interactional problems owing to several factors. These include the inability to give clear, consistent cues; easy fatiguability; interaction with multiple feeders; aversive oral experiences; and the lack of normal oral feeding sequences.

Additionally, caregivers may have difficulty bonding to an infant who does not provide good feedback and from whom they may have been separated by multiple hospitalizations. Caregivers may, further, feel a pressure to make their infant gain weight in order to help overcome his or her illness by growing new lung tissue or to meet weight requirements for a corrective surgical procedure. As a result of this pressure, caregivers may resort to force feeding or feeding at every opportunity, thus never establishing a regular feeding pattern.

Guidelines for Feeding Observation

The Nursing Child Assessment Feeding Scale (NCAFS) provides a model for a thorough assessment of feeding behaviors (Barnard [1979]; copies may be ordered from NCAST, University of Washington, WJ-10, Seattle, Washington 98195). The NCAFS assists the nurse to look at the behavior of the feeder, the behavior of the infant, and the infant–feeder interaction.

If a standardized tool such as the NCAFS is not used, certain aspects of feeding should be part of the nurse's observation. These include the time and length of feeding, types and amount of food offered, rate of feeding, food preferences, and aspects of both caregiver and infant behavior, described below:

- *Caregiver behaviors*—The nurse should observe the caregiver's behaviors antecedent to feeding, such as verbal or physical prompts to eat (coaxing, holding the chin or head), and the caregiver's consequent behaviors, such as verbal or physical reinforcement (praise, pats, smiles) or punishment (Iwata, Riordan, Wohl, & Finney, 1982).
- *Infant behaviors*—Infant behaviors to include as part of the observation are as follows: the ability to give hunger and satiety cues; response to presentation of food (head turns, acceptances, hands to mouth, crying, spitting); and response to the caregiver.
- *Interactions*—It is important to determine both if the parents are aware of the infant's cues and if they base their feeding actions on these cues. This can be assessed by asking the caregivers both how they decide when to initiate or end a feeding and what cues their infant gives. The nurse should also observe for parental interactions around feeding that may be overstimulating to the sensitive preterm infant and lead to aversive behaviors (Gardner & Hagedorn, 1991).

COMMON FEEDING AND NUTRITIONAL INTERVENTIONS

The nurse should share both normal and abnormal findings from the nutrition and feeding assessment with the family, in terms that they will understand. Any questions family members have should be answered. Generally, parental concerns and goals should be foremost in determining the intervention plan for nutrition and feeding. The parents will be carrying out the plan, and, therefore, it is essential that they are involved in its development. In some cases, the nurse may identify problems that differ from those of concern to the family. She should explain her concerns. Then the nurse and family should discuss their priorities to develop a common set of goals and priorities for intervention. Frequently,

Table 9–5 Recommended Intake for Term Infants Based on Age

Age (months)	Kcal/kg	Protein g/kg	Fluid mL/kg	Feeds/day	Ounces/feed	Solids
0–1	120	2.0–2.5	150	8–10	2–3	None
1–3	110	2.2	150	6–8	4–5	None
4–6	110	2.2	125	5–6	5–8	Cereal
7–9	100	1.6	125	4–5	8	Cereal, fruit, vegetables, meats
10–12	100	1.6	125	3–4	8	Semisolid table food, finger food, juice from a cup

Note. Premature infants need special formula with increased protein, calcium, and phosphorous until weight is approximately 2 kg and the lab value for calcium phosphate (CaPhos) is within normal limits and alkaline phosphatase (AlkPhos) is less than 300.

Source: Courtesy of Amy Purdy, MS, RD, Children's Hospital National Medical Center, Washington, D.C.

an infant's feeding and growth problems stem from multiple factors; all areas should be considered in planning care for the infant. Often, certain problems, such as increasing calories, changing positions, and improving the feeding schedule can be addressed by the nurse and family working together.

Increasing Calories

While meeting the recommended daily allowance (RDA) for the infant (see Table 9–5) will allow for normal growth, additional calories must be provided above and beyond the RDA to promote "catch-up" growth. Energy and protein needs for catch-up growth can be calculated as described in Exhibit 9–2.

The simplest method of increasing an infant's caloric intake is to increase the volume or frequency (or both) of feedings. For some infants, this may not be possible, and the caloric density of feedings will need to be adjusted; a physician's order is required for nurses to change the concentration of feedings. If an infant or toddler is unable to take adequate feedings by mouth to produce a positive curve on the growth chart, tube feeding may be considered (see Chapter 10).

Frequency of Feedings

In reviewing the diet record, it is important to note the frequency and amount of feedings. A rigid schedule may be appropriate in the hospital, but may not be effective for infants at home. Most infants can be allowed to feed on demand. Initially, the infant's schedule may be erratic, but as the infant takes more volume, spacing of feeding should increase (Gardner & Hagedorn, 1991). Some parents may need assistance in recognizing their infant's hunger and satiety cues. In this regard, infants should not be repeatedly offered more when they are indicating fullness, even though parents may feel nutrition is a primary need. Ignoring the infant's cues increases the likelihood of negative interactions, which can then adversely affect feeding behaviors.

As a related matter, for chronically ill infants, energy conservation is a primary need. Prolonged crying, especially prior to feeding, should be avoided. Additionally, feedings should be kept to approximately 20 to 30 min in length.

Volume

For infants who are fluid restricted, or those who are unable to take large volumes due to oral motor problems or food refusal, increasing the volume of feedings may not be an appropriate way to increase calories.

Caloric Density

More concentrated formulas can be used to increase the caloric content of feedings without increasing the volume. The physician or a dietitian can assist the nurse in determining what caloric supplement would be most appropriate. Most infant formulas (except "premie" varieties) contain 20 cal/oz. A 24 cal/oz formula can easily be made by mixing a 13 oz can of concentrated formula with 9 oz of water. If the formula needs to be even more dense in calories, commercial supplements such as Polycose or Moducal can be added to achieve a caloric concentration of 26 to 30 cal/oz. In very exceptional cases, a concentration of more than 30 cal/oz may be required; such concentrations are often prepared by the addition of vegetable oil or microlipids. Table 9–6 describes various calorie supplements and will assist the nurse in understanding the appropriate choice(s). Caution should be exercised when adding supplements in order to maintain an appropriate distribution of calories between fat, carbohydrate, and protein. Adding too much fat and carbohydrate can lead to protein, vitamin, and mineral deficiencies.

Infants with intestinal problems may not be able to tolerate highly concentrated formulas. As more concentrated formulas are used with an infant, prolonged diarrhea will signify inability to accept the formula density. If Polycose or Moducal is not accepted, microlipids, available through a pharmacy, or vegetable oil can be tried. Sometimes a combination of supplements, although more difficult for parents

Table 9–6 Calorie Supplements for Infants

Supplement	Cal/tbsp	Comments
Carbohydrate		
Polycose (Ross Labs)		May increase stool frequency
Powder	23	and loosen texture of stools
Liquid	30	Available at drug stores or by order through pharmacist
		Easy to mix into formula; can be mixed into entire batch
Moducal		
(Mead Johnson)	30	Similar to Polycose
Fat		
Microlipids	68	Stays in suspension for tube
(Sherwood Medical)		feeding or formula
		Available through a pharmacy
Vegetable oil	115	Floats in formula, so, to ensure that infant gets all of oil, best to put into 1 oz of formula and give as the first part of each feeding

Source: Courtesy of Amy Purdy, MS, RD, Children's Hospital National Medical Center, Washington, D.C.

to mix, can afford the highest caloric value without causing diarrhea. Concentrated formula can also cause constipation in some infants. In infants with gastroesophageal reflux, calories should be limited to 30 cal/oz, and no oil should be added to the formula because of the risk of aspiration.

Breastfed Infants

In breastfed infants, caloric intake may be augmented by increasing the frequency of feedings or by supplementing the feedings by using a Lact-Aid or supplemental nursing system (available from J. L. Avery, Inc., P.O. Box 6459, Denver, CO 80206, telephone 303/377-5325 or Medela, Inc., P.O. Box 660, McHenry, IL 60051, telephone 800/435-8316). These nursers consist of a plastic or disposable bottle hung on a cord between the mother's breasts. A thin tube runs from the bottle; the other end of the tube is placed against the mother's nipple. The infant is then able to suck the tube and nipple at the same time. Expressed breast milk or formula can be placed in the bottle (Gardner & Hagedorn, 1991). Offering a bottle after feedings is not an energy-efficient method to increase the breastfed infant's intake.

Honey

Corn syrup is a frequently recommended supplement. However, research suggests honey may contain botulinum spores (Arnon et al., 1979). While the spores pose no apparent risk of botulism for older children, a number of cases of

infant botulism have been associated with the ingestion of spore-containing honey. The spectrum of botulism in infants is uncertain but may range from constipation to failure to thrive; botulism has been associated with sudden death. For this reason, it is recommended that honey not be fed to infants under 1 year of age.

High-Calorie Table Foods

In an infant or toddler accepting some baby or table foods, high-calorie foods, including cheese and ice cream, should be encouraged, if there is no dairy allergy. Homemade baby foods usually contain less water than the commercial varieties and, therefore, are more dense in calories. Butter, margarine, or oil can be added to foods for extra calories, and powdered milk can be added to liquids, yogurt, puddings, and cereal. Each time the child eats, calorie-dense foods should be offered. For example, crackers with cheese, rather than plain crackers, can be offered for a snack.

Vomiting

A thorough feeding history and observation should evaluate the amount and frequency of vomiting in relationship to feeding amounts. Data to obtain includes frequency of feedings and types of food, as well as positioning and feeding techniques. In unusual circumstances, infants may vomit in stressful situations. Therefore, it may also be important to evaluate the environment in which the vomiting occurs. Common causes of vomiting include overfeeding, inadequate burping, and gastroesophageal reflux (GER).

Overfeeding

Overfeeding of the infant may contribute to vomiting. If overfeeding is suspected on the basis of history and observation, a detailed feeding schedule can be worked out with parents. Parents should also be informed that it is not necessary to feed the infant in response to every cry. In this situation, continued assessment and support by the professional may be helpful.

Burping

Inadequate burping may also cause vomiting. Discussion of the importance of burping should be followed by a demonstration, by the nurse, of proper technique. The infant's behavior should guide the frequency of burping. If the infant stops nursing or feeding or in some way indicates discomfort, the parent should then try burping the infant. Gently placing the infant on the parent's shoulder and rubbing the infant's back is an effective technique. Clapping the back or jostling the infant is not necessary. As part of teaching, parents, or whoever regularly feeds the infant, should give a return demonstration of proper burping. Review and reinforcement of proper techniques over several home visits can be helpful.

Gastroesophageal Reflux

GER refers to the unprovoked passage of stomach contents into the esophagus, which may, in some cases, lead to vomiting. This is a normal physiologic process (Shannon, 1993). However, severe GER can contribute to poor growth, so appropriate assessment and intervention is important. GER ranges from infrequent emesis with no pathologic sequelae to severe reflux with more frequent episodes of vomiting and sequelae that may include failure to thrive, aspiration pneumonia, increased respiratory problems, and esophagitis. Infants who appear to exhibit pain with emesis or feeding may have esophagitis. Pain with feeding may cause the infant to refuse feedings, further compromising his or her nutritional state.

In most cases, GER resolves spontaneously by 12 to 18 months of life (Shannon, 1993). However, if the vomiting is significant in amount or frequency, a medical assessment is indicated. Generally, conservative treatment is utilized first. The infant is positioned prone, with shoulders higher than feet by approximately 30°, for 1 to 2 hours after each feeding, and during sleep. Proper positioning can be accomplished by tipping the mattress in the infant's crib. Previously, placing the infant in the supine upright position such as in an infant seat was recommended, but this position has been shown to increase reflux and is no longer used. Also, frequent small feedings can be used. Formula can be thickened by the addition of rice cereal in the proportion of 1 to 3 tsp/oz of formula. The nipple hole may need to be widened to allow thickened formula to pass through. Breastfed infants can be offered thickened expressed breast milk through a nursing supplementer. Medications, such as metoclopramide and cisapride, may also be prescribed for the treatment of reflux.

If reflux vomiting is not controlled with the above treatments, surgical intervention may be indicated. A common procedure is the Nissen fundoplication, which wraps the fundus of the stomach around the distal esophagus to tighten the juncture.

Disorders of Feeding: Skills and Behavior

When it is suspected that difficulties with feeding skills are affecting nutritional intake, a feeding specialist—often a speech pathologist, occupational therapist, or pediatric dietitian—should be consulted. Following the assessment, therapy to help improve the dysfunction is usually initiated. The feeding intervention should build on any normal patterns the infant has and should proceed at the infant's pace. Whenever a feeding program is developed for an infant, the nurse can

work with the feeding specialist. The nurse is then able both to provide follow-up instruction and demonstration of positions and techniques for the parents and to assess the infant's progress. Close coordination between the nurse, therapist, and family will be important to ensure optimal benefits of the intervention program.

Common interventions are described below.

Positioning

In infants with feeding problems, positioning is important. Generally during feeding, the infant should be flexed with his or her chin tucked slightly downward and forward, and arms and legs flexed close to the body. In infants with an active startle reflex, swaddling may be helpful.

If the infant is breastfeeding, his or her whole body should be turned toward the mother so the head and trunk are in alignment (Gardner & Hagedorn, 1991).

Choice of Nipple

A frequent feeding intervention for the high-risk infant involves choice of the appropriate nipple for bottle feeding. Nipple choice should be evaluated if the infant's suck is weak or ineffective, if the infant tires easily, or if there are abnormalities in the oral-motor structures (e.g., cleft palate). In the absence of severe neurological deficits, proper choice of the size, length, and consistency of the nipple for the bottlefed infant is important for developing both an effective suck and coordination in the suck-swallow-breathe pattern.

A soft and small nipple can be used for a very young infant with a weak suck. For an older child, formula flows too rapidly through the soft nipple, and coordination of suck and swallow becomes difficult. A cross-cut nipple is more firm and encourages a suck. Other nipples, such as the "natural" nipple, can be experimented with as necessary to meet the infant's needs. While there is variation from one manufacturer to another, in general, orthodontic nipples are easier to suck than "premie" nipples, and regular (also called *standard*) nipples are the hardest. In addition, for a stressed infant, nonnutritive sucking (e.g., of a pacifier) is much easier than nutritive sucking and can be encouraged.

Facilitating the Suck-Swallow-Breathe Pattern

Other therapeutic techniques can be used to facilitate a smooth suck-swallow-breathe pattern. These include the following:

- positioning the infant with neck in a neutral midline position, out of hyperextension, or slightly flexed
- using the feeder's thumb and finger to promote jaw stabilization, thus allowing more free movement of the tongue and lips

- facilitating lip activity by providing jaw support, a combination of inward external pressure on the cheeks and upward pressure on the lower lip, and straw drinking as the infant progresses.

Lethargy

For the lethargic infant, there are several therapeutic possibilities. These include the following:

- minimizing activity before the meal (e.g., chest therapy, suctioning)
- keeping the infant cool during feedings (e.g., hold slightly away from parent's body)
- using the infant's vestibular system (through movement such as gentle rocking or bouncing) to increase awareness.

Food Refusal

For the infant exhibiting overt food refusal, therapeutic techniques include the following (Morris & Klein, 1987):

- daily digital stimulation of oral tissues to desensitize lips, gums, and tongue (distinct from feeding time)
- emphasis on gradual acceptance of pleasurable oral experiences
- use of pacifier, if accepted
- consistency in the person who feeds the infant.

Behavioral Interventions

When behavioral components play a major role in feeding problems, intervention may require attention to many aspects of the feeding program. A feeding specialist—often a speech pathologist, occupational therapist, or behavioral psychologist—should be consulted. Additionally, a referral to a child psychologist specializing in feeding may be beneficial. A team effort involving the specialist(s), nurse, and parents is essential for success. Specific interventions, described below, will address some aspects of behavioral feeding problems.

Regular Schedule and Routine

Infants should be assisted to develop a regular schedule by feeding them when they are fully alert and give cues that they are hungry. A pause for a diaper change or face washing midfeeding may help to alert the lethargic infant in order to complete the feeding. As the child begins to take more "meals," a regular meal schedule including snacks and breast or bottle feedings should be developed. The child should not be allowed to snack between feeding time. Some-

times even a few bites or sips of water are enough to decrease the child's appetite.

Environmental Considerations

When behavioral issues complicate feeding, the child should have a specific place for meals and, if possible, a chair that provides appropriate support but allows the child to be independent. The place for feeding should not be used for other procedures the child might find aversive, such as taking medications or treatments.

Environmental distractions should be reduced as much as possible during feedings. Television, music, or toys should not be part of mealtime. Interruptions should also be minimized since lengthy pauses are antagonistic to sustained feeding behavior (Wolff & Lierman, 1994).

Structured Mealtimes

Mealtimes should be limited to 20 to 30 minutes. Generally, after that, only minimal intake occurs. When the mealtime has elapsed or the child has refused food three to four times, the meal should be ended. The food should be removed in a businesslike manner without coaxing or scolding. Coaxing gives the child attention for not eating and should not be part of any feeding program.

Behavioral Principles

Two behavioral procedures frequently used for increasing intake include the Premack principle and positive reinforcement (Wolff & Lierman, 1994). The Premack principle can be summarized as "Grandma's Law": "First you eat your green beans, then you get your ice cream." This is applied to feeding problems by requiring the child to take a specified amount of a nonpreferred food before receiving the preferred food item. Positive reinforcement is probably the most frequently applied treatment. Parents are taught to smile, pat, or praise the child when he or she eats but to turn away or not respond when the child is not eating. With this method, the child receives attention for the appropriate behavior.

CONCLUSION

The community health or home care nurse is in an excellent position to assist in the management of the infant with nutrition and feeding problems. Early recognition of the problem(s) in conjunction with a thorough assessment provides the nurse with the necessary basis to offer appropriate intervention. In some cases, early intervention may prevent more severe problems. At other times, the nurse may recommend referrals to additional services. However, the nurse's role will remain crucial both in assiting the family in management of the infant's nutritional and feeding concerns and in providing the family with support as they deal with the ongoing special needs of their infant.

REFERENCES

Arnon, S.S., Mitura, T.F., Damus, K., Thompson, B., Wood, R.M., & Chin, J. (1979). Honey and other environmental risk factors for infant botulism. *Journal of Pediatrics, 94,* 331–336.

Barnard, K. (1979). *Nursing child assessment feeding scale* (NCAFS). Seattle, WA: Nursing Child Assessment Satellite Training Project.

Gardner, S., & Hagedorn, M. (1991). Physiologic sequelae of prematurity: The nurse practitioner's role. Part VI. Feeding difficulties and growth failure. *Journal of Pediatric Health Care, 5,* 306–314.

Groh-Wargo, S. (1990). Nutritional care of the premature infant after hospital discharge. *Pediatric Nutrition, 13*(2), 1–4.

Guo, S., Roche, A.F., Fomon, S., Nelson, S.E., Chumlea, W.C., Rogers, R.R., Baumgartner, R.N., Ziegler, E., & Siervogel, R.M. (1991). Reference data on gains in weight and length during the first two years of life. *The Journal of Pediatrics, 119*(3), 355–362.

Iwata, B., Riordan, M., Wohl, M., & Finney, J. (1982). Pediatric feeding disorders: Behavioral analysis and treatment. In P.J. Accardo (Ed.), *Failure to thrive in infancy and early childhood.* Baltimore, MD: University Park Press.

Morris, S.E., & Klein, M.D. (1987). *Prefeeding skills: A comprehensive resource of feeding management.* Tucson, AZ: Communication Skills Builder.

Peterson, K.E., Washington, J., & Rathbun, J.M. (1984). Team management of failure to thrive. *Journal of the American Dietetic Association, 84*(7), 810–815.

Pinyerd, B. (1992). Assessment of infant growth. *Journal of Pediatric Health Care, 6,* 302–308.

Satter, E. (1992). The feeding relationship. *Zero To Three, 12*(5), 1–9.

Shannon, R. (1993). Gastroesophageal reflux in infancy: Review and update. *Journal of Pediatric Health Care, 7,* 71–76.

Wolff, R.P., & Lierman, C.J. (1994). Management of behavioral feeding problems in young children. *Infants and Young Children, 7*(1), 14–23.

Nutrition and Feeding of the Healthy Infant

Margaret Wilson, MS, OTR, and Elizabeth Ahmann, ScD, RN

The infant having no nutritional problems will require approximately 110 cal/kg (50 cal/lb) per day to maintain normal growth (see Table 9–5). Breast milk or commercial formula with a caloric concentration of 20 cal/oz will supply the infant with all nutritional requirements if iron, fluoride, or both are supplemented as indicated by the health care provider. Feeding time for the healthy infant will provide a warm and close interaction between parent and child, establishing a trusting bond.

The ability to eat can be influenced by early reflexes, movement and positioning of the lips and tongue, jaw control, orofacial anatomic structures, general respiratory changes, sensory awareness of the oral area, and overall body postural tone. Many premature or full-term babies with various neurologic, neuromuscular, or physical impairments may have difficulty with oral motor functioning and consequently with feeding. It is often the nurse who, through careful observation, first becomes aware of feeding difficulties or the potential for oral motor skill delay.

The earliest oral motor skills seen in the normally developing infant are mainly reflexive and are outlined in the accompanying table, "Oral Motor Reflexes." As these reflexive skills mature and become more automatic, they are integrated into the child's oral motor repertoire and are no longer simply reflexive. The reflexive and subsequently integrated developmental pattern of sucking, swallowing, and then chewing should also be observed as the infant develops.

Early sucking is characterized by movement of the tongue back and forth from a position between the gums, creating a rhythmic licking motion on the nipple that is synchronized with jaw opening and closing. There is often loss of liquid from the mouth since the lips are only loosely sealed around the nipple. As oral motor control progresses, a rhythmic raising and lowering of the tongue independent of jaw movement, tongue tip elevation, reduced jaw motion, and a firm lip seal around the nipple are noted.

Early on, the sucking pattern triggers swallowing. A smooth coordination of suck-swallow-breathe will be observed in a normal newborn. As the infant develops, jaw stability, lip coordination, and control of tongue movement progress, and swallow eventually becomes independent of suck, allowing cup drinking to begin. Cup drinking can usually be introduced between 6 and 12 months of age.

The introduction of soft and then semisolid foods frequently depends on parental or physician preferences and on the infant's level of hunger. Developmentally, around 5 or 6 months of age, with the maturation of lip and tongue control, the infant progresses from scraping food off a spoon with the upper gums to active participation of the upper lip and tongue in the acceptance of foods. With practice, the infant will also learn to grade the amount of jaw opening needed to get the food from the spoon. By 5 to 6 months, with tongue movements maturing, the healthy infant will progress to accepting solid foods, and at 6 to 7 months, with the improvement of jaw control, to chewing.

The chewing motion of the jaw is initially vertical; it then becomes a side-to-side motion, followed by refined rotary motion, which is usually seen after the first year of life. Over time, the development of grasping and sitting skills encourages self-feeding, and by 2 years of age the infant with no nutritional problems will be cup drinking and self-feeding a wide variety of table foods.

Oral Motor Reflexes

Reflex	Age at Acquisition	Age at Integration	Description
Rooting	Birth	3 months	Turning of face toward a touch stimulus in search of nutrition
Suck-swallow	Birth	2–5 months	Automatic lip closure around food source with several repeated sucks followed by a swallow
Gag	Birth	Diminishes but remains throughout life	Protective mechanism stimulated by touch at back of tongue
Bite	1 month	5–6 months	Rhythmic pattern of bite and release following stimulation of lips or gums

Source: Courtesy of Children's Hospital National Medical Center, Home Health Care Services, Washington, D.C.

Feeding/Nutritional Assessment for the Infant

Patient's name _____ DOB _____

Diagnoses _____

Physician or Dietitian prescribing feeding:

_____ Phone _____

formula_____ cal/oz_____

amount/feed_____ frequency _____

how mixed_____

other foods (types, amount, and frequency): _____

_____

_____

_____

supplements _____

_____

dietary restrictions_____

_____

_____

_____

HISTORY

birth weight _____ length_____ head circumference _____

feeding history: TPN_____ duration_____

                   GT _____ duration_____

                   NG _____ duration_____

age at first p.o. feed _____

reflux _____

problems feeding _____

_____

CURRENT FEEDING PATTERNS (Parent Report)

formula _____ cal/oz _____

amount/feed _____ frequency _____

how mixed _____

other foods (types, amount, and frequency): _____

_____

supplements _____

_____

(Continued on next page)

source of iron _____

medications affecting diet (see accompanying list) _____

_____

TPN _____   GT _____   NG _____

self-feeding skills _____

cues to hunger _____

hungry at feeding time? _____

how long feeding takes _____

position during feed _____

reflux: amount _____   frequency _____

stool: type _____   color _____   frequency_____

problems: sucking _____   chewing _____   swallowing_____

                   vomiting _____   diarrhea _____   constipation _____

                   food allergy _____   anemia _____

Parental concerns regarding feeding:

_____

_____

PHYSICAL EXAM

overall appearance _____

_____

     actual weight _____   length _____   head circumference _____

     NCHS% weight _____   length _____   head circumference _____

weight/length (NCHS%) _____

Present 24-hour intake schedule (obtain *record*, not recall)

Time	Food	Amount	Time	Food	Amount

was this a normal day?_____

total 24-hr volume intake: _____

total 24-hr calorie intake: _____

ideal 24-hr calorie intake (ideal wt(kg)* _____ × 115 cal/kg†): _____

*The weight at the 50th percentile (NCHS) based on actual length.

†May need more if lack of weight gain related to high energy requirements.

FEEDING OBSERVATION

suck _____   suck-swallow _____

coordination with breathing_____

mouth closure on nipple _____

tires with feed _____

(Continued on next page)

Summary of observation (see accompanying guidelines): _____

_____

_____

_____

_____

Assessment: _____

_____

_____

_____

_____

_____

_____

_____

Plan: _____

_____

_____

_____

_____

_____

_____

_____

Completed by _____   Date _____

Nutritional Assessment

Guidelines for Feeding Observation

1. Child's position—safety, contact, comfort, eye-to-eye contact.
2. Parent's response to cues—hunger cue, satiation, distress, pauses.
3. Parent's responsiveness to infant—contingent verbal and facial responses, plays, rocks, talks with infant (note negative interaction).
4. Clarity of infant cues—clear hunger and satiation cues, positive response to feeding.
5. Infant's responsiveness to parents—contingent response to parents' smile or verbalization; infant smiles, verbalizes, or touches parent.
6. Is this feeding normal for this child/was parent uncomfortable because of observer?

Recommended Caloric Intake		Expected Normal Weight Gain	
Age(mo)	*cal/kg ideal wt*	*Age(mo)*	*oz/day*
0–6	115	0–3	1
6–12	105	3–6	2/3
12–36	100	6–9	1/2
		9–12	1/3
		12–24	1 1/2/week

Caloric Content of Foods

Premie formula	24 cal/oz
Regular formula	20 cal/oz
Baby fruit	70–120 cal/jar (pears, applesauce are lowest)
Baby vegetables	40–90 cal/jar (sweet potatoes are highest)
Strained plain meats	90–140 cal/jar
Baby cereal (dry)	10 cal/tbsp
Mixed dinners and desserts	less nutritious/cal

To increase calories

Concentrated formula:
24 cal/oz: 13-oz can of formula concentrate + 9 oz of water
26 cal/oz: add 1 1/2 tbsp polycose to 24 cal/oz mixture
28 cal/oz: add 3 tbsp polycose
30 cal/oz: add 4 1/2 tbsp polycose

Choose high-calories baby foods
Feed more frequently
Use supplements:
Polycose = 30 cal/tbsp, Vegetable oil or margarine = 40 cal/tbsp

Source: Courtesy of Children's Hospital National Medical Center, Home Health Care Services, Washington, D.C.

Chapter 10

Home Care of the Infant or Child Requiring Tube Feeding

Revised by Virginia C. Gebus, RN, MSN

Good nutrition is necessary to sustain life and achieve developmental milestones. However, the seemingly simple but actually quite complex task of oral feeding comes at great risk and effort to children with certain medical disorders. For these children, achieving the goal of good nutrition is a major undertaking requiring both parental commitment and effort and the assistance of various health care providers.

If an infant or child cannot accept adequate nutrients or calories by mouth, the use of tube feeding to provide sufficient intake may be necessary. The purpose of this chapter is to describe the various methods of tube feeding and to provide practical guidance regarding the care of these children in order to facilitate parental independence in managing the care of their child with special needs.

REASONS FOR TUBE FEEDING

Inadequate oral intake may result from a variety of problems. Infants initially maintained on gavage feedings gain little sucking experience in the nursery. Such infants commonly have poorly developed orofacial musculature or, because of lack of appropriate desensitizing oral stimulation, may have hypersensitive oral tissues, leading to ineffective sucking or food refusal. Infants and children with cardiac or respiratory compromise may not have the strength to consume the calories and nutrients necessary for adequate growth. Children with neuromuscular disorders,

such as cerebral palsy, may not have the oral skills to consume adequate nutrient intake safely. Infants or children with gastroesophageal reflux or other disorders causing frequent vomiting may be unable to retain enough formula or food to satisfy calorie needs.

Tube feedings have become adjunctive therapy in many acute and chronic diseases of children. Tube feedings are used to ensure adequate nutrient and caloric intake. Depending on the nature and severity of the underlying problem, tube feeding may either supplement or replace oral feedings. Tube feeding may be a short-term intervention or a lifetime endeavor.

TUBE-FEEDING OPTIONS

Parents or caregivers who will be involved in the child's daily care and feeding should participate with the nurse and the physician in deciding upon the most appropriate methods of tube feeding. They should be informed of the options as well as the risks, benefits, and practical details regarding alternative choices. The child's needs, parental preferences, and safety factors must all be considered in the choice of a home tube-feeding plan. In addition, the plan must take into consideration daycare and school issues.

There are several methods of tube feeding:

- Nasogastric tubes are relied upon for intermittent or short-term feeding but are also gaining acceptance for long-term use (see Plan of Care, NG-Tube Feeding, Appendix 10–A).

- Gastrostomy tubes are widely accepted for long-term tube feeding (see Plan of Care, G-Tube Feeding, Appendix 10–B).
- Nasojejunal and jejunostomy tubes are used less commonly and are fraught with care issues. However, they are being used increasingly as an interim method of feeding.
- Orogastric tubes are rarely used and are the least safe at home; they will not be discussed in this chapter.

Exhibit 10–1 lists abbreviations for the types of feeding tubes.

Nasogastric Tubes

In choosing the appropriate nasogastric (NG) tube for home use, several factors must be considered: size, material, safety, parental comfort in inserting, and cost. Comfort and safety should be given greatest weight in dictating the choice.

Size

The smaller the lumen of the feeding tube, the more comfortable it is for the child. However, formula passes slowly through a tube with a very small lumen, making feeding times unreasonably long. Feeding tubes are now manufactured with polyurethane that offers a large internal diameter. A 6 French polyurethane tube is now the preferred choice; however, a lumen size of 8 French may still be used.

Material and Safety

A second consideration is that available feeding tubes are made of several types of material. Selecting feeding tubes made with either polyurethane or silicone should be given serious consideration. The majority of currently manufactured feeding tubes for long-term use are polyurethane; pediatric tubes are available in polyurethane in varying lengths and lumen sizes. Silicone tubes are by far the most comfortable and should be used when feasible. They are an ideal choice for the older child who can independently place his or her own tube by swallowing it into position.

Exhibit 10–1 Abbreviations for Types of Feeding Tubes

NG	nasogastric
GT	gastrostomy
NJ	nasojejunal
JT	jejunostomy
GJ	gastrojejunostomy
PEG	percutaneously placed gastrostomy
PEGJ	percutaneously placed gastrostomy/jejunostomy

Polyvinylchloride (PVC) tubes are less safe than silicone or polyurethane when used as long-term indwelling feeding tubes; there is a greater risk of gastric perforation with these tubes since the plastic changes quality and stiffens after indwelling 1 to 3 days. Because a stylet is required for insertion, Silastic tubes are not practical for use at home.

Parental Comfort

It may be helpful to try several tubes to determine the type that the parents are most comfortable inserting. Since they will be caring for the child at home, their comfort, competence, and confidence in the insertion procedure is key to successful tube feeding.

Cost

If tube feeding is expected to be long term, the cost of supplies and the likelihood of insurance coverage may be a consideration in choosing a tube for home use. However, safety concerns should not be outweighed by minor cost differences.

Gastrostomy Tubes

Historically, only two types of tubes were available for gastrostomy feeding: (1) the Malecot self-retaining gastrostomy tube, which has a basket-type end for holding the tube in place, and (2) a Foley catheter, which has a balloon tip that holds the catheter in place. The Malecot is still used as the initial feeding tube placed at surgery when the open placement procedure (an abdominal midline surgical incision) is used. However, in the last decade, many advances in gastrostomy tubes have occurred. In response to previous complications associated with gastrostomy tubes, changes have been made both in the procedures for placement and the design of the tubes.

Placement options now include a PEG tube, which is a gastrostomy tube placed percutaneously with the use of endoscopy. This method of placement avoids open gastrostomy placement and the associated complications of ileus and wound infection. A side benefit is a decrease in hospital length of stay.

The redesigning of gastrostomy tubes addressed many long-standing problems. These included skin irritation secondary to tape; tube migration and outlet obstruction (the blocking of the pylorus valve, interfering with gastric emptying); balloon rupture and tube dislodgement; and last, but not least, cosmetic concerns. Currently, two new types of tubes are available and widely used: (1) a Foley catheter type with an antimigration device and (2) an entirely new category of tube, called *skin surface devices*. There are advantages and disadvantages to each.

Foley or "Balloon" Catheter Type

The new Foley or internal balloon catheter type gastrostomy tube (G tube) has an antimigration disk or ring that prevents the tube from moving inward and causing an outlet obstruction. The antimigration device secures the tube without the need for tape; a wonderful benefit for those with allergies or sensitivities to tape.

Skin Surface Types

Skin surface gastrostomy devices are commonly referred to as gastrostomy "buttons." Two prototypes are available: (1) a Malecot-type button that requires an obturator for placement and (2) a balloon-type button. Gastrostomy buttons are less obtrusive than a catheter and are well concealed under clothing. Parents almost uniformly prefer the button to the traditional gastrostomy tubes, either the Foley/balloon or Malecot.

Nonetheless, there are several disadvantages to the button devices. Feeding, giving medications, or venting through these tubes requires an additional step not required with the catheter tubes. A feeding extension set or decompression tube must be attached in order to open the button's one-way valve to either administer the feeding or to vent gas or emesis. Further, the small internal diameter of the venting or decompression tube limits the expulsion of gas and emesis. As a result, caution must be exercised in the use of these devices with children who require frequent venting after feeding. In children who have recently undergone a Nissen fundoplication surgical procedure to reduce the risk of gastroesophageal reflux, the gastrostomy button is safely used only when frequent venting is no longer needed.

Jejunal Feeding Tubes

Feeding directly into the jejunum is never taken lightly. It is usually considered when feeding into the stomach would place the child at risk of aspiration. The most common indication for jejunal feeding is gastroesophageal reflux (GER) when medical management is not fully effective in controlling symptoms and surgery is contraindicated.

The approach to the jejunum may be accomplished by any one of four methods. Two of these methods entail placing a small catheter into the jejunum, usually with the assistance of fluoroscopy or endoscopy. This may be done either through the nose (nasojejunal [NJ]) or through an existing gastrostomy stoma (gastrojejunal [GJ]). The third method is the surgical creation of a feeding jejunostomy (J-tube). The last method is the placement of a jejunal feeding tube during the initial placement of a percutaneous gastrostomy tube (PEGJ). The PEGJ consists of a gastrostomy tube with a J-tube "tail." The gastrostomy port of the PEGJ tube is used for gastric decompression during simultaneous feeding through the jejunal port. Currently, use of the PEGJ tube is limited in pediatrics due to the unavailability of appropriately sized tubes; however, appropriate tubes are likely to be available in the not-too-distant future.

All methods of jejunal feeding share common problems and frustrations. The problems fall into two categories: (1) mechanical and (2) feeding intolerance. Mechanical problems include inadvertent dislodgement and maintenance of tube patency. To correct this problem, many centers are successfully utilizing the gastrostomy button as a jejunal feeding device (Gorman, Morris, Metz, & Mullen, 1993). The button is ideal because it is stationary; does not require securing the position with tape; and rarely occludes, due to a large opening. By design, the button eliminates many problems related to human error. Perhaps if this method becomes the standard in jejunal feeding, jejunal feeds will be more easily managed and will not be viewed only as a last resort.

Feeding intolerance, demonstrated by diarrhea, is common with jejunal feedings. Many of the symptoms can be controlled by the use of an enteral feeding pump and the controlled delivery of formula. Formula selection for jejunal feedings remains controversial.

It is essential that parents and other caregivers understand and adhere to both diligence in securing techniques and a strict flushing regimen to prevent problems with the tube itself. Diarrhea can be controlled by both using an enteral feeding pump and limiting bolus feedings. Despite the inherent problems of jejunal feeding, with diligent care and attention to detail, parents can achieve success in its use in the home.

FEEDING METHODS AND EQUIPMENT

When tube feeding an infant or child, serious thought must be given to selecting the optimal feeding method: bolus feeds, gravity feeds, and continuous feeds. The key factors determining the selection include the indications for tube feeding and the history of vomiting due to tolerance of limited volumes and diarrhea due to dumping syndrome or rapid gastric emptying.

Bolus Feeding

The simplest and least costly method is the bolus feed. Bolus feeds are used when the child has no history of problems with vomiting or diarrhea. Bolus feeds are commonly used in two circumstances: (1) as supplemental feedings for infants who fatigue with oral feedings and (2) for children who are tube fed for long periods. It is believed that the bolus method most closely simulates natural feeding.

For bolus feeding, the formula is directly administered either through a 30 cc or 60 cc straight-tip syringe into an NG tube or through a 60 cc catheter-tip syringe into a gastrostomy tube. The feeding is delivered over a period of 15 to 20 minutes, and the flow is regulated by elevating or lowering the syringe.

Gravity Feeding

If bolus feedings fail as a result of vomiting or diarrhea, gravity feeding is an alternative. Gravity feeding controls the symptoms of vomiting and diarrhea by slowing down the administration time, preventing gastric distension and/or dumping. Gravity feeding is usually defined as a feeding delivered over a period of 45 min. A special gravity feeding set is used to accomplish this. The set consists of a plastic baby bottle with a cap attached to infusion tubing. The bottle is suspended in a plastic sleeve, attached to an intravenous (IV) pole, and the flow is regulated by a clamp. While the caregiver can still be present during a feeding, he or she does not actually deliver the formula.

Enteral Feeding Pump

The final and most costly method of tube feeding is the use of an enteral feeding pump. Despite costs involved, enteral feeding pumps are generally easy and safe to use in the home. They definitely contribute to improving the quality of care for children requiring enteral support in the home.

The use of an enteral pump is ideal when a slow, accurate infusion is indicated. A classic indication for the use of an enteral feeding pump is the infant with failure to thrive secondary to gastroesophageal reflux. The use of the pump allows the child to ad lib. small quantities during the day while ensuring adequate calories by a continuous overnight feed. The use of a pump prevents overfilling of the stomach, limiting the risk of vomiting.

Many brands of enteral feeding pumps are available, most with similar features. Enteral pumps used in the home are usually selected by the hospital discharge planner or the infusion company. An important criterion to consider is that the simpler the pump is to use, the better off everyone will be. Two additional questions should also be considered:

1. Is a stationary pump sufficient, or will portability be necessary? Generally, a stationary pump is appropriate for infusions limited to 12 hours during the night. If infusions of longer than 12 hours are required to maintain adequate calorie and fluid intake, portability will allow the child and family mobility and will free the child from the crib.
2. Will feeding rates change by 1 cc or 5 cc increments? Most children can tolerate rate changes of 5 cc at a time. Exceptions include children who are fluid-sensitive (e.g., those with bronchopulmonary dysplasia [BPD] or heart disease [CHD]) and children with short

bowel syndrome during the transition from parenteral to enteral feeds.

Criteria to consider in pump selection are included in Appendix 11–1.

During the last 10 years, the use of enteral feeding pumps has expanded. For some children, the goal is to transition completely to bolus feeds when feeding is better tolerated. For others, the feeding pump is needed for the duration of an illness. For example, children with short bowel syndrome need a slow, accurate infusion to maximize absorption; the pump is usually used during the bowel adaptation phase. For many neurologically impaired children, bolus feeds are uncomfortable, and frequent small bolus feedings soon exhaust parents. In these circumstances, the use of an enteral feeding pump ensures comfort and compliance.

When a child has an enteral feeding pump, the home care nurse should periodically evaluate the use of the pump and whether or not bolus feedings should be reconsidered as an option.

HOSPITAL DISCHARGE AND TRANSITION TO THE HOME

If an infant is discharged with tube feedings prescribed, it is important to help the family members assess their ability to continue the feedings at home. It is also important for the community health nurse to be familiar with the hospital's teaching program, the parents' skills and abilities, and any problems or concerns that may have arisen. Optimally, the parents will have demonstrated full responsibility for feeding for a 24-hour period prior to discharge. In addition, at the time of discharge, it is important that the parents have a list of all the supplies needed for the child's feeding, as well as information about where and how to obtain them.

An all-too-common recent scenario is for the initial teaching to be done in the home. This may occur as a result of the current trend toward limited lengths of hospital stay or because the therapy is considered safe enough to start at home. There are risks and benefits to initiating tube feeding instruction in the home. The decreased length of hospital stay required may be less disruptive to the family, and cost-savings to third-party payers may be significant. However, risks include readmission due to complications resulting from the treatment or to limitations of the caregiver's ability to administer the prescribed feeding regimen safely or appropriately. Careful screening of the child and family must be undertaken to minimize the risks. Some children are particularly vulnerable and require close monitoring during the initiation of continuous night feeds. Children who should be admitted to the hospital for a test of therapy may include those with the following:

• a known history of vomiting

- severe GER
- severe malnutrition
- diarrhea
- fluid-sensitive conditions (e.g., BPD, CHD).

ROUTINE HOME VISITS

Assessment of Growth and Feeding

On the first and on every subsequent home visit, the infant's growth parameters should be obtained, and both total daily intake and tube feeding intake should be determined. It is helpful for parents to keep a record of formula or food intake for 3 days prior to the clinic visit. This usually gives a good representation of the overall intake. It is important to note that if tube feedings are needed for supplemental feeding only, intake through the tube may vary daily with the ability to accept oral feeds. Weight discrepancies, such as weight loss or excessive weight gain (gaining at twice the expected rate), should be noted, discussed with the family, and communicated to the physician overseeing the child's nutritional care. There is always a concern about excessive weight gain resulting in feeding intolerance, often exhibiting as gagging, vomiting, or food refusal. Additionally, since tube feedings are forced feedings, the child cannot communicate satiety and is therefore at risk for nausea and vomiting.

Abdominal Symptoms

Vomiting, diarrhea, and abdominal distension or cramping may result from incorrect tube feeding techniques. Inquiry about the occurrence of these symptoms should be a part of every home visit. Many times, these symptoms result from overconcentrated formula; problems with concentration may result from the improper use of measuring devices. For this reason, it is important for the nurse to assist the family in ensuring that the formula is being prepared and stored properly. To do this, the nurse can request that parents demonstrate formula preparation. Any errors in measuring should be corrected. If formula is being prepared properly, but symptoms of vomiting, diarrhea, and abdominal distension or cramping are present, parents or the nurse can discuss options for intervention with the physician and nutritionist. Table 10–1 reviews common tube feeding problems and interventions.

Skin Care

Skin care is an important part of routine care for the child being tube-fed.

Nares

If the infant has an NG tube, the nurse should assess the nares on each home visit. During the visit, parents should be able to demonstrate appropriate assessment and care of the nares. Usually, if the tube is taped securely at both the nares and on the cheek, little irritation will occur. Cleansing with a wet cotton swab or washcloth, and changing the tape regularly, will also limit the risk of irritation. A tape that ventilates well, such as Micropore tape, may be helpful. Transparent surgical adhesive dressings (e.g., Opsite or Tegaderm) are routinely used. Tape or dressing changes should occur twice a week.

As a routine, NG tubes are electively changed every 4 to 6 weeks. However, retaping of the tube usually needs to be done several times a week. At the time of retaping, the skin at the nares and cheekbones needs to be carefully examined for irritation. If irritation is present, changing the tube position to the other nostril can sometimes alleviate the problem. The irritated area should be cleansed carefully with water and patted dry. An antibiotic ointment should be applied only if a secondary skin infection is suspected. If irritation persists and tape allergy is suspected, the application of a skin barrier, such as Duoderm or Replicare, to the cheek area may help. The tube is placed on and taped to the barrier, preventing contact of tape and skin.

Gastrostomy or Jejunostomy

If the infant or child has a gastrostomy or jejunostomy, the stoma should be inspected on each nursing visit. Parents should be able to demonstrate appropriate care and assessment of the site for irritation, rashes, or granuloma formation. Routine care of the peristomal area should be accomplished daily. This consists of cleansing the area with soap and water. Peroxide should only be used in diluted preparations for a short period of time. A cotton swab may be used to remove any encrustations from the tube. After the skin is rinsed and dried thoroughly, it should be inspected carefully for redness, swelling, and skin breakdown or granulomas.

At each visit, tube placement should be checked. If the child has a balloon-type gastrostomy tube, placement can be ensured by gently pulling the balloon snug against the skin wall. The tube can best be secured by the use of an antimigration ring or a Hollister clamp. Using tape may not prevent the risk of tube migration. Occasionally, the tube may slip when tape is wet and poorly adhering. If a gastrostomy button or a PEG tube is in place, it should be rotated 360° to ensure proper position. Jejunostomy tubes are secured with either tape or transparent dressings. Their position should be noted by the use of marker tape placed at the point of insertion; it should alert the parents and nurse if the tube is slipping out. Tip placement can only be confirmed by radiograph. Any concerns about possible malposition of these feeding tubes should be communicated to the child's physi-

Table 10–1 Common Tube Feeding Problems and Interventions

Problem	Cause(s)	Intervention(s)
Tube site irritation	Movement of tube back and forth Skin irritation under tape	Tape tube securely. Change position of tape every 1–2 days; assess site for infection or granuloma.
Constipation	Inadequate fluid Lack of bulk in the diet Inactivity	Increase water. Feed prune juice; feed puréed fruits or vegetables. Consult physician for use of a laxative. Encourage activity.
Diarrhea	Feeding too fast Concentrated formula Allergy (intolerance) to an ingredient Side effect of medications given with feedings Flu or gastroenteritis Feeding formula contaminated by bacteria, or "spoiled" formula Lack of bulk in the diet. (This does not really cause diarrhea but can make stools so loose as to cause diaper rash.)	Feed more slowly if gravity feeding; check rate with physician if feeding by pump. Consult dietitian or physician. Divide medications into smaller, more frequent doses if possible. Consult physician. Stress care in daily cleaning of supplies; clean preparations and refrigeration of feedings. Consult with dietitian about adding a bulky food such as puréed vegetables or fruit.
Abdominal cramping **IF SEVERE, CALL PHYSICIAN.**	Feeding too fast Concentrated formula Gastrostomy allowing air into the stomach	Slow the rate of bolus feedings; if using a pump, check the rate: if at the prescribed rate, consult with physician about changing rate. Consult with dietitian. Consult with physician.
Vomiting	Feeding too fast Feeding tube in the wrong place	Feed slower if bolus feeding; consult with physician if feeding by constant drip. Check tube position; tubes in stomach (especially G tubes) may slip out and block the outlet into the intestine.
Aspiration	Tube not inserted fully Associated with vomiting	**STOP FEEDING; CLEAR AIRWAY;** call physician. (*Always* check tube placement before feeding.) Keep head of bed elevated; position infant on stomach to avoid aspiration.
Plugged tube	Contents not flushed completely through	Prevent by rinsing tube with water after feeding (formula or medications) and before clamping the tube.

Source: Adapted from *Tube Feeding Your Child at Home* by J. Ward, S. Robbins, and L. Riggs, pp. 16–17, with permission of Children's Hospital National Medical Center, Clinical Nutrition Group, Washington, D.C., © 1983.

cian. Tables 10–2 and 10–3 provide a guide to assessment of possible problems at the gastrostomy site.

THE FIRST HOME VISIT

All aspects of routine visits are, of course, incorporated into the first home visit. The nurse should ascertain that the necessary supplies and equipment are available in the home (See Exhibit 10–2). In addition, parental preparation to provide safe and appropriate care must be determined. Nurses are further reminded that assessment of the care of the tube-fed infant or child should be made in conjunction with an evaluation of nutritional status, including efforts to ensure

that nutritional needs are being met. In this connection, a thorough nutritional history should be obtained on the first visit (see Chapter 9).

Parental Skills

On the first home visit, assessment of the parents' readiness to provide safe and appropriate feeding is important. This is best achieved by observation. The nurse should also assess the parents' confidence in performing the procedures and their comfort in caring for the child during feeding times. It may take time for confidence and comfort to grow, and frequent encouragement during the first several weeks

Table 10–2 G-Tube Site Care: Possible Problems, Causes, and Interventions

Problem	Causes	Interventions
Formula leakage	Tube migration	Confirm placement. Gently reposition tube against skin wall. Use a tube with antimigration ring, or use a Hollister closing.
	Balloon deflation/rupture	Check water in balloon. If balloon is ruptured, replace tube; if balloon is deflated, reinflate with 2–5 cc water.
	Abdominal distension	Caution: Persistent leakage may be a sign of bowel obstruction. Other care: Protect skin with a skin barrier. *Do not* place a larger tube; instead downsize.
Rash or skin excoriation	Tube migration Balloon rupture Monilia infection Tape allergy	Refer to tube migration. Refer to formula leakage. Contact physician to start antifungal agent. Confirm what type of irritation. Acid burn: Contact physician to initiate use of H2 blocker and prokinetic agent. Other care: Do not cover with gauze. Use skin barrier cream, if acid burn. Wash only with water. Do not use peroxide. Pat dry, no rubbing.
Granuloma at G-tube site	Tube movement	Consider use of G-tube with antimigration ring, Hollister clamp, or a G-button.
	Response to foreign body	Apply silver nitrate carefully. Do not allow tube to dangle.
Tube migration	Tube not secured well	Check placement regularly by gently pulling on tube. Use a tube with antimigration device or a Hollister clamp. Consider a button.
Dislodgement	Balloon rupture	If within 2–4 weeks postsurgery, take child to health care provider immediately.
	Dangling tube Self-removal	Post weeks: Reinsert new tube. Parents should always have a spare tube at home, when traveling, or at school.

at home can be helpful. Providing instruction as needed is essential as well. During this time, if at all possible, the nurse should be available to visit or to offer telephone consultation should any problems arise.

NG-tube Insertion

If a child has an NG tube, the nurse should watch as the parent inserts the tube and checks its position prior to a feeding. The placement can be checked in two ways: (1) by aspirating for stomach contents and (2) by placing a stethoscope over the infant's stomach and, while quickly injecting 3 cc of air into the NG tube, listening for a popping sound, which indicates correct placement. If not in place, the tube should be removed and repositioned before feeding; a tube placed incorrectly can result in aspiration of formula.

Positioning

Correct positioning of the infant during tube feedings is important. It is best for the infant or young child to be held by the parent during bolus feeding. If the infant is not being held, he or she should be positioned prone or on the right side, with shoulders higher than feet by at least 30° to facilitate flow of formula through the alimentary tract and to pre-

vent reflux. Generally, a sleeping infant or child can be placed either prone or on the right side, propped, if possible, by at least 30°. The position should be maintained for 20 to 30 minutes after the feeding. Children who are fed via an NG, PEG, or GT tube without a Nissen fundoplication must be fed using reflux precautions, as described. While jejunal feedings are considered safer, tube position can change, and reflux precautions provide an added measure of safety.

Duration of Feeding

If the infant or child is fed by intermittent bolus, feeding should take approximately the same amount of time as for an oral feeding, namely, 15 to 20 minutes. If a pump is not being used, the feeding should run in by gravity. In this case, the rapidity of the feeding will be determined by the height of the syringe or bottle. Generally, an appropriate height is 4 inches above the abdomen, although more height may be needed with thicker formulas. The height is important because if the tube is held too high, formula may enter the stomach too fast, causing vomiting, diarrhea, or even overfill of the stomach with resulting aspiration. If the parent wants both hands free to hold the child, the feeding apparatus can be either hung on a hanger or taped to the wall or crib. Because of the risk of aspiration, it is important that the

Table 10–3 Gastrostomy Button: Problems, Causes, and Interventions

Problem	Causes	Interventions
Leakage of formula through one-way valve	One-way valve in open position	Reposition valve by gently inserting Q-tip. Flush with carbonated beverage. Make sure CAP is well secured. Persistent leakage will cause a skin acid burn, so protect skin with skin barrier such as Ilex cream.
Leakage of formula around G-button shaft	Abdominal distension Coughing/intermittent illness Constipation Malposition Balloon rupture	Rule out bowel obstruction. Treat underlying cause. Correct constipation. If unable to rotate button 360°, contact physician. If balloon type, check water and replace if needed. Other care: Protect with skin barrier. Replacing with a larger button will not solve the problem.

parent not leave the infant unattended during bolus or gravity tube feedings.

Oral-motor Program

On the first home visit, the nurse should review with parents the recommended oral-motor program and any instructions for oral feeds, sham, or simulated feeds.

Use of Pump

If continuous infusion feedings are used, the first visit is an appropriate time to review with parents the instructions for routine operation of the pump and appropriate responses to alarms. (Sample home care discharge instructions for a Kangaroo feeding pump are included in Appendix 10–C.) The following five principles are important:

1. Positioning, as discussed earlier in this section, will limit the risk of aspiration.
2. To prevent unnecessary infusion of air with the feeding, the drip chamber should be half filled with formula, and the entire feeding line completely filled before the tube is attached to the NG or G tube.
3. To prevent contamination, formula should only be hung for 12 hours at a time. Careful hand-washing is essential to prevent contamination.
4. All possible alarms should be reviewed with parents: low battery, occlusion, and run-away infusions. Emphasis should be placed on corrective actions for the occlusion and run-away infusion alarms. Responses to alarms are based on the type of pump; manufacturer instructions should be reviewed with parents. The pump should be kept plugged into an electric outlet in order to keep the battery charged.
5. Parents should be within hearing range of the feeding pump alarm; an intercom can be used if the child is in a different room.

Each brand of pump has a specific feeding bag. In this regard, reuse and proper measuring should be addressed with parents. Standards for reuse of the bag vary. If feeding bags are to be reused up to a total of 24 hours infusion time, they must be stored in the refrigerator between infusions to limit bacterial growth. Additionally, parents should be instructed to measure the enteral formula accurately by using a measuring cup or by specifying the number of cans to be added to the bag; the numerical markings on the feeding bag are an inaccurate way to measure formula.

Aspiration

Aspiration is a serious risk with any tube feeding. Steps to prevent aspiration, as well as symptoms and interventions, should be reviewed with parents on the first home visit. During tube feedings, appropriate positioning during the feeding (as described previously in this section) is important to prevent aspiration. If at any time during the feeding the child exhibits any signs of aspiration, the feeding should be stopped. Signs and symptoms of aspiration include the following:

- color change
- inability to make noise
- choking
- coughing
- difficulty breathing
- tachycardia
- tachypnea.

With an NG tube, determining proper placement before each feed is also crucial. If the NG tube is accidentally pulled out during the feeding, or if correct placement is uncertain, the parent should both reposition the tube before the feeding is resumed and should remain alert for the signs of aspiration just described. Of course, if aspiration occurs, the physician should be contacted.

Exhibit 10–2 Supplies for Home Tube Feeding

NG and NJ Feedings	**Gastrostomy Button**
• transparent tape	• extra gastrostomy tube
• syringe	with antimigration device
• extra NG tube	• feeding adapter
• stethoscope	• decompression tube
• lubricant	• catheter tip syringe
• measuring cups	• 6 cc syringe
• Pedialyte	• lubricant
	• Pedialyte
GT and PEG Feedings	
• extra gastrostomy tube	**Jejunal Feeding**
with antimigration device	• straight tip syringes
• catheter tip syringe	• transparent tape
• lubricant	• skin barrier
• tape	• Pedialyte
• Hollister clamp	
(if new stoma)	**Traveling Supplies**
• 5 cc to 6 cc syringe	• spare tube
• Pedialyte	• tape
	• syringe
	• lubricant
	• stethoscope

SUBSEQUENT HOME VISITS

On each subsequent home visit, it is important to assess the infant's nutritional intake, obtain growth parameters, and, as necessary, observe and review feeding techniques. A history should be obtained regarding any episodes of vomiting, diarrhea, distension, cramping, or aspiration, and the skin should be assessed for signs of irritation at the nares or at the gastrostomy or jejunostomy-tube insertion site. Any parental concerns should also be elicited and addressed. Any problems related to equipment and supplies should be investigated. Additional assessment and teaching should address the following issues.

Normalizing Feedings

Assisting the family to normalize the feeding experience, as much as possible, may be important in the prevention of long-term feeding problems. Age-appropriate feeding skills are described in Appendix 9–A. Two aspects of normalization can be reviewed with caregivers. First, in order to assist in maintaining an organized and effective suck and to prevent later oral refusal, parents or other caregivers can have the infant suck on a bottle or pacifier during the tube feeding. A pacifier can be used when nutritive sucking is contraindicated or when it is too tiring for the infant. An effective oral-motor program, developed in collaboration with an occupational and/or speech therapist, in conjunction with the introduction of age-appropriate oral feeds for the child who can tolerate them will provide the child with the best long-term assurance of eventual full oral feeding.

A second aspect of normalizing the feeding experience involves the psychosocial component of feeding. Normal patterns of attachment should be encouraged during each feeding, including holding, cuddling, and talking gently to the infant or young child. (Chapter 9 provides further discussion of the psychosocial component of feeding.)

Residual Stomach Contents

There are many opinions regarding the value of and indications for checking residual stomach contents prior to a feeding. The best indication may be if either vomiting or gastric distension presents a problem. Otherwise, checking for residuals is not routinely recommended.

Parents should be instructed in how to check for residual stomach contents should the need arise. (It will not be possible, however, to assess accurately stomach residuals when a small-bore NG tube is used.) The nurse should describe and demonstrate the procedure for checking the residual and then watch as caregivers demonstrate the techniques, to ensure adequate knowledge. To check stomach residuals, the infant should be placed in the supine position. A 20 cc syringe is attached to the end of the NG, G, or J tube. It is best to check for residuals by allowing the aspirate to drain by gravity rather than pulling back on the syringe. (If residuals must be checked via a button, a decompression tube made for checking residuals must be used.) The volume of stomach contents in the syringe is called the *residual volume;* this amount is noted, and the contents are then allowed to flow back into the stomach by gravity. Refeeding the residual prevents loss of fluid and electrolytes. If large volumes of residual remain 1 to 2 hours after a feeding, the next feeding should be delayed. If large-volume residuals persist, a change in formula or in volume of feedings may be indicated.

Flushing the Tube

If medications are given through the feeding tube, or if feedings are intermittent, clogging of the tube may become a serious problem. To prevent this, several measures must be taken. Gentle flushing of the feeding tube with 2 cc to 5 cc of water (infant) is important both before and after giving a medication and immediately after completing a feeding. This is particularly true of gastrostomy and jejunal feeding tubes. Viscous medications should be diluted with water prior to administration. Medication tablets must be *thoroughly* crushed and diluted in water. Water flushes may be given by gravity or by gentle injection into the tube. If resistance is met, force should not be exerted for fear of rupturing the tube. If the infant is on a fluid-restricted diet, any water used to flush the tube should be counted as part of the total daily intake.

Unclogging an Obstructed Tube

There is no failsafe method for unclogging an obstructed feeding tube. The best method is *prevention*, and this means reinforcing the importance of consistent efforts to maintain tube patency. Parents should always carry water and a syringe in case they need to give medications or a feeding when away from home.

If the tube does occlude, changing the NG or G tube is usually the best option. If the child has a jejunal feeding tube, methods for unclogging the tube should be discussed with the child's physician. Several methods for unclogging the tube can be tried, although they generally meet with limited success. These include carbonated beverages, cranberry juice, fresh pineapple juice, meat tenderizer, and pancreatic enzyme with sodium bicarbonate.

ONGOING CONCERNS

The child's normal daily activities need not be curtailed owing to the use of a feeding tube. In order to prevent accidental dislodgement during play, NG, G, or J tubes can be taped securely to the skin or wrapped inside clothing. Using a dressing such as surgiflex, made into a belly binder, helps prevent tubes from dangling and being accidentally pulled out. Other than careful positioning during and after feeding, the infant can be allowed full freedom of movement. The child with a G tube should not be uncomfortable in the prone position, and play in this position should be encouraged. Bathing and tub play are also safe for the infant with the G tube, although parents may need encouragement to be comfortable with this activity.

The ultimate goal for the child who is tube-fed is twofold: (1) a safe transition from hospital to home and (2) age-appropriate independence in activities of daily living, including the progression of oral-motor development and oral feeds if appropriate. The goal of all nutrition is to maintain health and maximize full potential. A tube feeding is merely a tool to achieve wellness in a child who would otherwise fail to thrive. There are many pressures on families of children with special needs. Nurses can promote wellness by assisting parents in developing confidence in their skills for managing the child's special needs at home. The home care nurse can ensure parental confidence by being diligent in teaching parents the necessary skills related to tube-feeding their child.

REFERENCE

Gorman, R., Morris, J., Metz, C., & Mullen, J. (1993). The button jejunostomy for long-term jejunal feeding: Results of a prospective randomized trial. *Journal of Parenteral Enteral Nutrition, 17*(5), 428–431.

ADDITIONAL RESOURCES

Beckert, B., & Heyman, M. (1993). Comparison of two skin-level gastrostomy feeding tubes for infants and children. *Pediatric Nursing, 19*(4), 351–354.

Bockus, S. (1991). Trouble shooting your tube feedings. *American Journal of Nursing, 91*(5), 24–30.

Ekvall, S. (1993). *Pediatric nutrition in chronic diseases and developmental disorders.* New York, NY: Oxford University Press.

Gauderer, M.W.L., Picha, G.L., & Izant, R.J. (1984). The gastrostomy "button"—A simple skin-level, non-refluxing device for long-term enteral feedings. *Journal of Pediatric Surgery, 19,* 803–805.

Huddleston, K., & Ferraro, A. (1991). Preparing families of children with gastrostomies. *Pediatric Nursing, 17*(2), 153–158.

Marcuard, S., & Stegall, K. (1990). Unclogging feeding tubes with pancreatic enzyme. *Journal of Parenteral and Enteral Nutrition, 14*(2), 198–200.

Powell, K., Marcuard, S., & Farrior, E. (1993). Aspirating gastric residuals causes occlusions of small-bore feeding tubes. *Journal of Parenteral and Enteral Nutrition, 17*(3), 243–246.

Shike, M., Wallace, C., Gerdes, H., & Herman-Zaidris, M. (1989). Skin-level gastrostomies and jejunostomies for long-term enteral feedings. *Journal of Parenteral and Enteral Nutrition, 13*(6), 648–650.

Steele, N. (1991). The button: Replacement gastrostomy device. *Journal of Pediatric Nursing, 6*(6), 421–424.

Home Care Plan: NG-Tube Feeding

Date _____   Case manager _____

Name _____ Hosp # _____ DOB _____

PROBLEM: **NASOGASTRIC FEEDING**

GOALS/OBJECTIVES	METHODS	STAFF/REVIEW
Child will receive prescribed NG feeding.	Assess NG feeding plan at each visit; confer with primary care provider and dietitian as needed.	
	Assist to obtain supplies needed.	
Caregivers will demonstrate appropriate safe technique for passage of tube and for assessment of correct position.	Observe caregivers pass tube and check position. Teach/reinforce skills as needed.	
Caregivers will demonstrate ability to give feeding in appropriate manner via tube.	Observe caregivers administer formula via tube; teach/reinforce skills and safety precautions as needed.	
If continuous infusion pump used, caregivers to describe use of pump and appropriate response to pump alarms.	Assess knowledge and teach/reinforce as needed.	
Caregivers will describe s/sx of appropriate interventions.	Assess knowledge and teach/reinforce as needed.	
Child will be held close and cuddled or otherwise attended to, during feeding.	Assess attachment behavior during feeding and encourage as necessary.	
Child will suck during tube feeding if indicated.	Assess caregivers' efforts to encourage sucking. Reinforce as necessary.	
Child's nares will be without excoriation. Caregivers will demonstrate ability to assess nares for excoriation and will describe appropriate care measures.	Assess nares each visit. Teach/reinforce care as needed. Contact primary care provider prn re: excoriation.	
Caregivers will describe/demonstrate appropriate plan for cleaning supplies.	Assess knowledge. Teach/reinforce prn.	

Source: Courtesy of Children's Hospital National Medical Center, Home Health Care Services, Washington, D.C.

Home Care Plan: G-Tube Feeding

Date _____ Case manager _____

Name _____ Hosp # _____ DOB _____

PROBLEM: **G-TUBE FEEDING**

GOALS/OBJECTIVES	METHODS	STAFF/REVIEW
Child will receive prescribed G-tube feeding.	Assess G-tube feeding plan at each visit; confer with primary care provider and dietitian as needed. Assist to obtain needed supplies.	
Caregivers will demonstrate ability to give feeding in appropriate manner via tube.	Observe caregivers administer formula via tube; teach/reinforce skills and safety precautions as needed.	
If continuous infusion pump used, caregivers to describe pump use and appropriate response to pump alarms.	Assess knowledge and teach/reinforce skills and safety precautions as needed.	
Child will be held close and cuddled or otherwise attended to, during feeding.	Assess attachment behavior during feeding and encourage as necessary.	
Child will suck during tube feeding if indicated.	Assess caregivers' efforts to encourage sucking. Reinforce as necessary.	
Caregivers will demonstrate appropriate routine stoma care and will describe signs of excoriation and appropriate interventions.	Assess stoma site at each visit. Observe caregivers providing routine stoma care. Assess knowledge of signs of excoriation and interventions. Teach/reinforce as needed. Contact surgeon or primary care provider as needed re: excoriation/granuloma formation.	
Caregivers will correctly describe technique for reinsertion of G-tube and for assessment of correct position.	Assess knowledge. Teach/reinforce as necessary.	
Caregivers will describe/demonstrate appropriate plan for cleaning supplies.	Assess knowledge. Teach/reinforce as necessary.	

Source: Courtesy of Children's Hospital National Medical Center, Home Health Care Services, Washington, D.C.

Sample Home Care Discharge Instruction Sheet: Kangaroo Pump

HOW TO OPERATE:

1. WASH hands well using soap from a pump dispenser. Dry hands with paper towel or a clean cloth towel.
2. Remove feeding bag from plastic wrap. Close roller clamp by rolling red wheel down.
3. Pour_____ formula into feeding bag.
4. Close lid to bag by pressing down on the middle of the lid with thumb to create a tight seal.
5. Hang bag on pole.
6. Prime tubing by hanging tubing straight down while opening roller clamp while holding the end of the tubing in the other hand. When milk gets to the end of the tubing, close roller clamp.
7. Place tubing on pump by inserting clip chamber into slot (slide chamber in from top of slot). Wrap stretchy part of tubing around the pump wheel. Insert tubing into "elbow" and close latch to keep tubing from falling out.
8. Take cap off end of tubing and insert red portion of tubing into your child's feeding tube.
   IF YOUR CHILD HAS AN (NG) NASOGASTRIC TUBE—ALWAYS CHECK PLACEMENT OF TUBE!!
9. Open roller clamp.
10. Press *ON*.
11. Set rate to _____ cc/hour.
12. PRESS *START/HOLD* BUTTON. You should see the wheel turn briefly and you will note a little red dot bouncing across the rate panel.

TIPS FOR THE ALARM PANEL

1. FLOW ERROR- (FLO ERR)	2. NO SET (NO SET)	3. HOLD ERROR (HLD ERR)	4. LOW BATTERY: (LO BATT)	5. SYSTEMS ERROR: (SYS ERR)
This means that the formula is not flowing properly through the tubing. Check the following: • Empty Feed Bag • Closed Roller Clamp • Overflow of Drip Chamber • Kinked Tubing • Kinked or Clogged Feeding Tube	Tubing not set on pump correctly. Fix problem quickly because this causes milk to free flow into your child. Wrap tubing tightly around wheel, insert into groove above wheel. If you can't do this quickly, close roller clamp to stop flow.	Pump has been in hold pattern for more than 2½ minutes. Press start/hold one time to continue hold pattern; two times to restart pump infusion.	Pump has lost battery charge; plug into electrical outlet.	Pump is broken. Call Caremark to replace pump.

*To stop the "beeping" press the START/HOLD button. After you correct the problem press START/HOLD button again. This will restart the infusion.

Remember to flush your child's tube with 3–5 cc water after all feedings. If you need to give a medicine during the feeding, flush the tube before and after giving the medicine. This will prevent tube blockage.

Source: Courtesy of Children's Hospital National Medical Center, Home Health Care Services, Washington, D.C.

Chapter 11

Home Care of the Infant with Short Bowel Syndrome Requiring Nutritional Support

Kathi Huddleston, RN, MSN

Home care nurses have an opportunity to become increasingly involved in the care of infants with short bowel syndrome (SBS) on home parenteral nutritional therapy (HPN). Unfortunately, many of the infants who have SBS may also have suffered from other sequelae of prematurity. Prolonged hospitalization, dependence on technology, and the uncertain future nutritional needs may overwhelm the most confident of parents. The home care nurse can support family members through the emotional peaks and valleys and provide the education, support, and care coordination necessary to assist them in resuming control over their lives and clarifying their role(s) as parents of a child with SBS (Thompson, 1994; Warner & Zeigler, 1993).

The nurse caring for infants or young children with SBS and requiring HPN must have many areas of clinical proficiency. These include nutritional support, vascular access device management, enteral access device management, skin care, fluid/electrolyte assessment, and assessment and intervention related to oral-motor skills and stimulation. The care of children with SBS and requiring HPN may present unique and challenging problems that require a home health nurse to have a basic understanding of pathophysiology, be aware of the potential complications of therapy, and be creative to assist the family in integrating the complex care and technology necessary to care for this child into home and family life (Czyrko, Delfin, O'Neill, Peckham, & Ross, 1991; Weber, Tracy, & Connors, 1991).

This chapter provides information on short bowel syndrome and subsequent bowel adaptation, home parenteral nutrition, and venous access devices. Both the plan of care and nursing care priorities are discussed. Care of infants with SBS requiring HPN benefits from a strong multidisciplinary team and requires the attention of many specialists. The home care nurse is strategically positioned to assist the family in coordinating care and ensuring that both the health care needs and needs related to growth and development are addressed.

SHORT BOWEL SYNDROME

A growing number of infants are surviving problems that require massive bowel resection. Reasons for removal of significant portions of the small bowel in infants and children can be divided into two categories:

1. congenital anomalies, such as intestinal atresia, complicated abdominal wall defects, and vascular abnormalities
2. acquired processes, such as ischemic or inflammatory bowel disorders.

Among infants, necrotizing enterocolitis is the most common cause of short bowel syndrome.

Symptoms

The term *short bowel syndrome* (SBS) is used most frequently to describe a set of certain clinical signs and symptoms of malabsorption and malnutrition resulting from small bowel resection. Common symptoms are rapid intestinal transit, inadequate digestion, and the inability to allow absorption of nutrients. These result in the malnutrition associated with SBS. Aggressive nutritional management is necessary to enable infants and young children to survive and adapt to extensive resection of the small bowel (Thompson, 1994).

There is a continuum of the symptoms of SBS. The severity of the disease is determined by a number of factors:

- length of bowel
- location of bowel remaining
- functioning of remaining bowel
- presence/absence of ileocecal valve (ICV)
- mucosal integrity of the bowel.

The amount of bowel that has to be removed before a child starts to have significant malabsorption varies greatly with the age of the child and the location of bowel involved. Understanding the basic physiology of the gastrointestinal tract can assist in identifying potential problems (Warner & Zeigler, 1993).

Physiology

The small intestine is continuing to grow and develop during the last trimester of pregnancy. The small bowel doubles in length from the period between 19 to 26 weeks and 36 to 40 weeks gestation. Premature infants have approximately 115 cm of jejunum, whereas full-term infants have 250 cm (Wise, 1992). The infant who undergoes massive bowel resection can resume intestinal mucosal growth and develop "new" small bowel tissue, unlike older children and adults. Therefore, infants have a more favorable prognosis and are better able to "adapt" than older persons.

Each section of bowel is responsible for a specific absorptive function; therefore, the absence of certain portions of bowel will produce different clinical symptoms. In the infant, healthy functioning bowel tissue will adapt to "take over" the absorptive function of an absent section. Specific absorptive functions of the intestines depend on the overall function of the gastrointestinal tract (Purdum & Kirby, 1991). Table 11–1 describes the functions of different portions of the gastrointestinal tract.

Physiological Response to Intestinal Resection

Small bowel adaptation is the term used to describe the clinical course and the process of intestinal adaptation to bowel function after massive bowel resection. The adaptation process may take up to 3 years before optimal intestinal

Table 11–1 Functions of Specific Areas of the Gastrointestinal Tract

Area	Function
Stomach	The functions of the stomach include digestion of gastric contents by the secretion of acid and pepsin; regulation of the delivery of contents to the small bowel; maximization of the mixing of secretions with food; and the production of intrinsic factor. While it is possible to survive without a stomach, the lack of intrinsic factor will result in vitamin B_{12} deficiency.
Duodenum	Biliary and pancreatic enzymes mix in the duodenum, and these agents appear to be responsible for villous height and growth through the small bowel. The villi are finger-like projections and are responsible for the absorption of nutrients; they provide an absorptive surface 600 times larger than the actual bowel length.
Jejunum	The primary role of the jejunum appears to be transport and absorption of nutrients. In most cases, the loss of jejunal tissue does not impair the absorption of carbohydrate, protein, fluid, or electrolytes. The distal small bowel is very capable of adapting and compensating for the loss of the jejunum.
Ileum	The ileum is approximately 100 cm in length, and its primary function is to reabsorb bile salts; vitamin B_{12}; and fat-soluble vitamins such as A, D, E, and K. Massive resection (over 75%) will lead to steatorrhea and biliary cholestasis.
Ileocecal valve	The ileocecal valve is a specialized muscle that functions as a one-way door from the ileum to the colon. It prevents colonization of the small intestine with colonic bacteria from the lower intestine. It also slows the intestinal transit time from ileum to colon, thus increasing the length of time nutrients are exposed to the intestinal mucosa and facilitating absorption of nutrients. The loss of the ICV results in greater severity of the disease process and more frequent complications.
Colon	The major functions of the colon are to reabsorb sodium and water, excrete potassium and bicarbonate, and control fluid losses. It also assists in the adsorption of oxalate, which prevents the formation of kidney stones.

function is achieved. Many people with SBS never fully return to normal bowel function; as a result, they may require specialized nutritional support for a lifetime.

Controversy exists over the amount of small bowel necessary to survive and adapt to full enteral (i.e., gastrointestinal) feedings. In the past, the presence or absence of the ileocecal valve was thought to be a determining factor. It is conservative opinion today that infants with at least 10 cm to 15 cm of small bowel can survive and may be able to adapt eventually to enteral feedings (Weber et al., 1991). A three-phase adaptation response, described by Rombeau and Rolandelli (1987) occurs; infants and children are hospitalized until stabilized in the second or third phase of adaptation.

Phase 1

Phase 1 after intestinal resection involves the immediate postoperative course and is characterized by major fluid and electrolyte losses from massive diarrhea and fluid shifts within the body. After resection of bowel, the infant will have a functioning stoma (the proximal end) and mucous fistula(s) (the distal portion). During this period, nutritional support must be provided by total parenteral nutrition (TPN). Although necessary, TPN itself has been associated with bowel atrophy, further complicating the process of nutrient absorption. Atrophy can be prevented by exposing the bowel to small amounts of enteral feeding, thereby stimulating the bowel mucosa and normal cellular function. The enteral feeding may also be given through the mucous fistula in order to stimulate bowel growth to the distal segment.

The first phase of adaptation is often characterized by a roller-coaster course and can be very stressful for families. This stress may manifest later if problems arise in home management.

Phase 2

Phase 2 involves the gradual increase of enteral feeding and the transition from parenteral nutritional support to full enteral feedings. This process may take from weeks to years. This phase of adaptation is characterized by stabilization of the diarrhea and successful increase in enteral feeding. Enteral feedings stimulate the gut mucosa and promote the adaptive hyperplasia of small bowel tissue. Tolerance of enteral feedings is a great hallmark of small bowel absorption and function, as well as an indicator of small bowel mucosal growth.

Continuous feedings are better tolerated than oral or bolus feedings during adaptation after small bowel resection. Enteral feedings can be slowly advanced and well controlled if delivered via a continuous infusion pump. Feedings are advanced by alternately increasing caloric density and volume: calories are usually increased first, followed by an increase in feeding volume. Advancing the enteral feedings is a slow and often tedious process for the infant and family.

Despite careful advancement, the infant may have large stool outputs and require a regression of the feeding regime—sometimes back to the original strength and volume. Setbacks occurring during Phase 2 of adaptation can also be quite stressful for families.

Successful adaptation of the bowel is signaled by a decrease in stool volume, stool pH greater than 5, and the absence of reducing substances in the stool. When this occurs, the infant can be taken back to surgery for the reanastomosis of the intestines. Once intestinal continuity is reestablished, the infant will have the opportunity to use the distal segment of small bowel, should be much more stable in fluid and electrolyte balance, and will be more easily able to advance his or her nutritional status.

Phase 3

Phase 3 of intestinal adaptation after resection involves the tapering of TPN and the advancement of continuous enteral feedings to a more "normal" diet pattern, to eventually include oral solid foods and bolus feedings. Some children never complete Phase 3 and remain on some form of long-term parenteral nutrition. Children with SBS receiving long-term parenteral nutrition have many long-term needs and are at risk for ongoing complications.

HOME PARENTERAL NUTRITION

Just 20 years ago, TPN and reliable pediatric vascular access made survival after extensive small bowel resection possible. However, at that time, mortality rates of 80% to 90% were reported with such disorders as gastroschisis and intestinal atresias. Now, solely due to the ability to provide nutrition directly to the body, the survival rates are above 90% (Testerman, 1989).

The goals of parenteral nutrition include providing sufficient nutrition to meet both basal energy requirements and the increased metabolic needs of stressed patients; replenishing malnourished patients; and, for the pediatric population, promoting growth and development (Dorney, Amant, Berquist, Vargus, & Hasalle, 1985).

Parenteral nutrition involves administering nutrients intravenously via the bloodstream. Peripheral parenteral nutrition (PPN) can be delivered only at glucose concentrations of 12.5% or less. TPN solution is more concentrated. It contains water, carbohydrate, protein, lipid, seven major electrolytes, minerals, and 13 vitamins and trace elements; this concentrated solution must be delivered via the central circulation (Orr, 1989; Testerman, 1989).

Components of TPN Solution

The nurse and family should be familiar with the components of the TPN solution. These include fluid, calories, protein, fat, electrolytes, and minerals. The important areas of assessment and monitoring related to these solution components will be described below. When laboratory studies are recommended, the frequency of monitoring is determined by the discharging physician and is based on the stability of the infant's laboratory studies during hospitalization.

Fluid

Fluid is usually the first component of a child's TPN solution to be calculated. Water constitutes greater than 80% of the body weight in an infant. Fluid requirements are generally those needed for maintenance or one and a half times maintenance. If the infant has had problems with high stool output, greater than 20 cc/kg/day, then fluid requirements will be greater. In an infant with an ileostomy, careful attention to fluid requirements is essential as rapid dehydration can occur. When an infant is sick with a fever, for every degree in temperature elevation, there will be a 10% greater fluid need. This can be accomplished through increased oral intake or by the physician ordering additional intravenous solution, as appropriate for the child. Weight, stool output, hydration status, and temperature during an illness are important factors to monitor.

Calories

Calories given parenterally are usually are 5% to 10% less than those required for enteral feeds. In times of increased metabolic needs (such as infection or high stool output), the infant may need additional calories. However, overfeeding—giving too many calories or giving an unbalanced delivery of calories—can contribute to liver problems and will be an additional stressor on the infant's metabolic system. The distribution of calories should be balanced with the main source of energy being carbohydrate (30%–50%), protein should provide approximately 15% of calories, and calories from fat should be less than 60%. Weight gain of the infant can greatly influence the formulation of TPN. For this reason, the weight of the infant or young child must be obtained at least weekly.

Carbohydrate

Glucose is the main source of calories for infants; 1 g of glucose equals 3.4 cal. Without sufficient glucose, infants quickly become hypoglycemic. Blood sugar and urinary sugar are both valuable monitoring tools.

Protein

Amino acids are given for growth; protein is a poor source of calories. A brand of amino acids called *Trophamine* is generally used in the HPN solution because it is a pediatric preparation and contains taurine, an essential amino acid for infants and children. Protein needs will

increase with an increase in metabolic demands, such as losses from wounds, the inflammatory response, or sepsis. Blood urea nitrogen, bicarbonate, ammonia, and albumin will be monitored for protein losses.

Fat

The delivery of fat, 2 cal/cc, is usually accomplished as Intralipid 20%. Of the calories of the HPN solution, 40% to 60% will come from lipids; 4% of the daily caloric intake will be linoleic acid to prevent essential fatty acid deficiency. Triglycerides will be monitored closely to assess lipid metabolism.

Metabolites

The quantity of electrolytes and minerals in the HPN solution will vary with each individual child. Calcium and phosphorous are problematic and will be closely monitored with infants who have SBS. Acetate may be added to prevent acidosis. After 6 to 8 weeks selenium and iodine are usually added. Trace elements are also added, and copper and zinc will also need frequent monitoring (Bendorf & Lyman, 1993; Grant & Kennedy-Caldwell, 1988).

Home TPN Solutions

In the hospital, lipids are often administered in a separate bag from the other components of the TPN solution. Some infants will be discharged to home care with this arrangement, as some providers feel it is optimal for ensuring solubility of calcium and phosphorus. However, infants and children may be discharged from some institutions on what is called an "all-in-one" or "three-in-one" HPN solution. The "all-in-one" solution, which combines the glucose, amino acids, and lipids into one bag, has been found to be safe and successful in infants and is often preferred in home care. It requires the use of only one pump and one set of tubing, therefore decreasing the cost and making the infusion of the solution much easier and more convenient to administer.

Total parenteral nutrition in pediatrics requires a higher concentration of calcium and phosphorous than that in adults. Unfortunately, solubility constraints dictate the amounts of calcium and phosphorous actually allowed in the solution. If the concentration of calcium and phosphorous are increased, then precipitations may occur. The higher the calcium and phosphorous concentrations, the more increased the chance of incompatibility with medications. In fact, there have been deaths associated with inappropriate admixtures (Virginia C. Gebus, personal communication, May 1995). The all-in-one solution is creamy white in appearance and has a thicker viscosity due to the addition of the lipids. The amount of calcium and phosphorous added to the all-in-one solutions needs to be assessed, as the white precipitate that may occur would not be visible with the lipids added to the solution. Hypocalcemia can result in resorption of calcium from the bone, resulting in rickets. If any questions arise, the physician and pharmacist should be consulted (Bendorf & Lyman, 1993; Hennessy, 1989).

It is important to define the responsibility for monitoring and reporting the TPN laboratory studies. It may be the home infusion company nurse, the community health nurse, or the extended hour home care nurse who draws the blood for laboratory studies and takes it to the laboratory for analysis. When drawing blood from infants and young children, the nurse must be conservative and should draw the smallest amount of blood possible. Frequent blood tests can lead to anemia. It is imperative that the physician report the results of the studies to the pharmacy and that the infusion company share the results with the home care nurse and family in a timely fashion.

Choice of a Pump

The careful choice of pump for the administration of TPN is important. The right pump will assist parents in maintaining a somewhat normal lifestyle. It will allow for mobility of the child and flexibility in activities the child and family choose. The home health nurse needs to be aware of choices available on the market, and their advantages and disadvantages, in order to both educate the family in what is available and be an advocate for the family in negotiations with the insurance company (Bendorf & Lyman, 1993; Cedy & Yoskioka, 1991). Often, the choice of pump is made by the third-party payer. A list of criteria to consider in pump selection is included in Appendix 11–A.

Preventing Complications of TPN

Cycling TPN

Long-term parenteral nutrition generally should be infused over a period of 12 to 18 hours to allow the child's body a period of fasting. This method of cycling TPN may help to lower circulating insulin levels during rest periods and allow for lipolysis and fat mobilization from the liver, thus controlling fatty liver infiltration, a possible risk of TPN. Both overfeeding and high glucose infusions of greater than 5mg/kg/minute have been associated with liver abnormalities (Thompson, 1994).

Enteral Feeding

Cyclic TPN, appropriate nutrition, and the administration of enteral feeding will decrease the risk of liver complications. Use of the gut whenever possible, even if total enteral support is not attainable, will also prevent the atrophy and loss of function of the small bowel (Amarnath, Fleming, & Perrault, 1987).

Hypoglycemia

To prevent hypoglycemia, it may be recommended to decrease the HPN infusion rate hours before discontinuation in each cycle. Although recent studies have shown that, in children over the age of 2 years, tapering is not necessary, and abrupt discontinuance of HPN is safe (Werlin, Wyatt, & Carnitta, 1994), tapering is still routine under the age of 2 years. If tapering is requested in the care of an infant or child on HPN, an important factor in pump selection will be the presence of a tapering feature.

MANAGEMENT OF CENTRAL VENOUS ACCESS

Types of Central Lines

During hospitalization, the child may have had various types of central venous lines, but for home infusion of TPN, it is necessary that a "Broviac" type catheter—a silicone long-term central venous catheter with a Dacron cuff—is in place. The catheter is usually placed in the subclavian, internal, or external jugular vein and advanced to the superior vena cava. The proximal end of the catheter is pulled through the subcutaneous tissue, so that the cuff is implanted under the skin, and the catheter exits on the chest. The cuff is usually palpable and should be felt in the middle of the skin tunnel. The cuff adheres to the skin and seals off the tunnel, which then functions as a barrier to infection. The catheter may be single or double lumen and may be of various sizes, from 4 to 9 French (Huddleston, Ferraro-McDuffie, & Wolfe-Small, 1993).

Preventing Problems with the Central Line

The identified hospital expert in the care of central venous lines (CVL) should be available to guide both the home health nurse and the family if problems arise in care of the central line. The most frequent problems are infection, catheter rupture, occlusion, dislodgement, and irritation of the skin at the catheter exit site. Parents and nurse should routinely observe for swelling, discharge, and/or redness at the catheter exit site. Catheter rupture must be repaired immediately.

Both aseptic dressing changes and catheter flushes, if ordered, can be important in preventing problems with the central line. Protocols for aseptic dressing changes and flushing of the catheter vary from one institution and agency to another. It is important that the nurse learn how the parents have been instructed to carry out these procedures in order to minimize confusion by introducing yet another method. Hand-washing technique should be reviewed with parents since it is the most effective measure for preventing nocosomial infections.

Infections

Infants requiring HPN have a higher rate of infection than do older children. Aseptic technique is critical for this population since they are dependent on these catheters for their nutritional support. If the catheter is identified as a source of the infection, and the contamination cannot be cleared with antibiotics, the CVL will have to be removed. As a preventive measure, the nurse should attempt to minimize the number of times the central line is entered (e.g., draw all daily labs at one time), as each break in the closed system will increase the risk for infection.

A high index of suspicion for central venous catheter infections is appropriate with these infants and young children. Routine care should include blood cultures if the infant or child has a temperature of 101 °F (38.5 °C) or greater. Cultures should be done from each lumen of the central venous line and from a peripheral vein. If the blood cultures are positive, then all attempts are made to treat the infection with antibiotics. Cultures can be drawn by the home care nurse and antibiotics administered at home, thereby avoiding hospitalization in most instances.

If at all possible, any antibiotic used should be compatible with the TPN solution so that the nutrition does not need to be stopped 1 hour before and then during antibiotic administration. If the antibiotic and TPN solution are not compatible, the infusion of the antibiotic needs to be administered with a high dextrose solution to avoid drastic shifts in blood glucose.

If the central venous catheter has a double lumen, the positive cultures need to be evaluated to see whether both lumens of the central venous catheter harbor organisms. To treat only one lumen of the catheter will leave the organism in the untreated lumen, thus reinfecting the child after antibiotics are completed. A rotation schedule should be developed so that the TPN solution and the antibiotic are alternated between the two lumens of the catheter.

It may also be of value to treat an infected line with a thrombolytic agent such as urokinase if thrombus or clot is suspected (Duffy, Kerzner, Gebus, & Dice, 1989).

Occlusion

Closely related to infection is the significant problem of catheter occlusion. The rate of occlusion may be greater in children due to the smaller lumen size of the catheters, the smaller vessels, or the high concentrations of certain minerals in the HPN solution.

A number of factors can lead to an occlusion (Crummette & Boatwright, 1991; Zahr, Heflin, LaRosa, & Damian, 1992), and questions to consider when occlusion occurs include the following:

- Was a medication just given prior to catheter occlusion?
- Was there a history of problems with blood withdrawal?
- Was there a problem in flushing the catheter recently?
- Did the child recently receive blood or blood products through the line?
- Has a new drug been started, or has the schedule been changed?

These events need to be evaluated in order to prevent recurrence of the clot when possible.

Drug precipitates, precipitates with lipids, precipitates due to the high calcium and phosphorous ratios in pediatric TPN, as well as occlusions due to thrombus or fibrin sheath development need to be treated. These can be treated at home by a nurse with a physician's order; standing CVL protocol orders may address these treatments.

Drug precipitates may be treated with different agents as follows (Bendorf & Lyman, 1993; Duffy et al., 1989; Testerman, 1989):

- Hydrochloric acid (HCL 0.1N) is used when a calcium/phosphorous precipitate is suspected or if the drug administered would cause a precipitate in the nature of a base (as opposed to acid).
- Sodium bicarbonate may clear a drug precipitate of an acidic nature; sodium bicarbonate cannot be administered with the TPN.
- Ethanol (70%) has been very successful in clearing lines that have a lipid sludge, sometimes caused by all-in-one TPN.

Many studies suggest that the process of line occlusion or problems with flushing and blood withdrawal can be precursors of the infectious process. The presence of a blood clot on the distal tip of a catheter may function as a "ball-valve" to prevent aspiration of blood; it may also serve as a nidus for infection. There have been studies that suggest that the routine administration of urokinase may decrease the incidence of both thrombus and infection (Dann, 1994; Duffy et al., 1989). Urokinase is recommended for catheters that have a long history of blood withdrawal problems, suggesting that a blood clot or thrombus may be involved (Dann, 1994). As with treatments for drug precipitates, this can be administered by a nurse in the home with a physician's order.

Catheter Dislodgement

Prevention of accidental dislodgement of the catheter will bring out the creative talents of any parent or home care nurse. The importance of the line is usually clear to the parents, and they need to be involved in designing methods to secure the catheter. Usually the catheter is looped and taped down securely. A one-piece outfit or similar clothing will help to keep the catheter out of the infant's grasp. There are several taping methods in the literature, and recommendations vary among institutions and agencies. Generally, whichever method parents prefer is acceptable. As the child grows and develops, new challenges may arise to securing the catheter (Huddleston et al., 1993; Zahr et al., 1992).

Irritation at the Catheter Exit Site

Routine care of the catheter exit site includes monitoring the area around the catheter exit site for redness, irritation, a rash, or any sign of infection or compromised skin integrity. The parents need to be able to change the type of dressing at the catheter exit site if skin irritation occurs. They also need to be independent in performing procedures for changing the the dressing and tape using protocols they have been taught.

DECIDING ON HOME CARE

Over the past decade, infants with extremely short segments of small bowel have had the opportunity to adapt due to advances in vascular access, parenteral nutritional support, specialized enteral formulas, and advances in home care technology and support. Nutrition support itself was among the first of the high-tech therapies to make the transition from hospital to home (Amarnath, Fleming, & Perrault, 1987; Thompson, 1994). The use of HPN requires an intensive discharge planning process; coordination with insurance companies and durable medical equipment companies; and the involvement of two multidisciplinary teams, one inpatient and one outpatient, that are willing to work with the family to bridge the chasm of hospital to home care.

In considering the feasibility of home nutritional support, several factors are important. Preparing for home parenteral nutrition (HPN) requires a thorough assessment of the child, family, home, and community. It also requires proper selection of equipment.

Stability of the Child

The relative stability of the small bowel adaptation process and the ongoing ability to maintain and progress the child's nutrition should be evaluated. The child should be medically stable for several weeks prior to discharge. Problems with high stool output and dehydration should not be an ongoing concern. The infant should be tolerating a consistent HPN solution, and frequent changes should not be anticipated.

Family Preparedness

The attitude of the parents toward caring for their child at home is important. HPN in infants is most often used as a supportive rather than curative therapy. Parents should be aware of the potential risks and benefits of home care and feel comfortable in accepting those risks that may occur at home. They should be informed of the responsibilities entailed. Central venous access will need to be closely assessed and evaluated. Complications and potential infection risks will require careful monitoring with an action plan in place. Usually enteral access, such as a gastrostomy, is present, but a nasogastric tube may need to be inserted. Nutrition support equipment will often include an infusion pump for the HPN at night and a portable enteral feeding pump for continuous enteral feedings. Some centers use only 12-hour night feedings and allow token oral feeds during the day. Parents must be comfortable knowing that they may be tied to technology and equipment of sorts, and must be willing to learn all the skills required for routine and emergency care.

Home Environment

A clean and well-organized space is necessary to care for the child receiving HPN. Running water, heat, air conditioning, a working refrigerator, and a telephone should be available. Usually a 1-week supply of HPN solution is delivered at a time. There will need to be a designated space in the refrigerator for storage of the solution, any additives, and medications needing refrigeration. In some cases, a separate refrigerator may be supplied by the infusion company. A clean area, such as an empty drawer or closet shelf, should also be designated for storage of supplies and necessary equipment.

Community Resources

A community support system will be necessary to make home care possible and safe for the child requiring HPN. Questions to consider include the following: What emergency medical support will this family have? Will the closest emergency department have the resources to repair a central venous line in an infant (Bendorf & Lyman, 1993)? Are there home health nurses with the appropriate skills and training to assist the family? Is there a company that can provide the equipment, supplies, and solution that the family will need to care for the child? What provisions are there for equipment malfunction?

Exhibit 11–1 Home TPN Supplies

Routine Care
- dressing supplies
- clamp, on catheter (ensure that it functions)
- replacement caps for catheter ends
- repair kit for catheter (correct type, size, lumen)
- 5 cc or 10 cc syringes (any smaller size exerts too much pressure, increasing the risk of catheter fracture)

Emergency Care
- thrombolytics, especially if the child has a history of clotting or drug precipitates
- hemostats with covered ends
- repair kit, *always available*

Selection of Equipment

Appendix 11–A offers criteria for pump selection. Other equipment and supplies that are needed in the home include those listed in Exhibit 11–1.

HOSPITAL DISCHARGE AND TRANSITION TO THE HOME

For many families, the infant's long hospitalization has been a frustrating experience, and the possibility of going home is eagerly anticipated. While the transition is welcome, it also may be greeted with some trepidation, as it is a big adjustment. The family has most likely developed a relationship with a primary nurse or clinical nurse specialist; these nurses can be instrumental in the transmission of information, trust, confidence, and support during the transition from hospital to home care.

Discharge Planning Process

Thorough and careful preparation is the cornerstone for a successful hospital discharge for the infant or child requiring home TPN. All of the knowledge and best of care will not compensate for poor discharge planning. In this regard, discharge planning is an active process that should begin at least several weeks prior to discharge. Effective planning requires collaboration between the hospital-based health care team, the home care team, and the family. A member of the hospital team should remain available for consultation with the parents and home care personnel after discharge.

Parental Training

As part of the preparation for successful home care, the parents or other caregivers, including an identified "backup" person, should be expected to demonstrate competency in managing the central line, the gastrostomy and enteral feedings, and the infusion devices and hanging the TPN solution. They also must be knowledgeable about strategies for oral stimulation and the promotion of infant development. These competencies and this knowledge should be attained prior to hospital discharge. Further, it is strongly suggested that families have the opportunity to provide care for at least 24 hours in the hospital setting, using the equipment to be used in the home. This will allow the family the opportunity to perform the care independently, while support is available if necessary, assuring both themselves and hospital staff of their readiness to assume full responsibility for care at home.

Emergency Preparations

Prior to discharge, it is imperative that emergency preparations be addressed. Potential emergencies include the following:

- central line fracture, or accidental removal
- accidental rapid infusion of TPN solution
- accidental removal of gastrostomy tube (See Chapter 10).

Caregivers in these potential emergency situations benefit from advance instruction and role playing. With adequate preparation, the parent should be able to state a plan of action for each scenario and indicate an appropriate response. Central line fractures should be repaired immediately. If the home care or infusion company cannot provide this service, parents should take their own CVL repair kit to the hospital emergency department for assistance.

Prior to hospital discharge, parents should be encouraged to post important and emergency telephone numbers by the telephone(s). It can be helpful for the family to visit the closest fire station with emergency support personnel. This visit should provide the emergency personnel with specific information regarding the potential transportation of the infant. (It may be useful to make this visit with cookies or donuts and a picture of the child.) Other emergency preparations include ensuring a telephone in the home and notifying the telephone and electric companies that the family needs to be on a priority service list. (See sample notification letters in Appendix 12–D.)

Transportation Plans

Plans for transportation home should be established prior to discharge. If the child can go without enteral feedings during the trip home, travel will be much less complicated. Similarly, TPN should be off during the trip home if possible, to prevent any potential problems with the functioning of the pump in the car. If TPN is necessary while in transit, a registered nurse (RN) escort should be considered.

Home Care Notebook

A notebook can be used both to assist parents in becoming organized for home TPN and to share information regarding care for the infant. The notebook can set in writing the infant's individualized health care plan. This notebook may include the material listed in Exhibit 11–2.

ROUTINE HOME VISITS

The home health nurse should expect the parents to be proficient in the care for the CVL, the gastrostomy, the hanging and discontinuing of the TPN, trouble-shooting of problems with the infusion pumps, proper organization and storage of supplies. Parents should also be knowledgeable about the child's daily schedule of care, signs and symptoms of infection, and utilization of emergency plans. At the same time, the nurse should be prepared to assess parental prepa-

Exhibit 11–2 Suggested Contents of a Home Care Notebook for a Child Requiring Home TPN

About SBS
- a few articles regarding the diagnoses of the infant
- a copy of the discharge orders and discharge summary

About TPN
- written policies or standards for care of the central venous line, the gastrostomy, and so forth
- the daytime and on-call telephone numbers of the equipment and infusion companies
- an emergency plan (a copy to be posted by the bed)

About the Physicians
- a list of the infant's physicians and their telephone numbers
- an outline of the physicians' roles and a brief description of who to call for which type of potential problems

Care and Schedule for the Day
- the infant's daily schedule: line flushes, medications, TPN start and stop times
- enteral feeding tolerance
- number of stools a day
- a growth chart with previous trends

Individual Needs and Tips
- developmental assessments to give anticipatory guidance
- tips on special care or needs of the infant, such as "you get an easier blood return from her central line if she is lying on her right side"
- skin care products that have worked in the past
- travel advice, including carrying a repair kit, storing solution, etc.

Exhibit 11–3 TPN Monitoring: Sample Initial Home Protocol

Growth
- weight: twice a week on a balance beam scale
- height: twice a month
- head circumference: monthly

Laboratory
- electrolytes, glucose, complete blood count (CBC): weekly for 2 weeks then monthly
- calcium, phosphorous, magnesium, triglycerides, alkaline phophatase, gamma glutumyl transferase, prealbumin: weekly for 2 weeks then monthly
- transferrin, zinc, copper, cholesterol, albumin, bilirubin, alanine amino transferase, vitamins A and D: monthly

Urine
- sugar, protein, and specific gravity: daily

---

ration in these areas and review and reinforce information and skills with parents as necessary.

A sample initial home protocol for monitoring the growth and nutritional status of the infant requiring TPN is included in Exhibit 11–3.

Physical Assessment

All home visits should include a physical assessment of the infant.

Vital Signs

Vital signs (heart rate, respiratory rate, and temperature) should be monitored regularly. An increase in temperature should be noted, discussed with parents, and brought to the attention of the physician. Fever can signal an infection of the central line; fever can also increase fluid requirements.

Growth Parameters

Special attention should be given to assessing growth parameters (weight, length, and head circumference) and reporting changes to the physician. (Growth parameters are discussed more fully in Chapter 9.) As the child grows and gains weight, TPN, enteral feedings, medication, and hydration orders will need to be recalculated.

Intake, Output, and Hydration

Intake, output, and hydration status should be assessed on each visit. Daily intake records should be maintained by parents or other caregivers and reviewed by the nurse. Any trends (increase/decrease) should be noted. If the infant still has a functioning ostomy, the output should be closely monitored. Ostomy output can be measured or weighed, and a diaper can be weighed. This infant should be closely assessed for signs of dehydration and metabolic acidosis. Deviations from the expected normal intake and output for this infant should be noted, discussed with the parents, and brought immediately to the attention of the physician. A small infant with an ostomy is at grave risk for rapid dehydration.

Feeding Tolerance

In addition, it is important to assess the child during the TPN infusion, during the discontinuation of the infusion, and during the enteral feeding (if continuous) or at the end of the feeding (if bolus) for actual/potential problems. These times are valuable for evaluating the infant's ability to tolerate the high fluid delivery and changes in serum glucose.

Progression to oral feedings should be assessed, and oral-motor behaviors should be evaluated by an occupational or speech therapist if aversive oral behaviors are noted. Chapter 9 describes the assessment of feeding behaviors in detail.

Skin Care

Skin care is a significant concern for the infant with SBS, a central line, and gastrostomy. Skin around the vascular access device needs to be assessed for infection. The color of the surrounding skin, any drainage, or tenderness should be noted. Care of the site should follow agency or institutional protocol compatible with instruction received by the parents.

If the infant has ostomies, the bag should periodically be removed and the peristomal skin assessed. Any skin irritation and breakdown requires close monitoring to prevent a progression to systemic infection. The use of a different appliance, and stoma-adhesive paste and powder, may be of assistance; an enterostomal therapist should be available for consultation as needed.

Skin at the enteral feeding site should also be examined. Often the infant with short bowel syndrome has a small stomach due to the continuous feedings and lack of bolus enteral feeds. If peristomal gastrostomy drainage is a concern after bolus feeding, it may simply be that the stomach is too small to hold the volume of feeding. Stomach capacitance will increase over time. If stomach drainage is a problem, several techniques may be of assistance: the feeding can be slowed down, so as to infuse over a greater amount of time; the infant can be fed right side down with the head of the bed raised at least 45°; and the volume of postfeeding water flushes can be minimized. Any drugs that are given in the enteral feeding tube may be able to be spaced, so that postmedication water flushes are spread throughout the day. Chapter 10 provides further information on skin care and other needs of the child requiring tube feedings.

Prior to reanastomosis of the bowel, the surgeon may recommend perianal skin preparation. This may include placing stool (the ostomy output) in the diaper of the infant to prepare the perianal skin for feces. If parents consider that procedure distasteful, then some surgeons will recommend "roughing up" the perianal skin by rubbing it with alcohol or a rough, air-dried wash cloth. Alternatively, barrier creams such as Ilex can be used. Skin care is a very important aspect of care in the infant after reanastomosis, and adequate preparation will help to minimize the problems. High stool output after reanastomosis increases the risk of perianal skin breakdown.

THE FIRST HOME VISIT

Family Priorities

On the first home visit, the nurse should ask the family what they see as their needs and care priorities. Possible questions to ask include, "What is the most important concern that I can help you and your family with?" and "What are your expectations of home care?" The family members' assessment of their own needs may change over the first 4 to 6 weeks of home care, as they increase in comfort and confidence in the care of their child.

Physical Assessment

All aspects of the physical assessment described for the routine home visit should be part of the first home visit. The well-baby care needs of the infant should be emphasized; the nurse can be available to assist parents in understanding and providing for the general care needs of this special infant (see Chapter 8).

Safety Measures and Emergency Preparations

Another primary concern on the first home visit is to ensure that basic safety measures and emergency care plans are in place. The care priorities for a child on parenteral and enteral nutrition should address:

- the risks of hypo/hyperglycemia
- fluid and electrolyte imbalances/disturbances
- risk of dehydration due to high stool output/vomiting
- skin care needs
- nutritional provision
- central venous and enteral access devices
- the signs and symptoms of infection.

Parents should be knowledgeable about these areas and about how to respond to potential problems. If parents need review, a learning contract between the nurse and parents can be established with learning needs, contracted teaching times, and outcome measures defined. A home visit should be scheduled in the near future to ensure that parents do not go without essential skills and information for the care of their child.

On the first home visit, emergency protocols and the plan to notify support personnel are also reviewed. Rehearsal of responses to emergency situations—such as a fractured CVL or accidental removal of the gastrostomy tube—should be conducted. A bag of the TPN solution should accompany the child on any visit to the emergency department; this enables the physician to know the TPN prescription should hospital admission be necessary.

Supplies and Equipment

The nurse should ascertain that all essential supplies and equipment are available in the home. An "emergency bag" should be available at all times, kept both near the infant's crib and in the diaper bag or a "fanny pack" for use on trips outside the house. Contents of the emergency bag are described in Exhibit 11–4.

On the first home visit, all equipment should be checked for proper functioning. The presence of trouble-shooting manuals for any equipment and a 24-hour number for the durable medical equipment (DME) distributor should be ensured. The equipment should also be checked for functioning alarms: the alarms should be loud enough to hear throughout the home or an intercom or baby monitor should be used to ensure parents and other caregivers can hear the alarms at all times.

Depending on the age of the infant or young child, and the presence of other children in the home, a tamper-proof panel should be setup to prevent accidental change of pump settings by curious hands. Usually, such a panel can be provided by the pump manufacturer or supplier.

Parents should be informed that in case of pump malfunction, the DME company should have personnel on call to assist in troubleshooting any problem. Parents and the nurse should know how long the child can go without parenteral feeds before problems with hypoglycemia arise.

For the infant with SBS requiring continuous enteral feedings, a method of gravity feeding can be used as a back-up if the enteral feeding pump fails. The enteral feeding pump should be checked, as some enteral pump systems do not allow for a gravity drip option. As with parenteral feeds, parents should know how long their child can go without enteral feedings before problems with hypoglycemia would arise.

TPN Solution

The nurse should ensure that parents and other caregivers are familiar with the infant's prescribed TPN solution. The

Exhibit 11–4 Contents of CVL Emergency Bag

• CVL clamp	• a 10 mL syringe
• replacement caps for catheter ends	• normal saline for CVL flushing
• gauze	• G tube
• tape	• packaged handwipes with disinfectant

parenteral solution will come from the infusion company weekly, and parents should be able to state the delivery schedule. Storage of TPN, medications, and additives should be in a clean, refrigerated space. If the infant requires continuous infusion of the TPN solution, there should be a back-up plan in case the solution is not delivered on time or a bag ruptures. Generally, a bag of IV fluid of the same dextrose concentration as the TPN preparation can be used; this should be kept available in the home at all times. Parents should know how long their child can go without parenteral feedings before developing problems with hypoglycemia.

SUBSEQUENT HOME VISITS

Assessment of the Infant

On each subsequent home visit, it is important for the nurse to assess the infant's nutritional intake, evaluating both the parenteral and enteral intake. The actual intake, documented by parents or other caregivers, should be compared with the prescribed intake to ensure the delivery of appropriate nutrition.

Growth parameters should be obtained regularly. It is important to communicate changes to the physician so that as the child gains weight, caloric intake and medication doses are increased appropriately.

Progressing to Oral Feeds

The readiness of the child to progress to oral feeds is determined by several factors:

- intestinal tolerance of increased enteral nutrition
- tolerance of bolus feeds
- the ability to take oral feedings.

A multidisciplinary team effort will ensure a thorough assessment of readiness, and a physician's order is required to begin or increase oral feeds. The progression to oral feeds is incremental and individual. It may proceed as 10 cc today, 20 cc next week, and 60 cc next month.

As with any child who is technology dependent and has had a long hospital stay, developmental and feeding milestones should be addressed periodically. Introducing pureed foods at the appropriate developmental moment helps to minimize texture refusal behaviors. It also adds pectin, which is known to help with diarrhea. For the child with nutritional complications, it is especially important periodically to review feeding techniques with the family and encourage them to continue efforts to develop the infant's oral-motor skills. As necessary, the nurse can observe the infant's feeding behaviors. (See complete description of a feeding assessment in Chapter 9.) Observations should be discussed with the family. The family can be assisted as necessary in arranging appointments with a speech or occupational therapist to assess or intervene further with the infant in the development of oral feeding skills. Any plan to introduce oral feedings must be a multidisciplinary effort because of the many complex and interrelated concerns for this child.

Long-term Concerns

There are three long-term concerns in the care of the infant with SBS: bacterial translocation and overgrowth, increased susceptibility to infection, and nutritional deficiencies. The home care nurse should observe for them as follows.

Bacterial Overgrowth

Bacterial overgrowth should be considered in the child who previously tolerated feedings with adequate weight gain but now experinces bloating, cramping, diarrhea, and GI blood loss. The symptoms of bacterial overgrowth may be similar to those of Crohn's disease with frank ileitis or colitis. Bacterial overgrowth causes malabsorption and increases the overall risks of infection. The physician should be notified if bacterial overgrowth is expected. The diagnosis will be made by a breath hydrogen test and/or by aspiration and culture of intestinal fluid. Treatment is with broad-spectrum antibiotics. Antimotility agents should be avoided during treatment for bacterial overgrowth.

Infection

The infant with SBS should present a high index of suspicion for infection if febrile, suddenly not tolerating enteral feedings, exhibiting lethargic or irritable behavior, demonstrating a sudden change in oral intake, or having an increase in output for no apparent reason. Careful assessment of the CVL is necessary, as bacterial overgrowth may "leak" gastrointestinal bacteria into the bloodstream and place the infant at a greater risk for infection. The physician should be notified immediately if infection is suspected.

Nutritional Deficiencies

Nutritional deficiencies associated with SBS and long-term TPN include iron, calcium, magnesium, copper, phosphorous, vitamins A and D, and zinc. Vitamin B_{12} is absorbed solely in the ileum and in the case of extensive ileal resection, vitamin B_{12} shots may need to be given monthly. When enteral feedings are started, there may be a loss of bicarbonate, and supplementation may be required. Once parenteral nutrition has been discontinued, malabsorption of the fat-soluble vitamins may occur. When TPN is discontinued, the pediatric GI team may no longer be following a child, and community pediatricians may be unaware of the need to monitor malabsorption. The home care nurse should educate parents about this possibility so that they can ensure appropriate laboratory monitoring as necessary.

Health Maintenance

Health maintenance needs in the infant with complex medical problems are often overlooked (see Chapter 8). The subspecialists may be used as the primary physician, and the family may need to be encouraged to seek out and utilize a pediatrician. The coordination of appointments may be necessary, since the family may need to see several subspecialists on a regular basis. One goal of home care for such a family may be to encourage family members to become case managers of their child. The nurse should be aware that taking on case management tasks is a process that takes time, assistance, and mentoring. When achieved, the family is confident in coordinating and providing the total care needs of the child.

ONGOING CONCERNS

Financial Concerns

The multiple stressors on the family of a technology-dependent child require creative and supportive interventions. Financial stress is a main factor for most families. Supplies and equipment are costly, and even if the insurance is compensating for most care, the additional out-of-pocket expenses for utilities, supplies (increased diaper needs due to diarrhea, skin care products, ostomy supplies), and transportation to physician visits can be stressful, especially if combined with lost wages due to missed time from work. Consultation with the hospital social worker or clinical nurse specialist who is aware of the available community resources may be helpful in developing a creative care plan that will provide some financial support, reallocation of resources, and family respite. (See Chapter 7.)

Promoting Normalization

While the above stressors are a continual reminder that this child is different, the family can be assisted to focus on promoting "normal" growth and development. (See Chapters 19 and 20.) Oral-motor and feeding skills have been compromised and often require specialists to ensure optimal development. It is not uncommon for children with SBS to have severe oral/feeding aversions and require intervention from a multidisciplinary feeding team.

Speech, occupational, and physical therapists are extremely helpful in assisting the family to focus on appropriate childhood activities. The infant can enjoy bath time and water play, as do all infants. Most surgeons will allow the child to swim in a pool (but not ocean, pond, or lake water as the bacterial count is much higher) after the CVL cuff has healed and the tract is secure. Encouraging the family to participate in infant stimulation and developmental programs will have benefits for the infant and may provide a period of supportive respite for the family. As the infant develops, parents will eventually have an opportunity to view their child as one who is growing and developing and who just happens to have short bowel syndrome and special nutritional needs.

REFERENCES

Amarnath, R.P., Fleming, C.R., & Perrault, J. (1987). Parenteral nutrition in chronic intestinal diseases: Its effect on growth and development. *Journal of Pediatric Gastroenterology and Nutrition, 6*(1), 89–95.

Bendorf, K., & Lyman, B. (1993). Transition from the hospital to the home for the infant requiring total parenteral nutrition. *Journal of Perinatal and Neonatal Nursing, 6*(4), 80–90.

Crummette, B., & Boatwright, D. (1991). Case management in inpatient pediatric nursing. *Pediatric Nursing, 17*(5), 469–473.

Czyrko, C., Delfin, C.A., O'Neill, J.A., Peckham, G., & Ross, A.G. (1991). Maternal cocaine abuse and necrotizing enterocolitis: Outcome and survival. *Journal of Pediatric Surgery, 26*(4), 414–421.

Dann, A.I. (1994). Central line sepsis in children with gastrointestinal disorders. *Gastroenterology Nursing, 16*(6), 259–263.

Dorney, S.F., Amant, M.E., Berquist, W.E., Vargus, J.H., & Hasalle, E. (1985). Improved survival in very short small bowel of infancy with use of long-term parenteral nutrition. *The Journal of Pediatrics, 107,* 521–525.

Duffy, L., Kerzner, B., Gebus, G., & Dice, D. (1989). Treatment of central venous catheter occlusions with hydrochloric acid. *Journal of Pediatrics, 114*(6), 1,002–1,004.

Grant, J.A., & Kennedy-Caldwell, C. (1988). *Nutritional support in nursing.* Philadelphia, PA: Grune & Stratton.

Hennessy, K. (1989). Nutritional support and gastrointestinal disease. *Nursing Clinics of North America, 24*(2), 373–382.

Huddleston, K.C., Ferraro-McDuffie, A., & Wolfe-Small, T. (1993). Nutritional support of the critically ill child. *Critical Care Nursing Clinics of North America, 5*(1), 65–78.

Orr, M.E. (1989). Nutritional support in home care. *Nursing Clinics of North America, 24*(2), 437–456.

Purdum, P.P., & Kirby, D.F. (1991). Short-bowel syndrome: A review of the role of nutrition support. *Journal of Parenteral and Enteral Nutrition, 15*(1), 93–101.

Rombeau, J.L., & Rolandelli, R.H. (1987). Enteral and parenteral nutrition in patients with enteric fistulas and short-bowel syndrome. *Surgical Clinics of North America, 67*(3), 551–571.

Testerman, E.F. (1989). Current trends in pediatric total parenteral nutrition. *Journal of Intravenous Nursing, 12*(3), 152–162.

Thompson, J. (1994). Management of the short bowel syndrome. *Gastroenterology Clinics of North America, 23*(2), 403–416.

Warner, B.W., & Zeigler, M.M. (1993). Management of the short bowel syndrome in the pediatric population. *Pediatric Clinics of North America, 40*(6), 1,335–1,350.

Weber, T., Tracy, T., & Connors, R.H. (1991). Short bowel syndrome in children. *Archives in Surgery, 126,* 841–846.

Werlin, S.L., Wyatt, D., & Carnitta, B. (1994). Effect of abrupt discontinuance of high glucose infusion rates during parenteral nutrition. *Journal of Parenteral and Enteral Nutrition, 124*(3), 441–445.

Wise, B.V. (1992). Neonatal short bowel syndrome. *Neonatal Network, 11*(7), 7–16.

Zahr, L., Heflin, H., LaRosa, P., & Damian, F. (1992). The short bowel syndrome: An update and a case study. *Journal of Pediatric Nursing, 7*(3), 189–195.

ADDITIONAL RESOURCES

DePotter, S., Goulet, O., Colomb, V., Lamour, M., Corriol, O., & Ricour, C. (1994). Longterm home parenteral nutrition in pediatric patients. *Transplantation Proceedings, 26*(3), 1,443.

McFarlane, K., Bullock, L., & Fitzgerald, J.F. (1993). A usage tool of total parenteral nutrition in pediatric patients. *Journal of Parenteral and Enteral Nutrition, 15*(1), 85–88

Rombeau, J.L., & Caldwell, M.B. (1990). *Clinical Nutrition: Enteral Tube Feedings.* Philadelphia, PA: W.B. Saunders.

Rosenfield, R. (1994). *Your child and health care.* Baltimore, MD: P.H. Brooks.

Wesley, R., & Corran, B. (1992). Intravenous nutrition for the pediatric patient. *European Journal of Medicine, 1*(3), 212–230.

Criteria for Selection of a Pump

Pump selection can greatly affect the compliance and effectiveness of the nutritional therapy. In evaluating which infusion devices are best for the child and family, the following criteria should be considered.

COSTS OF ENTERAL/PARENTERAL PUMPS

Enteral feeding pumps are usually significantly less expensive than parenteral pumps and should be used for the enteral feeding so as to minimize the potential for hooking up the enteral feed to the parenteral pump. If the parenteral pump is used for enteral feeding, then the tubing will be adaptable for the parenteral pump, and a grave error could be made (Huddleston, 1993).

SIZE

How large is the pump? Does it need to be on an IV pole, or can it sit on a table-top or be attached to a wagon?

WEIGHT

How heavy is the pump? Can a mother or nurse carry both the child and the pump?

PORTABILITY

How moveable is the pump? This is an important consideration especially if the child requires infusions for 20 hours/day.

ALARMS

Usually all parenteral infusion devices are similar, but check enteral pumps for dose limit and total volume alarms.

INFUSION RATES

Most parenteral infusion pumps will infuse at low rates, but check the enteral pumps to make sure the infusion rates can be increased in 1 cc increments for the small infant. Clarify with the physician the anticipated rate of feeding progression.

POWER SOURCE

Assess the battery back-up life, and evaluate the family's need for electric versus battery power.

COMPLEXITY OF USE

How easy is the pump to use? Can the family be taught to troubleshoot problems with the infusion device? Is there a 24-hour phone number, or will there be a knowledgeable staff person to answer any questions?

SERVICING

Is there a 24-hour service technician available? How long would it take to replace the pump in the home if there were a malfunction?

DELIVERY SYSTEMS

Could the tube feeding system be used without the pump? This feature can be helpful to free the family of the machine as bolus feedings are begun. Is there a "run-away" flow precaution for the parenteral infusion device?

RELIABILITY

It is important to "field-test" infusion pumps. Hospital biomedical technicians may be aware if any complaints have been noted regarding a particular device.

INSTRUCTIONS

Are the instructions clear? Are they appropriate for the family: reading level, language translation, clear use of pictures and diagrams?

SUPPLIER

If the nurse and family feel a specific pump would be best for the family (e.g., a small ambulatory pump for continuous TPN feeds or the pump used in the hospital), the supplier should be notified, as they often have access to different devices.

Source: Courtesy of Kathi Huddleston, RN, MSN.

Appendix 11–B

Home Care Plan: The Infant Requiring TPN

Name _____   Case Manager/Clinical Nurse Specialist _____

Date _____   DOB _____

PROBLEM: TPN

GOALS/OBJECTIVES	METHODS	STAFF/REVIEW
Will receive prescribed nutrition to achieve adequate nutrition	Obtain weight; chart on graph. Monitor I&O; notify physician of excess output (> 20 cc/kg/day). Administer TPN/gastric feedings, and assess parental ability to administer. Monitor labs. Observe for signs and symptoms of obstruction. Observe for cholestasis/liver failure. Provide oral stimulation.	
Will recieve prescribed hydration and be at minimal risk for dehydration fluid/electrolyte imbalance	Observe for dehydration. Monitor stool output (< 20 cc/kg/day). Monitor electrolytes. Administer antimotility/antidiarrheal as prescribed. Monitor for metabolic acidosis. Evaluate procedure for administration of TPN as needed, and assess child's response to TPN. Evaluate procedure for enteral and oral feedings, and observe as needed to assess child's response to feeding.	
Will remain infection-free	Assess vital signs daily, including temperature. Assess vulnerability to infection (immune and nutritional status). Assess for s&s of infection. Inspect skin around CVL, G-tube, ostomy, and perianal area.	

GOALS/OBJECTIVES	_METHODS_	_STAFF/REVIEW_
	Perform and model good hand-washing. Provide strict aseptic technique in CVL and avoid invasive procedures and breaks in the infusion system. Obtain cultures as ordered. Evaluate nutrition/hydration. Minimize exposure to infectious disease. Evaluate for bacterial translocation.	
Maintain skin integrity	Wash buttocks/perianal area and dry well with each diaper change. Assess skin care needs frequently. Change diapers frequently. Apply ointments/lotions as needed. Ensure adequate nutrition and vitamin mineral supplementation.	
The child will gain weight, height, and head circumference and developmental milestones	Monitor TPN and enteral feedings to ensure prescribed nutrition. Monitor growth parameters. Monitor laboratory parameters. Monitor developmental milestones. Consult with speech/occupational/physical therapy prn. Encourage family involvement and control of total care.	
Caregivers demonstrate competency with supplies and equipment	Assess knowledge of supplies and equipment, observe equipment use, teach/reinforce as needed. Evaluate for safe use of equipment. Ensure that safety/emergency measures are known by all caregivers. Ensure that health care resources are posted and utilized as needed. Assess knowledge of how to troubleshoot pump alarms. Assess plans for emergency care, interventions, notification.	

Source: Courtesy of Kathi Huddleston, RN, MSN.

Part IV

Respiratory Concerns

One Mother's Experience

Karen D. Dixon

Our son, David, was born August 4, 1983. He was premature, born at 28 weeks. He weighed 2 lb 7½ oz. It is frightening when your baby is born so early because you don't know why . . . or what the chances are he'll survive . . . or what his problems will be if he does survive.

David was born with immature lungs and required a tracheostomy, ventilation, and oxygen. He also had Pierre Robin syndrome (small chin and a complete cleft palate). He ended up staying 5 months and 9 days in the hospital.

When he came home, everybody came to see him, but they all shied away when I had to do his care. Before he came home, people would look at pictures of him and say, "He's so cute," but when he came home they didn't want to get near him. Friends and relatives gave me a lot of verbal support, but when I brought David to them they got glassy-eyed and would say, "No, I don't want to hold him—he's too small." Yet if any other baby came into the room, everybody would fight to be first to hold it. This was very frustrating to me. I cried over it many times. It is better now, though. Many of my friends have learned his care.

When David came home, I felt ready for him. I had been at the hospital every day or two and had gone through so much training in the nursery. (My husband, though, felt he shouldn't come home until he was more stable.) David came with the tracheostomy, a gastrostomy tube, lots of medicines, and all the equipment. I wasn't too concerned, though, because I knew the monitor would tell me if this or that went wrong . . . and I had learned all the care.

What was different, though, was having all the equipment and supplies in our apartment. At first we had the monitor; a suction machine; an air compressor; an aerosol machine; medicines; and catheters, tubing, and other supplies. Later, we also got oxygen. You see, a baby's dresser is usually decorated with baby items. My baby's is decorated with medical machines. I'd rather have lotions and powders instead of distilled water—but I had to have my own nursing station.

The other important thing about the equipment has been to keep it clean and have it always working. This is very time-consuming. Even the littlest things can make it work improperly. For example, the filter on the back of the air compressor needs to be cleaned every week. One time the compressor stopped working. I had the mechanic out here with a new machine before I realized I had forgotten to wash that filter. It was so embarrassing!

Well, David had been home for 3 weeks. He had been to see the doctor, and the nurse had been to visit once or twice each week. But in that third week, he became seriously ill, so we rushed him to the hospital. This kind of thing happened many times. It often gave me feelings of guilt. I thought I knew what I was doing, and he'd still get sick. I would think maybe there was something I did or didn't do that caused it . . . or I should have noticed it earlier. It helped a lot when the doctors or nurses would tell me that I didn't cause it. Sometimes, I would think he was getting sick and I'd take him to the hospital, but the doctors couldn't find anything . . . then, 2 days later he'd be sick, and they'd admit him. These babies with BPD [bronchopulmonary dysplasia] can get sick very easily, and mothers really know when something is wrong.

David's care has been a 24-hours-a-day job. At the beginning, it was helpful to have someone around just to watch David while I got organized to do all the little details of his care. It's also a good idea to have two or three people trained in the care so you can get a break now and then. Even when I finally get a break, get time to rest, I still feel uncomfortable, as if there were something I am supposed to be doing. For example, from 6 AM to 12 midnight David is getting medications or feedings or aerosol treatments at least every hour. He often needs suctioning in between. So all day I am very busy. Then when midnight comes, it is hard to fall asleep. Maybe by 3 AM I fall asleep. Then, I'm up again at 6 to start over. Even though he's been home for a year and a half, I still have this schedule.

His care is also demanding because I feel if I make a mistake, I risk his getting sick. For example, he was getting potassium. The dose was 3 cc twice a day. I read the bottle. It said 6 mEq.* For some reason, trying to be exact, I gave him 6 cc twice a day. When I found out, I was really upset. I was lucky he didn't OD on it.

I have had some nurses to take care of him, and that is very helpful. Still, it takes a lot of time to train them to do things the way you want them done for your baby. And if a nurse is sick and another one comes as a replacement, you have to start the training all over again. Some nurses have been really good with him, though.

Caring for a child like David can be a strain. It is very time-consuming, and both parents can get very tired and end up annoyed at each other because of the care they have to do for the baby. It also puts a limitation on your social life. You have to arrange anything you do for yourself between what the baby needs done (like feedings and medications). You have to be careful of the conditions you expose him to, so you can't take him everywhere you might want to go.

Another strain is the uncertainty. Once when David was in the hospital with a serious respiratory infection (from respiratory syncytial virus), the doctors and nurses held an important meeting with us. They told us he was doing very poorly and might not live. After that meeting, I went up to David's room and cried. Then I yelled at him to get himself together . . . and I prayed to God, saying we wanted to have David with us longer. The next morning, the doctor called me on the phone and said, "I don't know what you did to that boy, but he's looking much better today."

Another big uncertainty is his development. I have a goddaughter a year younger than David. When she was 6 months, she was sitting up. At that time, David was 1½ years old and was still lying there. It really hurt to see that. All parents look forward to the time when their babies walk. I knew that sitting up was a goal for David. Finally, when he was 16 months old, he sat up. Then he saw more, imitated more, played more, and developed much more quickly. He has found his own way of doing things. At 2 years, he is just starting to walk around, holding onto things . . . just beginning to express himself verbally (with his finger over the tracheostomy hole) . . . and although he still has the gastrostomy tube for feeding, he is starting to sample flavors. He is really fun now. At 14 months, his developmental scores ranged from 2 to 8 months. Now he is 2 and they are much higher. He'll be in school (a special program) in the fall, and I think he'll progress rapidly. The doctors are talking about maybe taking his "trach" out soon, too.

Working with David for the past 2 years has been very time-consuming, and I haven't had much time to myself. But it can't be all bad because I am due to have another baby any day now!

*6 mEq of potassium chloride is equivalent to 3 cc.

Cleaning Respiratory Equipment

Revised by Angela Jerome-Ebel, RN, MSN

Maintaining clean respiratory equipment is essential in preventing respiratory infections. A routine schedule of cleaning and disinfection is important, and the guidelines presented here are recommended for most respiratory equipment used in the home.

A cardinal principle is, of course, to clean equipment in a clean area. Cleaning should not be done under an open window or after vacuuming because of the risk of contaminating equipment with dust in the air. The sink should be thoroughly cleansed with a scrub brush prior to use. Hands should be washed before cleaning equipment. The screen-trap filter on the sink can be a breeding ground for Pseudomonas and should be removed.

While white vinegar can be used to disinfect equipment, Control III is the most widely used disinfectant for home care equipment. Insurance companies will often cover the cost of Control III but do not usually pay for vinegar. Control III comes as a concentrated liquid; one bottle will generally serve a family for several months. To prepare, 30 cc of concentrated Control III are mixed with 1 gallon tap water. (Families generally purchase two large several-gallon drums with lids to use for the Control III solution and rinse water.) Once mixed, the solution can be used for 14 to 15 days. Prior to cleaning equipment, the solution is checked with a test-tape that comes with the concentrate.

Dirty equipment is first rinsed, then soaked in Control III for at least 20 min, and finally rinsed in a fresh water bucket. All apparatus, after it is disinfected and allowed to dry, should be stored in jars or plastic bags to prevent contamination between uses.

RESUSCITATION BAG AND NEBULIZER

The outside of the resuscitation bag and nebulizer should be cleaned daily. Weekly, all parts should be disassembled; washed in warm, soapy water; disinfected; rinsed thoroughly; air dried; and reassembled. Resuscitation bags on "standby" and not used should be cleaned monthly. Disposable resuscitation bags that do not come apart should be replaced every 6 months.

SUCTION APPARATUS

If catheters are to be reused, aspirate saline through after each use; store in a clean, dry towel or bag; and use for no longer than 2 to 6 hours. Then, soak used catheters in warm, soapy water, and rinse well. A large syringe can be used to force water through the catheter. Every 2 days, soak the catheters in half-strength white vinegar solution or Control III for 20 min to disinfect, rinse thoroughly, and air dry.

The collection bottle contents should be emptied daily, and the bottle cleaned daily and disinfected weekly. To clean, aspirate warm, soapy water from a jar through the connecting tube, followed by warm, clear water. The collection bottle should then be washed in warm, soapy water, rinsed, and air dried. To disinfect, Control III or white vinegar can be used.

The connecting tubes, bottles, and rubber stopper should be washed daily in warm, soapy water and rinsed and should be disinfected weekly. To disinfect, fill the bottle with half-strength white vinegar or Control III, insert connecting tubing and used catheters, and soak the apparatus for 20 min, followed by a thorough rinse and air drying.

TRACHEOSTOMY TUBES

If plastic tracheostomy tubes are reused, the tube and obturator should be washed first with a mild soap with no lotion additives. Hydrogen peroxide can be used to remove crusted mucus. However, plastic tubes should not be soaked longer than 10 to 15 min in hydrogen peroxide, as the solution takes the "plastic" softness out of the tubes, leaving them brittle. If a pipe cleaner is used, care should be taken not to scratch the tube. After rinsing, the tube can be soaked in a half-strength white vinegar solution for 10 min, rinsed well in sterile water, and allowed to air dry. Alternatively, recent research (Jerome, McDonald, Tucker, Rogers, & Strope, 1991) suggests that soaking trach tubes in hydrogen peroxide and cleaning with a nonlanolin-based soap and tap water may be sufficient to prevent bacterial contamination.

If metal tracheostomy tubes are used, the inner cannula should be removed and cleaned daily with hydrogen peroxide and a small brush or pipe cleaner. Each week, the tracheostomy tube, inner cannula, and obturator should be cleaned with hydrogen peroxide and a small brush or pipe cleaner. Following this, sterilize by boiling the tube, jars, and lids for 10 min in a porcelain, Pyrex, or stainless steel pot. Remove apparatus from the pot, taking care to touch only the flange of the tracheostomy tube and the outside of the jars and lids. Allow to air dry. When it is dry, store the tracheostomy tube in a sterilized jar. Sterilize the tube again just before using.

VENTILATOR APPARATUS

The humidifier jar (e.g., cascade) and the tracheostomy swivel from the ventilator should be cleaned with Control III three times a week. The remainder of the circuit should be changed and cleaned weekly. This includes the ventilator tubing, water traps, and exhalation valve. To clean, completely disassemble the apparatus; wash in warm, soapy water; and rinse thoroughly. Then, soak overnight in Control III or half-strength white vinegar solution, and rinse thoroughly. Allow to air dry. Alternatively, after a first washing with warm, soapy water, ventilator apparatus can be disinfected in the dishwasher. Set tubes in the upper rack with their ends facing down, secure small pans to prevent floating during the wash and rinse cycles, and place the humidifier jar in the lower rack facing down. Regular dishwashing detergent and a normal wash cycle can be used. Thoroughly dry tubing by attaching to the aspirator or compressor for several minutes, followed by air drying. Ventilator tubing can be hung to dry over the shower curtain rod.

REFERENCE

Jerome, A.M., McDonald, K.K., Tucker, E.Z., Rogers, B., & Strope, G.L. (1991). Reusing tracheostomy tubes in ventilator-dependent children. *Respiratory Care, 36*(11), 1,286.

Chapter 12

Home Care of the Infant with Respiratory Compromise

Revised by Dorothy Page, MSN, RN-C

This chapter discusses principles and procedures applicable to respiratory compromise of any etiology. However, the general principles are illustrated by frequent reference to bronchopulmonary dysplasia, a lung disease commonly associated with prematurity.

DESCRIPTION OF THE PROBLEM

Many preterm infants are born with lungs insufficiently developed for ventilation and oxygenation. These infants may require mechanical support and supplemental oxygen. However, due to these life-saving measures, the lungs are subjected to high airway pressures and high concentrations of oxygen over a prolonged period of time. In the lung tissue of premature infants, these treatment modes can cause pathophysiologic changes, leading to diminished pulmonary function. The resulting complex of pathologic changes in the lungs of these infants is called *bronchopulmonary dysplasia* (BPD). The risk of BPD increases with lower birth weight and gestational age (Parker, Lindstrom, & Cotton, 1992). New therapies, such as surfactant, steroids, and high-frequency ventilation, have altered the picture of children with BPD. However, the overall incidence of BPD has changed little over the past 25 years due primarily to the survival of smaller infants (Abman & Groothius, 1994).

The changes of BPD do not occur all at once. Changes that occur in the lung over time can include anatomic changes, resultant physiologic changes, and ultimately alter-ations in pulmonary function. In some cases, the pulmonary disorder can also lead to cor pulmonale. Even when the lungs are growing and new portions develop, pulmonary physiology and function can remain abnormal. Some studies suggest that most children who have BPD will have abnormal findings on chest radiographs and/or pulmonary function tests into young adulthood (Blayney, Kerem, Whyte, & O'Brolovich, 1991; Northway, 1990, 1992). However, we have yet to see how the new generation of extremely premature infants, who have been subjected to new therapies, will fare as adolescents and young adults.

In planning home care for an infant with BPD, the following problems, for which summary treatment descriptions are provided, may need to be addressed.

Inflammation of Large and Small Airways

The use of nebulized bronchodilators may be necessary. The use of oral bronchodilators at home may not work as well as inhaled forms and may be associated with unpleasant side effects. Occasional use of steroids at home may be anticipated for the treatment of inflammation (Abman & Groothius, 1994; Bhutani & Abbasi, 1992; Ng, 1993).

Hypoxemia

Short- or long-term oxygen therapy may be required. (See Chapter 14.) Since the advent of the pulse oximeter, oxygen can be safely adjusted from the home care setting with pre-scribed guidelines. (See Appendix 12–A for description of the pulse oximeter.) Although there is no clear-cut standard for an optimum pulse oximetry reading, a reading in the 92% to 99% range is considered acceptable (Abman & Groothius, 1994; Bhutani & Abbasi, 1992; Cunningham, McMillan, & Gross, 1991; Hay, Brockway, & Eyzagueirre, 1989).

Retained Secretions

Chest physical therapy, suctioning, positioning, and humidity may be indicated treatments for retained secretions.

Infections

Infants with BPD may develop severe debilitating ill-nesses from respiratory viral illnesses, especially respiratory syncytial virus (RSV), adenovirus, and influenza virus. RSV is the most frequent pathogen, causing rapid progression from tachypnea and wheezing to hypoxemia and respiratory failure. The use of ribaviran, in the hospital setting, has altered the course of RSV for some children. Studies show that rehospitalization rates from viral respiratory infections in the BPD population range from 22% in the first 12 months of life (Bhutani & Abbasi, 1992; Cunningham et al., 1991) to 50% during the first 2 years of life (Abman & Groothius, 1994). The subviron influenza vaccine is gener-ally recommended for children with BPD. (See Chapter 8.)

Cor Pulmonale and Fluid Retention

Treatment includes the administration of oxygen, digoxin, diuretics, and sodium chloride. Fluid restriction may be necessary and can complicate the challenge of pro-viding adequate caloric intake for the infant with BPD. (Cor pulmonale is discussed in more detail later in the chapter.)

Growth, Nutrition, and Feeding

Altered growth and nutrition may adversely affect lung growth and development (Frank, 1992). Generally, infants with BPD, who receive adequate levels of oxygen therapy and nutritional support, grow at a constant rate (Groothius & Rosenberg, 1987). However, circumstances such as poor tolerance of dense formulas, fluid restriction, reflux, and oral aversion can complicate the child's progress (Abman & Groothius, 1994; Bhutani & Abbasi, 1992).

Neurodevelopmental Outcome

The incidence of neurologic and developmental abnor-malities among infants with BPD is variable, depending on many factors including gestational age of the infant, hospi-tal course, posthospital "wellness," and developmental ex-periences. Estimates of the incidence of cerebral palsy (CP) and neurodevelopmental problems range from 9% to 27%, depending on the population studied (Hack et al., 1994; Koops, Abman, & Accrso, 1984). Although the incidence of CP in very low birth weight (VLBW) infants with lung dis-ease is higher than among those without lung disease, neu-rological problems may be a result of extreme prematurity and are not necessarily related to lung disease (Luchi, Ben-nett, & Jackson, 1991).

HOSPITAL DISCHARGE AND TRANSITION TO THE HOME

Collaborative Process

The family and caretakers of the infant with respiratory compromise must be actively involved in all aspects of deci-sion making in the infant's transfer from the hospital to home. Prior to discharge, a coordination meeting should be held in which general guidelines are established that delin-eate both lines of responsibility and education needed and at which a potential discharge date is set. (See Chapter 5.) The attendees at this meeting should be the parents and care-givers, the hospital discharge team, pediatrician, primary home care nurse, durable medical equipment representa-tives, and specialty services. The parents should be encour-aged to invite a parent advocate to assist them if they feel that would be beneficial. A case manager to oversee the exe-cution of the plan, to assist the family in their advocacy for the child, and to help the family achieve independence in care of the child, should be assigned on mutual agreement.

Developing the Home Care Plan

The population of infants being transitioned from hospi-tal to home are much more fragile than they were 10 years ago. Several factors have influenced this trend: changes in medical technology, enabling the survival of increasingly premature infants; parental desire to have their infants home; payers' willingness to cover costs of home services; and the home care industry's development of safe, easy to operate home equipment. As a result of increasingly fragile infants going home, many infants now receive some level of daily skilled nursing care in the home during a transition period. A well-developed home care plan will assist the family through the transitions as the level of care for the infant changes. (See sample care plans: Appendixes 12–B and 12–C.)

The home care plan must reflect the individuality of the child and family and represent both the uniqueness of the home environment and the family's personal and cultural needs. The home care plan is a fluid document that reflects the changing needs of the child. It is vital that part of the care plan delineates how as well as when to transfer care entirely to the family. Termination of services is a reality for families and is dealt with better if discussed at the beginning of the home care experience.

Continuity of Care

Coordination between the parents, home care team, and the hospital staff is important to ensure continuity of care for the infant and family. The primary home care or community health nurse should obtain information about the infant's hospital course, baseline vital signs, discharge medications, care instructions, and plans for follow-up. In addition, information regarding parents' knowledge about the infant's condition and care, their level of confidence with providing care, and any further teaching and support measures recommended by hospital staff can assist in development of an appropriate home care plan.

Emergency Preparations

Coordination prior to discharge is also important to ensure that emergency preparations have been made. One important emergency preparation is having a telephone in the home. If a telephone cannot be obtained, an alternate plan for getting help in an emergency should be made. For example, if a neighbor is available during the day, the infant can be "football carried" to the neighbor's home during cardiopulmonary resuscitation (CPR), and the rescue squad called by the neighbor. It must be stressed, however, that this plan is not optimal, and every effort should be made to obtain a telephone in the infant's home. Creative solutions can be found to almost any dilemma. Occasionally, a charitable organization may pick up the cost of a pay phone in the home, so that the family will not be isolated. Also, a local telephone company may be willing to put in "911-only" telephone service.

The family members and caregivers should take a CPR course prior to discharge. It is helpful to have an emergency plan worked out in advance should the child need to be transported rapidly to a medical facility. Other preparations include making ready a bag of the infant's supplies and medications needed for a 24-hour period, providing parents with a summary of the child's most recent hospital stay, and listing all medications (including concentrations and dosages) and emergency telephone numbers. (See Exhibit 12–1.) It is also helpful to have the family members preplan who will care for the other children, who will be a backup in case the parent cannot drive, and the route they will travel at different times of day. They must be assisted to think through the

Exhibit 12–1 Emergency Telephone Numbers List

Post this information near each telephone in the home:
Rescue squad number _____
Fire department number _____
Emergency facility number _____
Location _____
_____
Physician number: Day _____
Evening _____
Physician name _____
Nursing agency number _____
Primary care nurse _____
Equipment supplier number _____
Contact person _____
Electric company emergency
number _____
Home address _____
_____
Nearest intersection _____
Home telephone number _____

possible events that may affect either care at home or emergency services (i.e., loss of power, snowstorm, etc.).

Another emergency preparation involves notification of community services that the family needs to be on a priority service list. These services include telephone, electricity, oil/gas company, department of public works, the family's local outpatient emergency medical service (EMS), pediatrician, local emergency department, and fire and police department. A copy of a sample notification letter should be given to the parents. The letter to the utility agencies should state the expectation that they will notify the family of any anticipated interruptions of service. Similarly, personal contact with rescue squad and emergency facility personnel accompanied by provision of written information can help to ensure prompt and appropriate emergency interventions, if necessary. Appendix 12–D contains sample form letters that can be used for each of these notifications.

Additional emergency precautions include posting CPR guidelines at the infant's bedside and a list of emergency telephone numbers and other important information near all telephones in the home, as shown in Exhibit 12–1. The home address and closest intersection or cross street should be included in case a nurse or babysitter must make an emergency call or parents panic and forget.

Other Issues

Prior to discharge, the family members should be able to perform competently all aspects of the care required for their infant or child. Additionally, several topics must be discussed with the family to ensure preparation for home care.

It can be most helpful for families if this information is put in writing. These topics include traveling with the infant (what, when, how, as well as a trial test for suitability of the car seat), infection control, developmental needs of the child, day care issues, primary pediatrician and specialist physicians (who to call for what), potential of rehospitalization, and anticipatory guidance regarding issues that arise from the multitude of services the child may require (i.e., who's in charge? I have no privacy! and others).

Parent-to-parent contact is vital as the family faces the challenges ahead. Parents can be informed of any pertinent local support groups. Some parents might benefit from individual contact with one or two other families in similar circumstances. Some parents may choose not to contact other parents or attend group meetings for a variety of reasons. However, most families do want to be included in receiving any newsletter or similar communication that may be available.

ROUTINE HOME VISITS

Assessment of the Infant

Vital Signs

On every home visit, temperature, pulse, and respiratory rate should be obtained and recorded. If there has been a concern regarding growth, hypertension, or fluid retention, then it is appropriate that the nurse also evaluate the head circumference, blood pressure, and weight. For the child with oxygen concerns, a pulse oximetry reading should be done at a variety of times, which will capture the total picture of the infant's oxygenation. Each infant will have unique baseline values for these vital signs. It should be noted that the respiratory and heart rate may increase after feeding, with changes in position, with activity or crying, and with fever. The respiratory rate and pulse will usually be lower during sleep times. The pulse oximetry reading may fluctuate during times of activity, sleep, and feeding. Often, oxygen saturation will drop during these times, but for some infants, it may increase. However, vital signs or pulse oximetry readings above or below the infant's baseline values, when not attributable to activity or emotional stress, may signify respiratory or cardiac compromise. It is the nurse's role to assist the caregivers in learning assessment of the infant as well as the importance of the vital signs. There will come a time that the family will need to assume the total care of the child and that preparation is best done from the start, particularly if they live in a rural area far from medical assistance.

Auscultation

Lung auscultation should be performed on each home visit. The stethoscope should be placed directly and firmly on the skin of the infant's chest to avoid the sound of skin or clothes rubbing. Auscultation should proceed from side to side and from top to bottom over the anterior, posterior, and lateral chest wall areas. Auscultation from side to side allows comparison of sounds in one lobe or area with those in the contralateral lobe or area.

The general quality of breath sounds, as well as the presence or absence of adventitious sounds, should be noted, as indicated in the following descriptions:

- *Quality*—During auscultation, the lengths of the inspiratory and expiratory phases should be compared. With BPD, the expiratory phase may be relatively prolonged. Decreased breath sounds and poor movement of air, in any or all lobes, may signal distress.
- *Adventitious sounds*—All lobes of the lung should be auscultated to assess for wheezes, rhonchi, and rales; these sounds are described in Table 12–1. Wheezes may be noted in the infant with hyperreactive airways disease and may be more pronounced during an exacerbation. Rhonchi are common in the infant with BPD and may signify increased or thickened secretions. Rales may signify pneumonia or edema and fluid overload.

Table 12–1 Adventitious Lung Sounds Common in BPD

Sound	Description
Wheezes	Continuous sounds or vibrations produced by airflow through smaller airways that are narrowed by constriction, mucosal swelling, secretions, and so on Generally high-pitched More prominent during expiration, but may also be heard during inspiration If mild, may clear with coughing
Rhonchi	Continuous sounds or vibrations produced by airflow through larger airways that are narrowed by mucosal swelling, secretions, and so on Generally low-pitched More prominent during expiration, but may also be heard during inspiration If mild, may clear with coughing
Rales	Discrete, discontinuous, bubbling sounds produced by moisture in the airways May be fine or coarse Usually heard during inspiration, and sometimes only in the dependent portions of the lung. (Note that in the infant, the dependent areas may not necessarily be the lower lobes.) If mild, may clear with coughing

Source: Compiled from *A Guide to Physical Examination*, 2nd ed., by B. Bates, p. 134, Lippincott-Raven, © 1973.

Some disagreement exists among published definitions of the terms *wheezes, rhonchi,* and *rales.* Therefore, for the purpose of effective communication with physicians and others involved in the care of the infant, it is important that the nurse use a consistent system of nomenclature and be able to describe clearly the adventitious sounds noted.

Each infant will have some unique characteristic lung sounds; auscultation during several visits will allow the establishment of a relative baseline. If caregivers desire, they can be taught to auscultate the lungs and to differentiate lung sounds.

Signs and Symptoms of Respiratory Distress

Signs and symptoms of respiratory distress should also be assessed on each visit. The infant's alertness and level of activity are important indicators of overall status. Retractions, nasal flaring, pallor, cyanosis, edema, or diaphoresis may signal distress. Irritability and loss of appetite should also be noted. Caregivers should be instructed to look for these signs and symptoms; they should also be given guidelines, developed in conjunction with the physician, identifying circumstances that require medical advice.

Respiratory Secretions

In addition, on each home visit, the infant's respiratory secretions should be assessed for amount, consistency, color, and odor. An increase in amount or viscosity of secretions, a yellow-green color, or a foul odor may signify infection. Caregivers should be instructed to contact the infant's physician should they notice any of these changes. (Measures that can be taken to limit the risk of infection are discussed later in this chapter.)

Medication Regimen

A further aspect of the infant's care that should be explored on each home visit is the medication regimen. Medications commonly used in the treatment of BPD are listed in Table 12–2. The nurse should regularly question the parent about and observe the infant for any medication side effects. Parental awareness of the purpose of each medication and of medication side effects is also important. Written information may assist caregivers in learning and remembering these details.

THE FIRST HOME VISIT

The first home visit may be scheduled for the day the infant arrives home or within 1 to 2 days thereafter. It is helpful to call or visit the caregiver after the first night at home with the child to provide support and problem solving and to assess when to make the next visit. If the home transfer of the infant is to be successful, it is important that the caregiver does not feel abandoned or left without resources.

Each visit to the infant's home should open with concern for the caregiver and how the caregiver is managing. Is he or she able to get out or away from the child at all? Are the services delivering supplies on time? How is the child doing?

On the first home visit, all aspects of the routine home visit should be addressed. In addition, parental provision of safe and appropriate care of the infant with respiratory compromise must be determined. Particular areas to address include medication administration, nebulized medications, chest physical therapy (CPT), and suctioning.

Medication Administration

On the first visit, and subsequently as necessary, all medications should be reviewed. Infants with BPD (or other respiratory compromise) may be on any combination of bronchodilators, digoxin, diuretics, electrolytes, and steroids. (See Table 12–2.) The dose and concentration on each bottle should be carefully compared with those prescribed. Since small errors can have a significant effect on an infant, the parents' ability to measure prescribed doses correctly should also be assessed. In this connection, labeling syringes for each medication with a piece of tape marking the dosage line can often aid in ensuring accuracy.

Medication schedules should also be reviewed with parents on the first home visit. Schedules may be complex since some infants with multiple problems may be on as many as 10 to 12 medications a day. Medication schedules at home should be tailored, as much as possible, to the family's daily schedule; minimizing nighttime doses and grouping medications at several times during the day can be very helpful. If the schedule is still unreasonable, it may be appropriate to help the parent to ask the physician to consider altering the frequency of doses or perhaps eliminating some medications if the infant has been stable for some time. Some parents may be assisted by a medication checklist, as illustrated in Exhibit 12–2.

Nebulized Medications

Parental techniques for administering nebulized medications should also be assessed, and the appropriate technique reviewed as necessary. Nebulized medications can be administered through a hand nebulizer or an electrically powered compressor. The compressor will provide the prolonged administration time that may be most effective in the very narrow airways of the infant.

For administration of nebulized medications with a compressor, the medication is inserted into the cup with the prescribed diluent, and the mask, T piece, or other delivery device is attached. The tubing is then attached to both the nebulizer and the source of air or oxygen. Baseline values

Table 12–2 Medications Used in the Home Management of BPD

Medication[a]	Use	Common Side Effects
Bronchodilators	For bronchospasm or hyperreactive airways disease (several bronchodilators may be used in combination)	
Xanthine derivatives (oral) Aminophylline Theophylline		Irritability, insomnia, palpitations, tachycardia, nausea, vomiting, anorexia
Beta-Agonists (oral, inhaled) Metaproterenol Terbutaline Albuterol		Insomnia, nervousness, tremor, palpitations, tachycardia (all side effects are transient with inhaled preparations); oral preparations may aggravate gastroesophageal reflux
Anticholinergics (inhaled) Atropine Ipratropium Bromide (Atrovent)	May be used in conjunction with or as a substitute for Beta-Agonists	Dry mouth, may irritate cough (If inadvertently sprayed in eyes, may irritate eyes or have transient visual effects)
Anti-inflammatories Cromolyn sodium (inhaled)	Improves lung function—not well studied for BPD	Rare—increased bronchospasm
Steroids (oral, inhaled)	Enhanced adrenergic response, may decrease severity of BPD	Irritability, hypertension, infection, growth alteration, gastric irritation
Digitalis	For cor pulmonale complicating BPD	Fatigue, muscle weakness, agitation, anorexia, nausea, cardiotoxicity
Diuretics Furosemide Chlorothiazide Hydrochlorothiazide Spironolactone	For fluid retention with cor pulmonale	Dehydration, electrolyte imbalances
Electrolytes	For electrolyte replacement during diuretic therapy, as indicated (sodium and potassium are those commonly required)	
Sodium		Gagging (because of taste), vomiting
Potassium		With overdosage leading to hyperkalemia, cardiotoxic effects, as well as nausea, vomiting, and abdominal pain

[a]For specifics on a particular medication, or for full range of side effects, contraindications, and drug interactions, consult the *Physicians' Desk Reference*.

for vital signs are obtained for the purpose of comparison with values obtained both several minutes after commencing treatment and when concluding treatment. (In general, a pulse of more than 230 in infants, or more than 200 in older children, or persistent tachycardia indicates a need to contact the physician.) The treatment may stimulate bronchospasm and cough. If the infant cannot clear secretions, it may be appropriate to stop the treatment and let the child rest and/or suction him or her. The treatment is continued until all of the solution has been inhaled, generally for 7 to 12 min. The bronchodilator is usually mixed with 2 cc of normal saline; more diluent will only prolong the treatment. If the infant is also receiving oxygen, the oxygen and the nebulized medication may be delivered simultaneously.

Chest Physical Therapy

In addition to giving medications to the infant with BPD, parents may be asked to provide regular CPT to ensure that secretions are not retained in the lungs. On the first home visit, the nurse should observe the parents while they administer CPT and, as necessary, should provide instruction in the appropriate positions, techniques, and schedule. Discussion followed by demonstration and parents' return demonstration may facilitate optimal routine performance of CPT. Accurate positioning during CPT is necessary to encourage the drainage of secretions from each lobe of the lung. (Positions are illustrated in Figure 12–1.) Percussing, or clapping with a cupped hand, will assist in loosening secretions;

Exhibit 12–2 Sample Weekly Medication Checklist

TIME	MEDICATION	SUN	MON	TUES	WED	THURS	FRI	SAT
6 AM	Quibron 5.5 cc							
	Metaprel Aerosol 0.15 cc in 2.5 cc NS*							
7 AM	Aldactazide 1.5 cc							
	Sodium Chloride 10 cc							
11 AM	Quibron 5.5 cc							
	Prednisone 3 mg							
	Ammonium Chloride 4 cc							
	Phenobarbital 4 cc							
12 NOON	Metaprel Aerosol 0.15 cc in 2.5 cc NS							
3 PM	Sodium Chloride 10 cc							
	Potassium Chloride 3 cc							
5 PM	Quibron 5.5 cc							
6 PM	Metaprel Aerosol 0.15 cc in 2.5 cc NS							
11 PM	Quibron 5.5 cc							
	Prednisone 3 mg							
	Ammonium Chloride 4 cc							
	Phenobarbital 4 cc							
	Aldactazide 1.5 cc							
	Sodium Chloride 10 cc							
12 MN	Metaprel Aerosol 0.15 cc in 2.5 cc NS							
*NS = normal (physiologic) saline								

percussing for 1 min in each position is generally recommended. CPT is provided as frequently as needed to clear secretions, usually after nebulizer treatments, before feeds, or both. CPT should be more frequent if the infant has a cold or respiratory distress with either increased or more viscous secretions.

Suctioning

Suctioning is another important component of care for the infant with BPD or other respiratory compromise. Caregivers' suction techniques should be assessed for both adequacy and safety, and instructions should be offered as necessary in appropriate techniques. If the infant is unable to clear his or her secretions, suctioning following CPT and nebulizer treatments may be indicated. In addition, suctioning should be done when secretions fill the oropharynx or nasopharynx; when secretions increase in amount or viscosity; when the presence of fluids is audible; or when the infant exhibits either respiratory distress or poor color. For some infants, a bulb syringe will be adequate for suction-

ing (see Figure 12–2). For this procedure, the syringe is squeezed before insertion into the nose or mouth and then slowly released to withdraw secretions. The syringe should be cleaned with a saline solution between each use.

Many infants will need deeper catheter suctioning to remove secretions. If a suction machine is in the home, its proper functioning should be determined on the first home visit. For this procedure, the catheter is first connected to the machine and then inserted gently into the oropharynx with no suction applied. The catheter is inserted only to the depth of the posterior oropharnx. (It is often helpful to hang up a suction catheter near the child's bed with a mark delineating the point to which the catheter may be safely inserted for that particular child.) Suction is applied with gentle rotation and slow withdrawal of the catheter for no more than 5 sec; harsh suctioning is avoided because of potential bleeding and tissue damage. The infant should be allowed at least three to five breaths, and color should be regained, between each pass of the catheter. The catheter is cleaned with saline between each pass, and suctioning is repeated until the oropharynx is clear. To maintain stable oxygenation, no more than three passes of the catheter

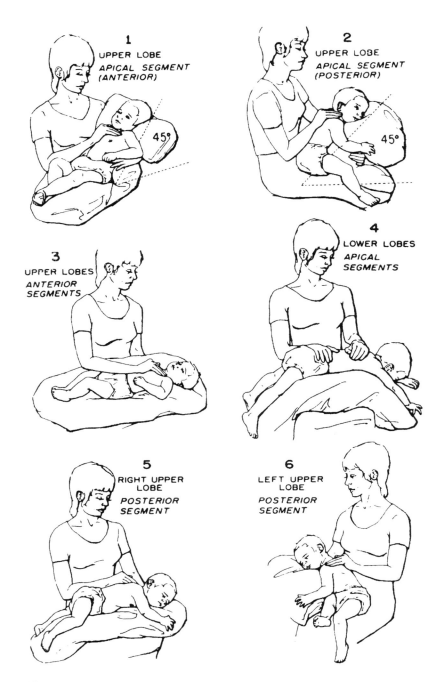

Figure 12–1 Chest Therapy Positions

should be used. The procedure may be repeated for the nasopharynx. A DeLee, or mouth, suction device should always be available in case of electrical failure, and caregivers should understand its use, as well as that of the suction machine. (The DeLee device is illustrated in Figure 12–2.)

SUBSEQUENT HOME VISITS

The initial weeks after hospital discharge are generally the most anxiety provoking for parents of an infant with res-

piratory compromise. Bonding may have been disrupted owing to prolonged hospitalization; degree of concern for the infant's safety and health is high; and fear of making mistakes in the infant's care is pronounced. Encouragement and support by the nurse during the initial weeks at home can help to build confidence in parents.

Home visits begin by addressing any problems or concerns identified by parents. It is helpful to ask open-ended questions that may trigger the caregivers' concerns. Parental concerns and needs must be addressed, or teaching will not be accomplished effectively. The nurse should use this opportunity to review the teaching care plan with the family

(continues)

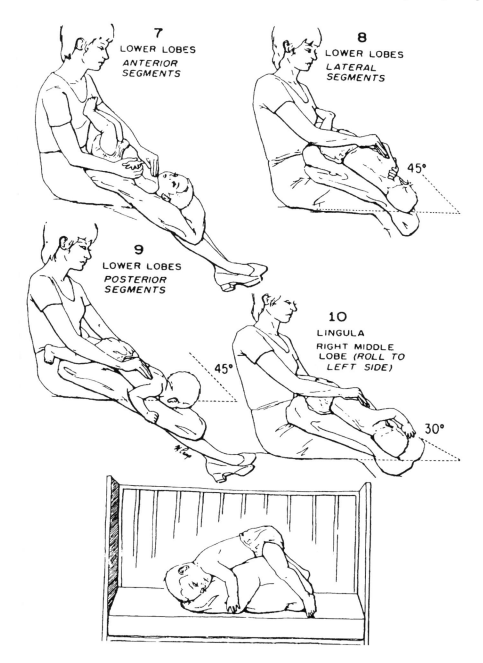

Figure 12–1 continued

Source: Courtesy of the University of Michigan Hospitals, Physical Therapy Division, Ann Arbor, Michigan.

and make additions and changes as determined by the family's needs. The plan should address not only those areas described for the first home visit and routine visits but also the following specific aspects of care: risk of infection, respiratory distress, general knowledge about BPD, nutrition and growth, and developmental issues.

Risk of Infection

Infants with BPD are at high risk for frequent infections throughout their first 1 to 1½ years of life, particularly if the disease is moderate to severe. This risk should be discussed with parents, in part to eliminate or minimize unnecessary guilt if rehospitalization does become necessary. In addition, simple principles for limiting the risk of infection can be reviewed. All caregivers, including the home care nurse and parents, should receive the yearly flu vaccine. Once the infant is 6 months old (chronological age), he or she can receive the flu vaccine. For the first dose, the vaccine is given in two divided doses. Only the split virus is given to children.

Other principles of infection control include: requiring meticulous hand-washing for anyone coming in contact with

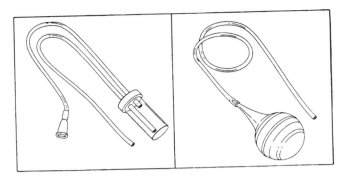

Figure 12–2 Portable Mouth Suction and Bulb Syringe

Source: Reprinted from *Home Care of Your Child with a Tracheostomy: A Parent Handbook* by P. Hennessy (Ed.), p. 9, with permission of Children's Hospital National Medical Center, Washington, D.C., © 1983.

the infant, limiting the infant's exposure to persons with an upper respiratory infection, avoiding crowds, and cleaning respiratory care equipment regularly and thoroughly (as discussed in the Special Issue, "Cleaning Respiratory Equipment"). Should the caregiver have an upper respiratory infection the advice should be: good hand-washing, limited face-to-face exposure with the child, and the wearing of a mask.

Of course, nurses should advise parents to observe the infant routinely for early signs of an infection: a change in secretions, respiratory pattern, or respiratory rate; irritability; a change in oxygen saturation; and a loss of appetite. The physician should be notified if these signs are observed.

Respiratory Distress

The nurse should also assist parents in assessing their knowledge of the signs and symptoms of respiratory distress: tachypnea, nasal flaring, retractions, tachycardia, grunting, wheezing, and cyanosis. Signs and symptoms should be reviewed as necessary, and, as discussed earlier in this chapter, caregivers should be given guidelines detailing what signs and symptoms indicate the need for medical consultation. Plans for emergency interventions should be assessed and assistance provided as necessary in developing appropriate plans.

As part of emergency planning, CPR technique should be reviewed regularly. Verbal recall is best supplemented by caregiver demonstration to ensure correct technique.

General Knowledge Related to BPD

Teaching on subsequent home visits should also be directed toward helping parents become knowledgeable about their infant's condition. Their knowledge of pulmonary anatomy and physiology and of the pathophysiol-

ogy, clinical manifestations, and clinical course of BPD, as well as the reason for each intervention (e.g., chest physiotherapy, suctioning), should be assessed. Any gaps in knowledge or understanding can be filled by teaching that includes discussion, drawings, written materials, and repetition, as necessary. In general, a knowledgeable caregiver is a more confident caregiver.

Nutrition, Growth, and Development

Nutrition and growth are often problem areas for infants with BPD. The nurse should perform an assessment of nutritional intake as well as growth parameters on all home visits (see Chapter 9). Because of the work of breathing, as well as feeding difficulties that may result from respiratory compromise, ensuring adequate calorie intake to promote growth may be a challenge. Parents will often be very concerned about poor growth patterns. The nurse should both assure them that slow growth is not uncommon with BPD and assist them to do whatever possible to encourage optimal nutritional intake in the infant. Chapters 9, 10, and 11 provide an in-depth discussion of nutrition and feeding. Breastfeeding is discussed in a Special Issue, "Breastfeeding the High-risk Premature Infant: Assessment and Management."

Encouragement and Support

Since many infants born prematurely will have developmental delays, it is important that the family be involved in an appropriate early intervention program. A screening assessment can be conducted by the home care nurse (see Chapters 19 and 20). The nurse can elicit information regarding the activities the infant is engaged in for developmental education, determine if the family feels the care is appropriate, and offer additional resources to the family if needed. At each visit, the nurse can offer praise and support for developmentally appropriate interventions that the family is using.

COR PULMONALE

Cor pulmonale is a form of heart disease in which the right ventricle becomes enlarged. Cor pulmonale can result from underlying pulmonary disease. Home care of the infant with cor pulmonale is based on plans for appropriate respiratory management, prevention of infection, and cardiac management. If cor pulmonale is present without congestive heart failure (CHF), cardiac management is aimed at reducing the overload of the right ventricle and improving its functioning. Diuretics, digoxin, and oxygen may be used, and fluid restriction may be necessary in some cases. The reader is referred to other resources for an indepth discussion of care of the infant with cardiac compromise. However, two aspects of care must be stressed here: (1) medication administration and (2) observation for signs and symptoms of CHF.

Exact measurement of medications is essential with infants owing to the small margin between therapeutic and toxic doses of both digoxin and diuretics. Observing parents administer medications on one or more visits provides the opportunity to access accuracy of dosage measurements. Unless the infant's cardiac condition is very unstable, it is generally unnecessary to have parents check the apical pulse prior to digoxin administration. However, guidelines for digoxin administration (see Exhibit 12–3) and signs of digoxin toxicity should be reviewed. In infants and young children, the earliest sign of digoxin toxicity is usually vomiting, often with a decreased appetite. The older child may complain of nausea. Although extracardiac signs can occur, they are less easily assessed in this age group.

The infant with cor pulmonale is always at risk of developing CHF. CHF occurs when the heart is unable to pump sufficient blood to the systemic circulation to meet the meta-

Exhibit 12–4 Clinical Manifestations of CHF

Cardiovascular	Respiratory
Tachycardia (sleeping, apical pulse of 140–160—infant)	Tachypnea
Precordial impulse	Dyspnea, orthopnea
Gallop rhythm	Retractions
Nasal flaring	Enlarged liver
Periorbital edema	Grunting respirations
Rapid weight gain	Fine rales
Peripheral cyanosis	Decreased pulse oxygen saturation level
Distended neck veins (rare)	

Related

Feeding difficulties, anorexia	
Diaphoresis	Irritability
Oliguria	Fatigability

Note: Some of these signs in isolation may resemble characteristics of the underlying respiratory problem; therefore, it is important to perform an overall assessment of the infant.

Exhibit 12–3 Guidelines for Administering Digoxin

1. Give digoxin at regular intervals, usually every 12 hours, such as 8 AM and 8 PM.
2. Plan the times so that the drug is given *1 hour before* or *2 hours* after feedings.
3. Use a calendar to mark off each dose that is given, or post a reminder, such as a sign on the refrigerator.
4. Have the prescription refilled *before* the medication is completely used.
5. Administer the drug carefully by slowly squirting it on the side and back of the mouth.
6. Do not mix it with other foods or fluids, since refusal to consume these results in inaccurate intake of the drugs.
7. If the child has teeth, give him water after administering the drug; whenever possible, brush the teeth to prevent tooth decay from the sweetened liquid.
8. If a dose is missed and more than 6 hours has elapsed, withhold the dose and give the next dose at the regular time; if less than 6 hours has elapsed, give the missed dose.
9. If the child vomits within 15 minutes of receiving the digoxin, repeat the dose *once*; if more than 15 minutes has elapsed, do not give a second dose.
10. If more than two consecutive doses have been missed, notify the physician.
11. Do not increase or double the dose for missed doses.
12. If the child becomes ill, notify the physician immediately.
13. Keep digoxin in a safe place, preferably a locked cabinet.
14. In case of accidental overdose of digoxin, call the nearest poison control center immediately.

Source: Reprinted from *Nursing Care of Infants and Children,* 2nd ed., by L.F. Whaley and D.L. Wong, p. 1325, with permission of Mosby-Year Book, © 1983.

bolic demands of the body. CHF can lead to, but is distinct from, true myocardial failure. Because of the risk of CHF, the nurse should observe for signs and symptoms at each home visit; these are listed in Exhibit 12–4. In addition, the nurse should assess parental knowledge of these signs and symptoms and then provide augmentative education as needed. Parents should also be instructed to seek medical attention at the first signs of CHF. Although mild CHF may be managed at home in some cases, CHF generally will require hospitalization during the acute phase.

ONGOING CONCERNS

Parents of the infant with BPD describe life after the infant's birth as a "roller-coaster ride." From birth, there is day-to-day uncertainty about the infant's survival, the need to digest complex information that can evoke terror, and emotions that run the range from joy to fear to guilt within a few hours. Coupled with this is the parental need to take care of themselves and perhaps other children, to work and sleep, and finally to resolve some of the issues so that they are not constantly living in a crisis. This "roller-coaster ride" does not stop once the parent takes the child home. In fact, the reality of the child's impairment may only become evident once the child is around other children who are healthy.

It is imperative to assist and support the family in developing realistic goals for the child. Although it is true that some infants may remain on oxygen or ventilatory support for years, and other children experience developmental sequelae, many children are able to wean completely from the oxygen over time. If developmental sequelae are present, for most children they will be mild and not handicapping (see Chapters 1, 19, and 20).

Many infants who have BPD continue to have some degree of airway obstruction and airway hyperreactivity as adolescents and young adults. This means that they will probably need to take "asthma-like" medications for symptomatic control. It is not currently known how the infants who are born today will fare in the future given both new therapies and the extreme prematurity of some of the survivors (Bhutani & Abbasi, 1992; Northway, 1992).

REFERENCES

Abman, S., & Groothius, J. (1994). Pathophysiology and treatment of BPD. *Pediatrics Clinics of North America, 41*, 277–314.

Bhutani, V., & Abbasi, S. (1992). Long term pulmonary consequences in survivors with BPD. *Clinics in Perinatology, 19*, 649–671.

Blayney, M., & Kerem, E., Whyte, H., & O'Brolovich. (1991). BPD: Improvement in lung function between 7–10 years of age. *Journal of Pediatrics, 118*, 202–206.

Cunningham, C., McMillan, J., & Gross, S. (1991). Rehospitalization for respiratory illness in infants less than 32 weeks gestation. *Pediatrics, 88*, 527–532.

Frank, L. (1992). Antioxidants, nutrition and BPD. *Clinics in Perinatology. 19*, 541–561.

Groothius, J.R., & Rosenberg, A.A. (1987). Home oxygen promotes weight gain in infants with BPD. *American Journal of Diseases of Children, 141*, 992–995.

Hack, M., Taylor, G., Klein, N., Eiben, R., Schatschneider, C., & Mercuri-Minich, N. (1994). School-age outcomes in children with birth weights under 750 gram. *New England Journal of Medicine, 331*, 753–803.

Hay, W., Brockway, J., & Eyzagueirre, M. (1989). Neonatal pulse oximetry: Accuracy and reliability. *Pediatrics, 83*, 717–722.

Koops, B.L., Abman, S.H., & Accrso, F. (1984). Outpatient management and follow-up of BPD. *Clinics in Perinatology, 11*, 101–122.

Luchi, J.M., Bennett, F.C., & Jackson, J. (1991). Predictors of neurodevelopmental outcomes with BPD. *American Journal of Diseases of Children, 145*, 813–817.

Ng, P.C. (1993). The effectiveness and side effects of dexamethasone in preterm infants with BPD. *Archives of Disease in Childhood, 68* 330–336.

Northway, W.H. (1990). Late pulmonary sequelae of BPD. *New England Journal of Medicine, 323*, 1,793–1,799.

Northway, W.H. (1992). An introduction to BPD. *Clinics in Perinatology, 19*, 489–495.

Parker, R.A., Lindstrom, D.P., & Cotton, R.B. (1992). Improved survival accounts for most but not all of the increase in BPD. *Pediatrics, 90*, 663–668.

ADDITIONAL RESOURCES

Hack, M., Breslau, N., Weissman, B., et al. (1991). Effect of very low birth weight and subnormal head size on cognitive abilities at school age. *New England Journal of Medicine, 325*, 231–237.

Schnapp, L.M., & Cohen, N.H. (1990). Pulse oximetry. *Chest, 98*, 1,244–1,249.

The Pulse Oximeter

Dorothy Page, MSN, RN-C

The principle of oximetry is based on Beer's law, which states that the concentration of an unknown solute dissolved in a solvent can be determined by light absorption. When a pulse oximetry probe is placed on any part of the body (e.g., finger, toe, etc.), light passes through that part. The majority of the light is absorbed by the connective tissue, skin, bone, and venous blood. The amount of light absorbed by these is constant and does not vary with the cardiac cycle. However, with each heartbeat, there is a small increase in arterial blood, which results in increased light absorption. The light source consists of two wavelengths: one for oxyhemoglobin and the other for reduced hemoglobin. The resulting ratio gives the oxygen saturation (Schnapp & Cohen, 1990).

Points to Remember

- The partial pressure of oxygen is not the same as the oxygen saturation.
- The pulse must correlate with the pulse oximetry reading, or the result will be incorrect.
- Movement can affect the reading.
- The use of the proper probe size is crucial to obtaining a valid reading.

REFERENCE

Schnapp, L.M., & Cohen, N.H. (1990). Pulse oximetry. *Chest, 98,* 1,244–1,249.

Appendix 12–B

Home Care Plan: Respiratory Compromise

Date _____   Case manager _____

Name _____   Hosp # _____   DOB _____

PROBLEM: **RESPIRATORY COMPROMISE**

GOALS/OBJECTIVES	METHODS	STAFF/REVIEW
Child to be at minimal risk for respiratory distress	Assess pulse and respiratory rate each visit. Auscultate lungs. Observe for signs/symptoms of respiratory distress. Assess for appropriate use of medications, including nebulized treatments if prescribed; review/teach as necessary. Assist caregivers in arranging a workable medication schedule. Assess for side effects of medications and teach caregivers the same. Assess caregivers' skill with chest therapy; teach/review as needed. Assess caregivers' skill with suctioning; teach/review as needed. Observe for signs of fluid retention. If fluid restriction prescribed, review daily fluid intake each visit. Teach caregivers reason for fluid restriction and signs of retention.	
Caregivers to verbalize an understanding of BPD	Assess knowledge of pulmonary anatomy/physiology, pathophysiology of BPD, clinical manifestations, and clinical course of BPD. Teach/reinforce as needed.	
Caregivers to verbalize signs/symptoms of respiratory distress and to have appropriate plans for intervention	Assess knowledge of signs/symptoms of respiratory distress. Teach/review as needed. Assess plans for emergency intervention and assist in developing as needed.	

GOALS/OBJECTIVES	METHODS	STAFF/REVIEW
	Ensure that phone and electric companies, rescue squad, and emergency departments are aware of child's status.	
	Assess caregivers' ability to provide CPR competently; teach/review regularly.	
	Review with caregivers the indications for calling doctor and/or rescue squad.	
Infant will be at limited risk for congestive heart failure	Assess pulse, pulse oximetry, and respiratory rate each visit.	
	Assess for signs and symptoms of cardiac failure each visit.	
	If medications prescribed, assess for appropriate use and observe for side effects/toxic effects.	
	Teach precautions to prevent infection and importance of early intervention if signs of infection develop.	
Caregivers will verbalize accurate knowledge of s/sx congestive heart failure	Assess knowledge and teach/review prn.	
Caregivers will be prepared for possibility of frequent hospitalizations	Educate and provide emotional support related to possible need for frequent hospitalizations.	
Caregivers will be involved in planning and directing child's care	Seek parental input. Offer names of community support agencies. Support parental advocacy attempts. Facilitate parent-to-parent support.	
Child to have regular and prn follow-up by physician managing pulmonary status	Encourage regular and prn appointments. Communicate/coordinate with managing physician(s) on a regular basis and as needed for problems.	

Source: Courtesy of Children's Hospital National Medical Center, Home Health Care Services, Washington, D.C.

Home Care Plan: Cardiac Compromise

Date _____   Case manager _____

Name _____   Hosp # _____   DOB _____

PROBLEM: **CARDIAC COMPROMISE**

GOALS/OBJECTIVES	*METHODS*	*STAFF/REVIEW*
Child will be at limited risk for cardiac failure	Monitor vital signs, and monitor for signs and symptoms of cardiac failure each visit.	
If medications prescribed, caregivers will demonstrate correct administration of medications, will state knowledge of purpose, side effects, and toxic effects	Monitor for side effects/toxic effects each visit. Assess caregivers for correct administration of prescribed medications. Stress critical nature of exact doses. Review medication schedule for appropriateness for family schedule. Assess knowledge of medications including purpose, side effects, and toxic effects; teach/review prn.	
Caregivers will verbalize accurate knowledge of signs/symptoms of cardiac failure	Assess knowledge and teach/review prn.	
Caregivers will state suitable plans for emergency intervention	Emphasize posting cardiologist phone number for easy access. Assess caregivers' plans for emergency intervention; assist in developing prn. Ensure that appropriate rescue squads/emergency rooms have been notified of child's status.	
Child will be at limited risk of infection	Teach caregivers that cardiac failure can be precipitated by an infection. Review precautions to prevent infection (avoid exposure to persons with infections, handwashing).	

GOALS/OBJECTIVES	METHODS	STAFF/REVIEW
	Stress the importance of early intervention should any signs of infection develop.	
Child will demonstrate acceptable growth patterns	Assess growth parameters and nutritional status on regular basis. Assess feeding patterns for use of soft nipple with large hole and small frequent meals; reinforce, if necessary. Establish schedule that fosters child's development within medical parameters. If persistent inadequate growth, confer with dietitian/pediatrician/cardiologist re: increased calories and/or tube feeding, prn.	
Child will have regular cardiology follow-up	Encourage regular appointments with cardiologist. Coordinate/communicate with cardiologist prn.	

Source: Courtesy of Children's Hospital National Medical Center, Home Health Care Services, Washington, D.C.

Appendix 12–D

Sample Notification Letters

Rescue Squad Notification

TO: Rescue Squad or EMT Unit		DATE: _____

_____
Address

_____

FROM: _____   PHONE: _____
Address
_____   DOB: _____

RE: _____
Child

_____
Parents

_____
Address

This child is at home in your catchment area.
The child named above has the following medical problem(s):

Medications:

Treatments:

Please verify above information with parents to determine if it is up to date.
The child's health care providers are:

_____   Phone: _____

_____   Phone: _____

_____   Phone: _____

In the event of an emergency, please transport the child to _____
Hospital. If this is not possible, please share the above information with the receiving hospital.

Thank you.

Source: Courtesy of Children's Hospital National Medical Center, Home Health Care Services, Washington, D.C.

Telephone Company Notification

TO: Telephone Company, Customer Services

_____

_____

FROM: _____   Telephone: _____

_____

_____

RE: _____   Billing Party: _____

Address _____

_____

Telephone _____

The child named above has a severe medical problem requiring continuous telephone service in the home.

This child should be placed on your priority list. In the event of anticipated interruptions of service, the parents should be notified beforehand. In the event of unexpected interruption of service, this family should have their service reinstituted on a priority basis.

Thank you.

Source: Courtesy of Children's Hospital National Medical Center, Home Health Care Services, Washington, D.C.

Electric Company Notification

TO: Electric Company, Customer Services

_____

_____

FROM: _____   Telephone: _____

_____

_____

RE: _____   Billing Party: _____

Address _____

_____

Telephone _____

The child named above has a severe medical problem requiring continuous electrical service for the following equipment:

This child should be placed on a priority service list. In the event of anticipated interruptions of service, the parents should be notified beforehand. In the event of unexpected interruption of service, this family should have their service reinstituted on a priority basis.

Thank you.

Source: Courtesy of Children's Hospital National Medical Center, Home Health Care Services, Washington, D.C.

Chapter 13

Home Care of the Infant on a Cardiorespiratory Monitor

Revised by Margie Farrar-Simpson, RN, MSN, CPNP

Infants may require apnea and cardiac monitoring as a part of the management of a variety of problems: respiratory compromise of various causes; tracheostomy use; a family history of sudden infant death; and documented bradycardia or apnea (see Exhibit 13–1). Apnea is relatively common in premature infants and will be discussed in some detail in this chapter. However, the principles and procedures related to use of the cardiorespiratory monitor are applicable when the monitor is used for any reason.

DESCRIPTION OF THE PROBLEM

Apnea

The American Academy of Pediatrics Task Force on Prolonged Apnea defines apnea as the "cessation of breathing for at least 20 seconds or as a briefer episode of apnea associated with bradycardia, cyanosis, or pallor" (American Academy of Pediatrics Task Force on Prolonged Infant Apnea, 1985, p. 129). Apnea has been observed in 25% of low birth weight (LBW) neonates; the incidence varies inversely with fetal maturity to as high as 84% in extremely-low-birth-weight (ELBW) neonates (Aranda et al., 1983).

Apnea can be classified as central, obstructive, or mixed. In central apnea, no movement of the abdominal or thoracic respiratory muscles occurs, and air flow is absent. In obstructive apnea, there is movement of respiratory muscles but no air exchange. Mixed apnea is a combination of cen-

tral followed by obstructive apnea. All three types of apnea can occur in premature infants as well as term infants.

A number of physiologic, metabolic, chemical, and other factors can contribute to or provoke apneic events (see Exhibit 13–2). Apneic episodes may be accompanied by bradycardia, a rise and subsequent fall in blood pressure, decreased peripheral blood flow, hypoxemia, and hypotonia. While sleep apnea is rarely fatal, prolonged apnea without intervention may lead to respiratory arrest, brain damage, and death.

Periodic Breathing

Apnea should be differentiated from periodic breathing, a frequent finding in premature infants. Periodic breathing is defined as "a breathing pattern in which there are three or more respiratory pauses of greater than 3 seconds duration with less than 20 seconds of respiration between pauses" (National Institutes of Health, 1987, p. 293). Periodic breathing is not usually associated with cyanosis or bradycardia but may be associated with hypoxemia. It is often benign.

Bradycardia

Recent research has demonstrated that bradycardia may precede or occur simultaneously with central apnea in infants who die of sudden infant death syndrome (SIDS).

Exhibit 13–1 Diagnoses That May Indicate the Use of a Home Cardiorespiratory Monitor in the Infant

- apnea of prematurity, if not resolved by hospital discharge
- apnea of infancy
- ALTE (apparent life-threatening event)
- BPD (bronchopulmonary dysplasia, on home oxygen)
- GER (gastroesophageal reflux) if symptomatic with color change and tone change
- ISAM (infant of substance-abusing mother) if clinically symptomatic
- sibling of SIDS victim
- infant with a tracheostomy

Source: Adapted from Policy TM:2 with permission of Children's Hospital National Medical Center, Washington, D.C., © 1991.

Exhibit 13–2 Factors That May Provoke Apnea or Bradycardia Events

- extreme immaturity
- hypoxia or hypoxemia related to airway obstruction, pulmonary disease, anemia, or congestive heart failure
- central nervous system (CNS) disorders including intraventricular hemorrhage (IVH), seizures, and other pathologic conditions
- metabolic alterations disturbing CNS metabolism, including hypoglycemia, hypocalcemia, hyperbilirubinemia, and acidosis
- infections (including colds) and fevers
- Valsalva maneuvers
- vasovagal stimulation (e.g., insertion of a feeding tube)
- thermal instability
- GER (gastroesophageal reflux)
- drugs (illicit/recreational) and some prescription medications

For this reason, prolonged bradycardia may itself be a factor in SIDS deaths (Kelly, Pathak, & Meny, 1991; Meny, Carroll, Carbone, & Kelly, 1994). Although the etiology of prolonged bradycardia is unknown, it may be preceded by hypoxemia or obstructive apnea or may result directly from impaired brainstem control.

ALTE

An apparent life-threatening event (ALTE) is defined as follows: "an episode that is frightening to the observer and is characterized by some combination of apnea (central or occasionally obstructive), color change (usually cyanotic or pallid but occasionally erythematous or plethoric), marked change in muscle tone (usually marked limpness), choking, or gagging" (National Institutes of Health, 1987, p. 293). These episodes frequently require prolonged, vigorous shaking or mouth-to-mouth resuscitation to restore breathing

(Brooks, 1992). Infants with a history of an ALTE should be managed similarly to infants with documented apnea. In 1986, the NIH Consensus Panel recommended that previously used terms such as *aborted crib death* or *near-miss SIDS* should be abandoned because they imply a possibly misleading close association between these types of episodes and SIDS (National Institutes of Health, 1987).

SIDS

Sudden infant death syndrome (SIDS) and apnea are not synonymous, although apnea may increase the risk of sudden death. SIDS is defined as "the sudden death of an infant < 1 year of age which remains unexplained after a thorough case investigation, that includes performing a complete autopsy, examining the death scene and reviewing the clinical history" (Willinger, James, & Catz, 1991, p. 681). Although no clear cause has been determined for SIDS, numerous factors have been associated with a higher risk of SIDS. These include the following: maternal, socioeconomic, ethnic, prenatal, perinatal, and postnatal factors; cigarette smoking during pregnancy and exposure to cigarette smoke in infancy; infections; gender (male infants are more frequently affected); hypoxia; impaired ventilatory control; altered breathing patterns; the prone position; and prematurity (Carroll & Loughlin, 1993).

MANAGEMENT OF APNEA AND SIDS RISK

The management of apnea and SIDS risk includes three components: (1) proper positioning, (2) cardiorespiratory monitoring, and (3) the assessment and restoration of breathing. Anyone caring for the infant should be trained in each of these management strategies.

Proper Positioning

Proper positioning of the sleeping infant is an important precaution in preventing SIDS and should follow the recommendations of the primary care provider and specialty physicians. Research in Europe demonstrated a strong relationship between prone positioning and SIDS (Dwyer, Ponsonby, Newman, & Gobbons, 1991). As a result of this research, in 1992, the American Academy of Pediatrics Task Force on Infant Positioning and SIDS recommended that "healthy infants, when being put down for sleep, be positioned on their side or back" (American Academy of Pediatrics Task Force on Infant Positioning and SIDS, 1992, p. 1,120). The exceptions to this recommendation included "premature infants with respiratory distress, infants with symptoms of gastroesophageal reflux, infants with certain craniofacial anomalies or other evidence of upper airway obstruction, and perhaps some others" (American Academy of Pediatrics Task Force on Infant Positioning and SIDS, 1992, p. 1,125). For the infant with symptomatic gastroesophageal reflux, the premature infant with respiratory compromise, and those with craniofacial or upper airway anomalies the prone sleep position is often recommended (American Academy of Pediatrics Task Force on Infant Positioning and SIDS, 1992; Willinger, Hoffman, & Hartford, 1994). When the prone position is recommended, it is *imperative* to discuss safe bedding with the parents and other caregivers. The optimal sleeping position for the premature infant has not been resolved (Willinger et al., 1994); however, physicians in several countries are recommending the supine position for premature infants at discharge. If the infant has gastroesophageal reflux, reflux precautions, including proper positioning after feedings, should be observed. Reflux precautions are described later in this chapter.

Cardiorespiratory Monitoring

Cardiorespiratory monitoring assists in alerting parents or other caregivers to episodes of apnea, bradycardia, and/or tachycardia, according to the prescribed boundaries placed on the monitor for that infant. (However, it is important to note that an apnea alarm will not be triggered by episodes of obstructive apnea unless accompanied by bradycardia.) Cardiorespiratory monitoring will be discussed in detail later in this chapter.

Assessment and Restoration of Breathing

Appropriate intervention is used to assess and, when necessary, restore breathing. Intervention ranges from assessment of shallow but normal breathing, to tactile stimulation for mild apneic episodes, to vigorous resuscitation for severe episodes lasting 30 sec or longer and/or accompanied by signs and symptoms of respiratory insufficiency. At some centers, infants with severe problems are sent home with a resuscitation bag, mask, and "stand-by" oxygen.

HOSPITAL DISCHARGE AND TRANSITION TO THE HOME

Coordination and Data Gathering

Coordination with hospital staff at the time of discharge from the hospital is important. The nurse should ascertain what cardiorespiratory monitor is to be used and learn the prescribed settings for the infant. The pattern of the infant's apneic episodes in the hospital (frequency, duration, associated symptoms, need for resuscitation, and precipitating factors) should be identified. In addition, the home care nurse should learn what the parents have been taught about apnea

and bradycardia, the infant's condition, use of the monitor, responses to monitor alarms, cardiopulmonary resuscitation (CPR), home recordkeeping, follow-up schedule, and criteria for discontinuing the monitor, as well as what fears and concerns parents have expressed. This information will enable appropriate planning for follow-up teaching and support. (A sample care plan and a home assessment form for cardiorespiratory monitoring are included in Appendixes 13–A and 13–B, respectively.)

Monitor Selection

The home care nurse may be asked to offer advice on the selection of an appropriate monitor and an equipment vendor. Today, the recording, or memory, impedance monitor is most frequently used. This type of monitor stores data on use and documents apnea, bradycardia, and tachycardia events. A strip, similar to an electrocardiogram (ECG) strip, can be printed, allowing the health care provider and the infant's caregiver to visualize apnea and bradycardia events and to differentiate true from false alarms. The memory feature can also be used to examine monitor usage (compliance). The memory monitor is considered the safest and most accurate approach for home monitoring. Other factors to consider in choice of a monitor are discussed in Appendix 13–C. Factors important in choosing an equipment vendor are listed in Exhibit 5–1.

Emergency Preparations

Before the infant is discharged from the hospital, it is important to ensure that emergency preparations have been made. These include the following (see Chapter 12 for greater detail):

- ensuring a telephone in the home
- placing the family on the priority service list with the telephone and electric companies
- notifying the local rescue squad and nearest emergency department of the child's health status and special needs
- posting CPR guidelines at the infant's bedside
- posting emergency telephone numbers, the home address, and the closest major intersection or cross street near the home telephone(s) (see Exhibit 12–1).

Transportation Plans

Plans for safely transporting the infant home should be reviewed step by step with the parents. The monitor should be used during transport since infants are often lulled to sleep by the vibrations in the car. Some rechargeable monitors can run at least 24 hours without an electrical outlet; a battery pack is available for other monitors. While most monitors used today are portable, if the monitor is not, parents should be instructed in how to hand-monitor. During transport, it is ideal to have one adult always available to attend to the infant should an apneic episode occur. Either the infant should be transported by cab or bus, or the parent should be accompanied by a relative or friend who will drive. However, in situations where there is only one adult, the following precautions apply:

- The infant's car seat should be placed in the front seat of the car—if there is no air bag on the passenger side of the car.
- The driver should drive in the right-hand lane, so that safe stopping is possible if resuscitation becomes necessary en route.
- Interstate highways or other high-speed roads should be avoided.

Around-the-Clock Contact

Because having a child at home on a monitor can be anxiety-provoking, especially during the transition to home, parents should know who can be contacted, on a 24-hour-a-day basis, if questions or problems arise with either the equipment or the infant's health. Parents should be assured that it is fine to call with any question no matter how trivial it may seem.

ROUTINE HOME VISITS

Certain aspects of assessment of the infant on a cardio-respiratory monitor must always be incorporated into the nurse's routine. At the same time, on any home visit, questions and concerns of the parents and other caregivers should receive priority attention. These questions and concerns will guide some of the assessment and teaching done by the nurse.

Assessment

Physical Assessment

On every home visit, the infant's pulse and respiratory rate should be obtained and documented. Respiratory patterns should be observed and documented. The infant's color, especially the presence or absence of pallor or cyanosis, should be observed and documented. The presence or absence of hypotonia, a sign of hypoxia, should be noted. If these signs are noted by parents or nurses persistently or

recurrently, a medical evaluation is indicated. Finally, the infant's skin should be examined in the area of the electrode patches for irritation and breakdown.

Alarms and Associated Symptoms

On each home visit, history of the frequency and duration of any apnea or bradycardia alarms should also be obtained. The infant's status during alarms, any preceding symptoms, and the degree of stimulation needed for arousal should also be reviewed. Parents should be encouraged to keep a complete record of all apnea and bradycardia events. A convenient form for this purpose is provided in Exhibit 13–3.

If the infant has GER, the frequency and amount of reflux should be noted on each visit. (See also Chapters 8 and 9.)

If a recording monitor is used, it will have a light-emitting diode (LED) display of the monitor settings that can be "called up." Each monitor will have a mechanism or procedure the nurse can use to assess the monitor settings and to adjust them as prescribed. The settings should match those prescribed for the infant and will need to be changed as the infant grows. A representative of the durable medical equipment supplier can instruct the nurse in reading the display for a particular monitor; programming instructions may vary among monitors.

Teaching

Color Changes

Since frequent, short apneic episodes, even those not severe enough to set off monitor alarms, can lead to hypoxia and subsequent pallor, cyanosis, and hypotonia, parents can best care for their monitored infant if well informed about what to observe and why. When the nurse is observing the infant's color, pallor and cyanosis can be described to parents and pointed out if noticed. At the same time, parents should be reassured about normal color changes related to sleep, feeding, room air temperature changes, and stooling.

Alarms

While reviewing the frequency of apnea and bradycardia alarms, the nurse should be aware that frequent alarms can be anxiety-provoking to parents. For each infant, the specific criteria for concern are determined in conjunction with the physician and should take into consideration the frequency, duration, and type(s) of alarms and specific associated symptoms. Parents should also be encouraged to telephone the nurse or physician any time they have concerns about the alarms or the infant's status.

Frequent alarms in the absence of any associated symptoms can be a nuisance to the family and may lead to noncompliance with monitor usage. The nurse and parents can discuss alarm frequency with the physician and, when ap-

Exhibit 13–3 Cardiorespiratory Monitor Event Form

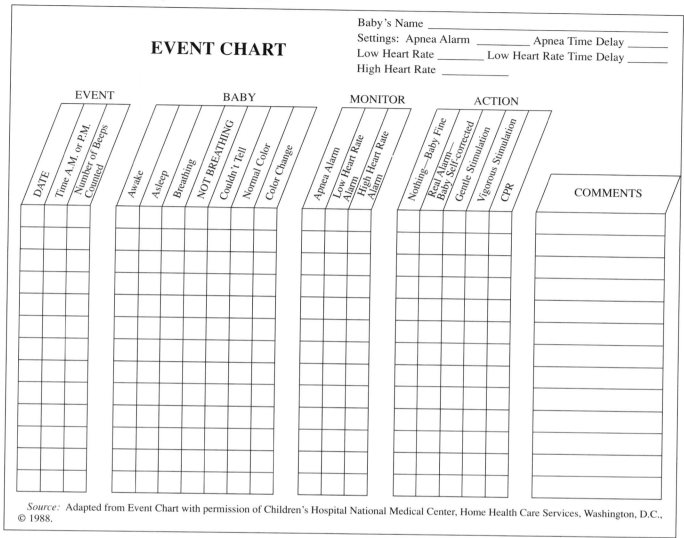

Source: Adapted from Event Chart with permission of Children's Hospital National Medical Center, Home Health Care Services, Washington, D.C., © 1988.

propriate, a change of alarm settings can be ordered to reduce the number of false, or true but trivial, alarms.

Appropriate responses to apnea, bradycardia, and false (or machine) alarms (described in detail in the section on the first home visit) can be reviewed as necessary. Parents and other caregivers should also be informed about factors other than serious apnea and bradycardia that can sometimes trigger alarms.

Bradycardia alarms may result from normal bradycardias caused by stretching, hiccupping, passing gas or a bowel movement, prolonged crying, and, in some cases, feeding. Frequent bradycardia alarms are of concern. They may signify the occurrence of many short apneas that are too short to be noted on the monitor but are leading to hypoxia. They can also be a sign of obstructive apnea, not directly detected by a cardiorespiratory monitor. As the infant grows older, the heart rate normally decreases, and increasingly frequent bradycardia alarms may indicate the need to change the monitor settings.

Apnea and bradycardia alarms may both be more frequent if the infant has a cold or fever. While this may be expected, an increasing frequency should alert the parents to potential major problems. Whether or not an increased frequency of apnea and bradycardia alarms is associated with immunizations is the subject of debate.

THE FIRST HOME VISIT

All aspects of routine home visits should be accomplished on the first visit. In addition, the nurse will want to review with parents the elements of safe and appropriate care for the monitored infant. Emergency precautions should be reviewed. Further, the equipment should be inspected and its appropriate use ensured. Both the rehearsal of responses to monitor alarms and a review of CPR procedures are additional components of a thorough first home visit.

Parental Assessment of the Infant

Parents' ability to assess accurately for pulse and respiratory movement can be ensured by instruction, demonstration, and return demonstration when necessary. Assessment of color and other characteristics can also be reviewed.

Safety and Emergency Precautions

Safety precautions for use of the monitor should be reviewed. These include the following:

- Never bathe the infant with the monitor on because of the risk of shock.
- Minimize the risk of strangulation by threading the monitor wires out the lower end of the child's clothing.
- For the older, active infant in a crib, the patient cable should be woven between the slats of the crib to reduce slack.

The nurse should also review emergency precautions with parents. These include the following:

- posting CPR guidelines near the infant's crib
- posting emergency telephone numbers and directions to the home (major cross streets/routes) near each telephone.

These precautions are described in more detail in Chapter 12.

Gastroesophageal Reflux

If the infant has gastroesophageal reflux leading to frequent vomiting, the nurse should review reflux precautions with parents. For some infants, feedings should be thickened with rice cereal. The infant should be held in an upright position during feedings, burped frequently, and not overfed. Finally, the infant should be positioned prone with shoulders higher than feet by 30° for 45 to 60 min after feedings. When the infant is placed prone, smooth, firm bedding should be used; the infant should not be placed on soft bedding such as a comforter or pillow. The frequency and amount of reflux should be noted on each visit. (See also Chapters 8 and 9.)

Equipment and Supplies

A systematic inspection of the equipment and supplies in the home is important on the first visit. First, since monitors differ in their sensitivity and controls, it is important to check that the monitor recommended in the treatment plan is the model actually in the home. In addition to the monitor, the following supplies should be available: lead wires (two sets minimum), disposable patches (four sets minimum), belt and permanent electrodes (optional), monitor manual with troubleshooting guide, and battery pack (optional). The monitor should be plugged into a grounded outlet, or a grounding adapter should be added. An extension cord should not be used.

It is also important to check the settings on the cardiorespiratory monitor. If there are other children in the home, the monitor should be kept out of their reach. A child-proof panel may be used to cover any knobs on the monitor so that curious fingers will not change the settings. (Panels are generally available from the manufacturer or supplier.)

The monitor should be placed on a hard surface at the infant's bedside with eight inches of ventilation space behind and above it. The monitor should not be placed on top of any other electrical equipment. It is important to ensure that the monitor alarms can be heard throughout the home; if they cannot, either a remote alarm or an inexpensive intercom system is recommended.

Electrode Placement

Electrode placement is also important to observe on the first visit. Electrodes should be placed symmetrically, as indicated in Figure 13–1. The electrodes may be repositioned

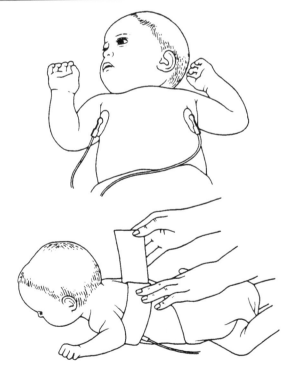

Figure 13–1 Placement of Monitor Electrodes

Source: Reprinted from *Home Care and Rehabilitation in Respiratory Medicine* by C.W. Bell et al., p. 261, with permission of Lippincott-Raven, © 1984.

to prevent skin breakdown, but they must always contact the sides of the chest wall in order to sense the movement of breathing. Electrodes should be replaced as their attachment becomes less secure and at least every 2 days. To prevent inaccurate monitoring, an electrode belt should not be used until the infant weighs more than 8 lb to 10 lb.

Responses to Alarms

As preparation for emergencies, parents should be confident in their knowledge of the appropriate response to each type of monitor alarm: apnea, bradycardia, and loose-lead or machine alarms. This aspect of the child's care, as well as CPR, should be reviewed with anyone who will care for the infant, including babysitters.

Apnea

The steps in response to an apnea alarm are as follows:

1. Observe and feel the infant for respiratory movement. If respiratory movement is noted, proceed to 2.a. If no respiratory movement is detected, proceed to 2.b.
2.a. If respiratory movement is felt, this indicates that the infant is breathing too shallowly for the monitor to note the movement. Shallow breathing is a normal variation.
2.b. If respiratory movement is ***not*** noted, or the infant appears lethargic, attempt to stimulate breathing by calling loudly to and then touching the baby, starting with a gentle touch and proceeding to a vigorous touch if necessary. If there is no response, proceed with mouth-to-mouth resuscitation and CPR if necessary.

Bradycardia

In response to a bradycardia alarm, stimulating the infant may be sufficient in some cases. However, if the alarm continues, or the infant looks unwell (poor color, lethargic), the following steps should be employed:

1. Stimulate the infant.
2. Ensure a clear airway by sweeping the mouth for objects and suctioning the airway.
3. Use oxygen, or increase the oxygen flow if the infant is already on oxygen.
4. Increase from gentle to vigorous stimulation.
5. If there is no response, proceed with mouth-to-mouth resuscitation and CPR if necessary.

It can be helpful to reassure parents that most infants will not require CPR. Nonetheless, maintenance of CPR skills,

with regular review, is crucial. Each person who will care for the infant should be asked to describe and demonstrate CPR; the nurse should observe for correct procedure and timing. In addition, it is important that each caregiver practices when and how to call for help and how simultaneously to manage CPR and call the rescue squad (e.g., "football carrying" the infant or dragging the infant along the floor). Previous practice using a dummy or doll makes coping with actual events less frightening. If teaching or review of CPR techniques is necessary, instruction followed by demonstration and return demonstration by parents, repeated as necessary, are recommended.

Loose-lead or Machine Alarms

Parents should also be instructed in how to respond to a loose-lead or machine alarm. A loose-lead alarm is a continuous alarm, in contrast to an intermittent alarm for bradycardia or apnea. This alarm may indicate any of the following: a loose electrode patch or belt, a dirty electrode, oil on the infant's skin, detachment of wires from the electrode or cable, malfunctioning wires that may alarm as a bradycardia event, a defective cable, or, more rarely, a monitor malfunction. Responses to loose-lead or machine alarms depend on the specific monitor. In general, the steps include changing the electrode patch and, if that does not work, changing the lead wires. A manufacturer's handbook or troubleshooting guide is usually supplied with each monitor. Review of these materials with parents can encourage a more thorough understanding of both the working of the monitor and troubleshooting strategies. Parents should be encouraged to contact the nurse, physician, or equipment supplier if needed as questions arise.

SUBSEQUENT HOME VISITS

Visits should generally begin by addressing any problems or concerns identified by parents. At the same time, the nurse should have a plan in mind for ongoing assessment and teaching. The plan should address not only those areas described for the first and routine home visits but also the following aspects of care.

Skin Care

Many parents are concerned about skin care. Electrode patches can generally be left in place for 2 days. The skin can be cleansed with soap and water as usual, but no oils or lotion should be applied in the area of the electrode patches, or the patches will not function properly. Some baby-bath products also leave a film on the skin and may lead to inappropriate alarms. If the skin under the patches becomes irritated, patches can be repositioned, but should remain in contact with the chest wall to ensure accurate monitoring.

Knowledge Gaps

It is important to help the parents assess their knowledge both about the child's condition and the reason for monitoring. If gaps in understanding are identified, instruction using discussion and written materials should be repeated as necessary. A thorough understanding of the condition and the reasons for monitoring will both encourage optimal compliance with a difficult care regimen and minimize parental anxiety.

Daily Patterns

For the family of a child on a cardiorespiratory monitor, daily patterns and normal household chores must often be reorganized to accommodate the need both to be within earshot of the monitor and to respond promptly when necessary. For example, vacuuming, going out to get the mail, going to the basement to do the laundry, and showering are not safe when only one parent is home with a monitored infant. The family may need assistance in identifying preferred daily patterns and in developing new ways to accomplish daily tasks and responsibilities without jeopardizing the infant's safety.

Babysitters

Despite the challenges involved, parents and other family members should be supported in their efforts to maintain involvement in their usual activities both inside and outside the home. The family may need assistance in finding qualified babysitters, because the child must never be left with someone unfamiliar with the monitor, apnea management, or CPR. Although parents may be anxious about leaving the child at first, support from the nurse or from other parents who have had an infant on a monitor may provide the needed encouragement. The strain of constant care and anxiety can wear heavily both on individual caregivers and on their interpersonal relationships.

DISCONTINUING USE OF THE MONITOR

The decision to discontinue monitoring an infant is a very individual matter. For a child with documented apnea, five general guidelines for discontinuation are used at Children's National Medical Center (Fink & Farrar-Simpson, 1994, p. 6). These are as follows:

1. The infant has not had any true and significant apnea or bradycardia events for 2 months.

2. The infant has endured a stressful event, such as a diphtheria-pertussis-tetanus (DPT) immunization or a respiratory illness without recurrence of apneic symptoms.
3. The infant has had one normal sleep study (off theophylline, caffeine, and/or oxygen) if on a recording (memory) monitor. If on a nonrecording monitor, the infant has had two normal sleep studies, 4 to 6 weeks apart.
4. Infant's weight is 10 lb or greater.
5. The infant's age is corrected to 4 months old.
6. Other criteria may be necessary for infants with GER, a tracheostomy, or other upper airway abnormalities.

Even when no further medical reason exists for monitoring, some parents may be reluctant to relinquish the monitor. Despite initial anxiety, most parents come to rely on the monitor for a sense of safety and security. A weaning program, allowing time to relinquish the monitor, may be necessary. Caregivers should also be helped to recognize the infant's stable condition and to view the infant as no longer "at risk."

ONGOING CONCERNS

In some cases, the parents of a child requiring a cardiorespiratory monitor may have concerns both about having more children and about whether subsequent children would also need monitoring. Parents should be encouraged to explore these concerns, with medical and nursing input offered as questions arise.

REFERENCES

American Academy of Pediatrics Task Force on Infant Positioning and SIDS. (1992). Position statement: Positioning and SIDS. *Pediatrics, 89*(6), 1,120–1,125.

American Academy of Pediatrics Task Force on Prolonged Infant Apnea. (1985). Prolonged infantile apnea. *Pediatrics, 76*(1), 129–131.

Aranda, J.V., Trippenbach, T., Turman, T., et al. (1983). Apnea and control of breathing in newborn infants. In L. Stern (Ed.), *Diagnosis and management of respiratory disorders in the newborn.* Reading, MA: Addison-Wesley.

Brooks, J.G. (1992). Apparent life threatening events and apnea of infancy. Apnea and SIDS. *Clinics in Perinatology, 19*(4), 809–832.

Carroll, J.L., & Loughlin, G.M. (1993). Sudden infant death syndrome. *Pediatrics in Review, 14*(3), 83–94.

Dwyer, T., Ponsonby, A.B., Newman, N.M., & Gobbons, L.E. (1991). Prospective cohort study of prone sleeping position and sudden infant death syndrome. *The Lancet, 337,* 1,244–1,247.

Fink, R., & Farrar-Simpson, M. (1994). *Home apnea protocols. Sleep apnea program.* Washington, DC: Department of Pulmonary Medicine, Children's National Medical Center. Unpublished.

Kelly, D.H., Pathak, A., & Meny, R. (1991). Sudden severe bradycardia in infancy. *Pediatric Pulmonology, 10,* 199–204.

Meny, R.G., Carroll, J.L., Carbone, M.T., & Kelly, D.H. (1994). Cardiorespiratory recordings from infants dying suddenly and unexpectedly at home. *Pediatrics, 92*(1), 44–49.

National Institutes of Health (1987). National Institutes of Health Consensus Development Conference on Infantile Apnea and Home Monitoring, September 29 to October 1, 1986. *Pediatrics, 79*(20), 292–299.

Willinger, M., Hoffman, H.J., & Hartford, R.B. (1994). Infant sleep position and risk of sudden infant death syndrome: Report of meeting held January 13 and 14, 1994, NIH, Bethesda, MD. *Pediatrics, 14*(3), 814–819.

Willinger, M., James, L.S., & Catz, C. (1991). Defining the sudden infant death syndrome (SIDS): Deliberations of an expert panel convened by NIH and human development. *Pediatric Pathology, 11*, 677–684.

ADDITIONAL RESOURCES

Ahmann, E., Meny, R., Wulff, L., & Fink, R. (1993). Home apnea monitoring and risk factors for poor family functioning. *Journal of Perinatology, 13*(4), 310–318.

Ahmann, E., Wulff, L., & Meny, R. (1992). Home apnea monitoring and disruptions in family life: A multidimensional controlled study. *American Journal of Public Health, 85*(5), 719–722.

Bass, J.L., Mehta, K.A., & Camara, J. (1993). Monitoring premature infants in car seats: Implementing the American Academy of Pediatrics policy in a community hospital. *Pediatrics, 91*(6), 1,137–1,141.

Cordero, L., Morehead, S., & Miller, R. (1993). Parental compliance with home apnea monitoring. *Journal of Perinatology, 13*(6), 448-452.

Desch, L.W., Corkins, M.R., & Blondis, T.A. (1990). Evaluation of changes made to an infant home apnea program in response to findings from a national consensus panel. *Journal of Perinatology, 19*(4), 701–761.

Guntheroth, W.G., & Spiers, P.S. (1992). SIDS and near-SIDS: Where we stand in 1992. *Journal of Respiratory Diseases, 13*(9), 1,280–1,294.

Hunt, C. (1992). Apnea and SIDS. *Clinics in Perinatology, 19*(4), 701–961.

Keens, T.G., & Davidson-Ward, S.L. Apnea spells, sudden death, and the role of the apnea monitor. *Pediatric Clinics of North America, 40*(5), 897–911.

Meadow, W., Mendez, D., Lantos, J., et al. (1992). What is the legal "standard of medical care" when there is no standard medical care? A survey of the use of home apnea monitoring by neonatology fellowship training programs in the United States. *Pediatrics, 89*, 1,083–1,088.

Miller, M.J., & Martin, R.J. (1992). Apnea of prematurity. Apnea and SIDS. *Clinics in Perinatology, 19*(4), 789–808.

Nobel, J.J. (1991). Apnea monitors. *Pediatric Emergency Care, 7*(5), 307–309.

Poets, C.F., Samuels, M.P., & Southall, D.P. (1994). Epidemiology and pathophysiology of apnea of prematurity. *Biology of the Neonate, 65,* '211–219.

Ruggins, N.R. (1991). Pathophysiology of apnea in preterm infants. *Archives of Disease in Childhood, 66,* 70–73.

Weese-Mayer, D.E., & Silvestri, J.M. (1992). Documenting monitoring: A turn of events. Apnea and SIDS. *Clinics in Perinatology, 19*(4), 891–906.

Home Care Plan: Cardiorespiratory Monitor

Date _____   Case manager _____

Name _____   Hosp # _____   DOB _____

PROBLEM: CARDIORESPIRATORY MONITOR

GOALS/OBJECTIVES	METHODS	STAFF/REVIEW
Child will be at minimal risk of life-threatening apnea episodes.	Obtain AP and RR each visit. Observe for pallor, cyanosis, shallow respirations, hypotonia. Assess caregivers for placement of electrodes, safe use of monitor; teach/review as necessary. Assess frequency of monitor use during all sleep times and when infant is out of sight. Assess number, type, and duration of alarms and associated symptoms each visit. Encourage family to keep careful record. Assess caregivers for appropriate response to each type of monitor alarm; teach as necessary. Review possible causes of false alarms with family. Assist family to recognize when to contact physician or apnea monitor supplier regarding concerns.	
Caregivers to verbalize knowledge about apnea and purpose of monitor.	Assess knowledge about apnea and purpose of monitor. Teach/reinforce as needed.	
Caregivers to develop appropriate plans for emergency intervention.	Assess caregivers' knowledge of when intervention is necessary. Teach/review as needed. Assess plans for emergency intervention and assist in developing as needed. Assess caregivers' ability to provide CPR competently; teach/review regularly.	

GOALS/OBJECTIVES	METHODS	STAFF/REVIEW
	Review with caregivers the indications for calling doctor/rescue squad.	
Child to be free from skin breakdown.	Observe areas of electrode placement for skin breakdown. Review skin care with caregivers including no oils or lotions and movement of patches, prn.	
Caregivers to adjust activities of daily living to allow for hearing monitor at all times.	Assess effect of home monitoring on caregivers' daily schedules. Assist family to develop new patterns of family member responsibilities, if needed. Assess effects of home apnea monitoring on other siblings. Advise as needed. Assist in developing safe travel plans, prn.	
If child has reflux, caregivers demonstrate appropriate reflux precautions.	Observe for use of appropriate reflux precautions; teach/reinforce as needed.	
Infant to have regular and prn follow up by managing physician.	Encourage regular and prn appointments and attention to need to change alarm parameters as infant grows. Communicate/coordinate with managing physician(s) on a regular basis and as needed for problems.	

Source: Courtesy of Children's Hospital National Medical Center, Home Health Care Services, Washington, D.C.

Appendix 13–B

Home Assessment: Cardiorespiratory Monitor

Name _____ Hosp # _____ DOB _____

Primary caretaker _____ Back-up caretaker _____

Address _____ Address _____

Telephone _____ Telephone _____

Date of hospital discharge _____ Start of service date _____

Discharging Hospital _____

Diagnoses _____

_____

_____

Reason for cardiorespiratory monitor: _____

Physician/Nurse Practitioner managing home monitor: _____

Hospital: _____

Telephone _____ Page _____

Type of monitor _____

Parameters/Settings: Apnea alarm _____ Apnea delay _____

Bradycardia _____ Bradycardia delay _____ Tachycardia _____

Equipment supply company _____

Telephone _____ 24-hour service telephone _____

EVERY VISIT: Assess number of apnea alarms, number of bradycardia alarms, number of "beeps" per alarm, patient status during alarms, frequency of use of monitor. Obtain AP, RR; and observe for pallor and cyanosis.

I. Equipment

	Date observed	N/A	Comments
Monitor type			
Leads (min. 2 sets)			
Patches (min. 2 sets)			

202

	Date observed	N/A	Comments
Belt			
Patches for belt			
Battery pack/charger			
Monitor manual or troubleshooting guide			

II. Emergency notifications

	Date sent	N/A	Comments
Letter to telephone co.			
Letter to electric co.			
Letter to rescue squad			
Personal contact with squad (opt)			
Letter to nearest emergency room			
Family given ER card			

III. Emergency information posted

	Date observed	N/A	Comments
Rescue squad number			
Physician's number day/evng/wknd			
Equipment supply co. number			
Power co. emergency number			
CPR guidelines			
Patient's name & address			
Written directions to home (major cross streets)			

IV. Emergency care

	Primary Caretaker Date	Back-up Caretaker Date	Comments
Describes response to alarms:			
a. Apnea			
b. Bradycardia			
c. Tachycardia			
d. Loose lead machine			
Describes emergency plan for:			
a. Respiratory failure			
b. Power failure			
Demonstrates CPR:			
Demonstrates use of ambu bag (trach)			

V. Routine care

	Primary Caretaker Date	Back-up Caretaker Date	Comments
State reason for apnea monitor			
Demonstrates set-up of leads and patches			
Demonstrates correct use of monitor			
States correct monitor settings			
States prescribed frequency of use of monitor			
Describes and demonstrates reflux precautions (opt)			
Medications (dosage, frequency, amt presently remaining)			

VI. Safety precautions

	Date reviewed	N/A	Comments
Monitor on hard surface			
Ventilation space on top			
Parents can hear from all locations			
Microwave/CB/color TV interference			
No use of extension cord			
8″ from wall in back			
Not on electrical equipment			
Parents cannot turn off during sleep			
Wires threaded out lower end of clothes			
Not to use in water			
Comments:			

Caretaker description of planning daily tasks to enable hearing monitor (e.g., vacuuming)

Primary caretaker _____

_____

_____

Back-up caretaker: _____

_____

_____

_____

VII. Describe caretaker/child interaction (overall interaction and with respect to monitor use)

_____
_____
_____
_____

VIII. Describe caretaker's overall confidence and concerns about apnea monitor

_____
_____
_____
_____

IX. Assessment of problems identified

_____
_____
_____
_____

X. Plan to address problems identified

_____
_____
_____
_____

Signature _____Date completed _____

Source: Revised with permission of Home Care Program, Children's National Medical Center, Washington, D.C., 1994.

Selection of a Cardiorespiratory Monitor

The selection of the most appropriate monitor for an individual infant and family depends on their situation and reasons for monitoring. In evaluating which monitor among several is best for an infant and family, the nurse considers:

TYPE: Is it an apnea or an apnea and bradycardia monitor? The type of monitor used is usually determined by the physician after identification of the cause of the apnea. Is it an impedance monitor? Does it have a memory chip?

SIZE: How large is the equipment? Determine if size will limit home use of a monitor.

WEIGHT: How heavy is the monitor? Determine if weight will limit a monitor's use in the home.

PORTABILITY: How movable is the monitor? This aspect may be more important for some parents, such as working parents with out-of-the-home babysitting.

TYPES OF ALARMS: What types of alarms does the monitor have? Common alarms sound in response to apnea, bradycardia, apnea and bradycardia, tachycardia, loose lead, and weak battery signals. Evaluate what types of alarms are best for each infant and family.

ALARM SIGNALS: What kinds of alarms does the machine have? Some monitors have visual alarms, others have auditory, and some have both. Evaluate how loud they are and how easily seen. For parents with deficits in either of these areas, this aspect may be critical. Does the monitor have a memory alert system? This system lets the parent know if an apneic and/or bradycardic event has occurred. If the infant begins to breathe again or if the heart rate picks up after the alarms have been activated, the audible alarm is silenced. However, the visual alarm will remain "on" until the reset button is pushed, informing the parent of the type of event.

SENSITIVITY: How sensitive is the machine? Is this variable factory preset, set by another piece of equipment, auto-matic, or dialed in by the human hand? Sensitivity can be a critical parameter in home use. Inappropriate activating of the alarms can lead to poor compliance.

POWER SOURCE: Evaluate whether an electric or battery-powered monitor is better for the family and the specific community. In areas of frequent power outages, battery back-up must be considered. Does the system have a battery recharger?

COMPLEXITY OF USE: How easy is the monitor to use? Is the equipment easy for parents to use? Can the family be taught to "trouble-shoot" the monitor? As this aspect varies from individual to individual, it requires careful assessment.

SERVICING: Is there a service technician available 24 hours a day? Are there regular service calls by the technician for periodic assessment of monitor functioning? Consider the background of the technicians: are they medically trained, for example, as respiratory therapists? Or are they trained as salespersons as well as monitor technicians? Determine if this aspect influences the situation.

ATTACHMENTS: What monitoring attachments are required? Is a belt used with fixed or movable electrodes? Or are electrodes placed directly on the infant's skin? Are these electrodes wet or dry? Assess the effect of these attachments on the infant's skin, movement, and other aspects of daily care and living.

COSTS: How much is the purchase or rental of the monitor? Prices vary among types of equipment. It is important not to let cost of the monitor dictate the type used. Funding is available through several sources. Private and state insurance companies will often pay part or all of home monitoring costs. State Children's Service Bureaus provide financial assistance if eligibility requirements are met. Philanthropic organizations also provide monies depending on the individual situation.

FLEXIBILITY: How flexible is the home monitor? Can the monitor record 24-hour tracings of heart and respiratory rates in the home? These pneumocardiograms are often used to monitor treatment. If they can be done in the home on the monitor the parents are already using, the need for additional equipment and possible hospitalization is eliminated.

RELIABILITY: It is important to assess reliability of the monitor. Evaluate manufacturer testing and field experience.

Determine if there have been any lawsuits regarding the monitoring equipment.

INSTRUCTIONS: Review monitor instructions. Are they adequate and clear?

SUPPLIER: Determine location of monitor company's headquarters. Validate availability of monitors in specific geographic areas and delivery time frame involved.

Source: Adapted from *Pediatric Nursing,* May–June, 1983, p. 179, with permission of Jannetti Publications, Inc., Pitman, New Jersey, © 1983.

Chapter 14

Home Care of the Infant Requiring Oxygen Therapy

Revised by Angela Jerome-Ebel, MSN, RN

Some infants with pulmonary or cardiac disorders will require oxygen therapy at home. A small number of infants with bronchopulmonary dysplasia will continue to need supplementary oxygen for some time (Abman & Groothius, 1994). This chapter discusses the variety of oxygen systems as well as factors relevant to both hospital discharge and home care of the infant requiring oxygen therapy.

CHOICE OF OXYGEN SYSTEM

Several factors influence the choice of oxygen equipment for use in the home. These include the prescribed liter flow or concentration, the need for portability (and duration of portability required), the requirement for continuous versus intermittent use, and humidity needs. In addition to considering the source of oxygen (concentrator, liquid, or cylinder), thought must be given to both the appropriate source of humidity and the optimal delivery method(s).

Source of Oxygen

Oxygen Concentrators

An oxygen concentrator is an electrical device that separates oxygen from the ambient (room) air and then concentrates that oxygen, finally delivering the more concentrated oxygen to the child (Sleeper, 1988a). Because it draws oxygen from the room air, the concentrator provides a continuous source of oxygen that is not depleted. Concentrators generally provide oxygen at delivery rates up to around 5 L per minute (Lpm). Humidity can be added to the system by the attachment of a bubble humidifier. If a concentrator is entraining oxygen into a tracheostomy collar, a cascade or other heated water system may be used to provide humidity. The filter on a concentrator requires cleaning with mild soap and water weekly.

Concentrators are cost-effective for the insurance company if used for continuous oxygen delivery at higher pediatric oxygen flow rates. However, families may face an increase in their electric bills. An additional consideration is that concentrators deliver oxygen under low pressure (as compared to oxygen cylinders) and as a result cannot be used with Venturi masks or medication nebulizers. The back-pressure from these delivery devices retards the flow of oxygen from the concentrator.

An oxygen concentrator is bulky, and the home should be assessed for available space prior to a decision to use one. Oxygen concentrators should not be placed in small storage areas since they generate extra heat, which could damage the unit and create a fire hazard. The oxygen concentrator should be placed 12 to 18 inches away from items that would block the inlet port. Most oxygen concentrators have an audible alarm that alerts the parents to a power failure. If a concentrator is used, a back-up oxygen system should be made available both for portability and in case of power failure or equipment malfunction.

Liquid Oxygen

Liquid oxygen is oxygen compressed into a cold liquid form (300°F below zero) and maintained under pressure (Sleeper, 1988a). It can be used with a nasal cannula, a tracheostomy collar, or a ventilator for home care. Liquid oxygen is a cost-effective method of oxygen delivery for continuous low-flow use. It is also the most efficient method of providing oxygen to children who are transported frequently, such as children who go to school daily. Relatively lightweight, easily carried portable units can be refilled as needed by caregivers in the home. Consideration should be given to how long the portable liquid oxygen in the tank will last based on the child's prescribed oxygen flow rate and the manufacturer's specifications. (See Exhibit 14–1 and footnote to the Exhibit.)

Like concentrators, liquid oxygen units do not provide the pressure and flow required to operate a Venturi mask or nebulizer. Further, a source of humidity must be added to the liquid system when stationary.

There are several important safety considerations when working with liquid oxygen in the home. The tank should be maintained in an upright position to prevent leaking of liquid oxygen. If there is spillage, the liquid should be kept away from the skin, eyes, and clothing. The "frosted" parts of the liquid oxygen tank should not be touched as liquid oxygen can freeze-burn the skin.

Exhibit 14–1 Duration of Use (days or hours) Based on Flow Rate: Liquid Oxygen
Approximate Hours/Days a Full System Will Last (Examples)[a]

Liters per minute	37 Liter Base Grandair	30 Liter Base Liberator 30	Portable 1.23 Liter Stroller/Liberator	Portable 1.08 Liter PulsairOMS-2
1.0	22.1 D	16.7 D	13 H	13.7 H
1.5	14.8 D	10.7 D	10 H	9.2 H
2.0	11.1 D	8.3 D	6.0 H	6.9 H
2.5	8.9 D	6.7 D	5.5 H	5.5 H
3.0	7.4 D	5.2 D	5.0 H	4.6 H
3.5	6.4 D	4.3 D	3.5 H	4.0 H
4.0	5.5 D	4.0 D	2.0 H	3.4 H

D = Days   H = Hours

[a]The duration of operation of liquid oxygen systems will vary depending on the size of the tank, the flow rate (liters per minute), and the manufacturer. Many additional portable units are reviewed in Lucas (1988) and, depending on the wait, duration of use at one liter per minute varies widely from as few as 5.5 to as many as 26 hours. Manufacturer specifications should be obtained for each individual unit used.

Source: Adapted from *Home Respiratory Therapy* by J. Lucas, J. Golish, G. Sleeper, and J. O'Ryan, eds., with permission of RCOD Publishing, Dayton, Ohio, © 1988.

Exhibit 14–2 Duration of Use (hours) Based on Flow Rate: Tank/Cylinder Oxygen
Approximate Hours a Full Tank Will Last

Liters per minute	C	D	E	H
1.0	2.5	5.0	10	105
1.5	1.7	3.5	7.5	75
2.0	1.2	2.5	5.0	52
2.5	1.0	2.0	4.0	43
3.0	0.75	1.5	3.0	35
3.5	0.5	1.2	2.7	30
4.0	0.5	1.0	2.5	26

Source: Adapted from *Home Respiratory Therapy* by J. Lucas, J. Golish, G. Sleeper, and J. O'Ryan, eds., with permission of RCOD Publishing, Dayton, Ohio, © 1988.

Cylinder Oxygen

Cylinder oxygen can be used with any nasal cannula, tracheostomy collar, ventilator, Venturi mask, or nebulizer if the appropriate regulator and connector are chosen. Cylinder oxygen is most cost-effective for low-flow use or for intermittent use up to 12 hr per day. A source of humidity must be added to the system.

Oxygen cylinders come in a variety of sizes. "H" cylinders are the largest usually used in home care; followed by "E" cylinders; and the most portable size, the "D" cylinder (Lucas, 1988). Portability can be achieved by use of a small "E" cylinder on a rolling stand or a "D" cylinder in a backpack. It is important for the parent and home care nurse to know how long a particular oxygen tank will last at the child's prescribed oxygen flow rate, particularly for purposes of portability (see Exhibit 14–2).

Both the home care nurse and the parent(s) should be capable of changing the tank regulator and checking the remaining oxygen level. For safety reasons, oxygen cylinders should ideally be kept in a secure, upright position once the regulator is attached. Some parents do lay cylinders down in a basket under the infant's stroller. If this is done, caution should be exercised to protect the regulator and its juncture with the oxygen cylinder. Tanks have been known to propel themselves quite a distance if the regulator is knocked too forcefully. Another safety precaution is to turn the oxygen off when not in use.

Humidification Devices

Adequate humidity is necessary to prevent drying of the airways when oxygen is used. Humidity can be delivered by jet nebulizer, cascade, bubbler, or other heated humidity system.

The jet nebulizer delivers an aerosol mist, which is actually particles of water suspended in air. As these particles enter the airways, they can stimulate hyperreactive airways such as those of the infant with bronchopulmonary dysplasia (BPD). In contrast, humidity provided by a cascade, bubbler, or other heated humidity system consists of molecular water in the air and generally does not stimulate hyperreactive airways.

Delivery Methods

Oxygen delivery methods include the following: tracheostomy collar, oxygen mask, Venturi mask, nasal cannula, tent, and ventilator. The choice of delivery method should involve consideration of the infant's age and corresponding developmental, visual, and mobility needs. Consideration should of course be given to the capacity to meet the infant's oxygen needs.

- A tracheostomy collar is generally the preferred oxygen delivery device for an infant with a tracheostomy, because it provides a directed flow of oxygen and humidity into the airway. If the collar is moved away from the tracheostomy tube at night as the infant turns, a chest belt with a Velcro anchor may be useful.

- Oxygen masks are bulky, restrictive, and generally inappropriate for use with infants.

- Venturi masks are used infrequently with infants.

- Nasal cannulas, although they can roll off easily during sleep, have distinct advantages for use during the waking hours of an infant without a tracheostomy. The nasal cannula provides oxygen while offering the least restriction for the infant's visual, auditory, and motor environments. If a nasal cannula is used, it can be held in place by a headband, Duoderm, tape, or a clear surgical adhesive dressing (e.g., Opsite or Tegaderm). If the cannula prongs do not fit the nares, as in a small infant, they can be clipped off (Jennings, 1982). Careful taping of the oxygen cannula usually maintains placement even through the night. In addition, as illustrated in Figure 14–1, other eyelet holes can be cut around the cannula to make oxygen available regardless of the cannula position under the nose. With the use of long tubing for the nasal cannula, caregivers can more easily take the infant from room to room. Long tubing is also useful for the toddler, who needs the opportunity to roam more freely. The physician should be asked to approve eyelet holes and the length of tubing as there may be some concerns about altered oxygen concentration.

- Oxygen tents are sometimes used with infants, but in most circumstances are less desirable than a nasal can-

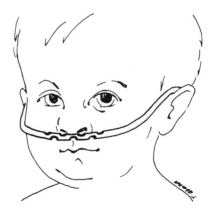

Figure 14–1 Nasal Cannula for Oxygen Delivery

Source: Courtesy of Teresa Ahmann.

nula because they restrict the visual and auditory environment so drastically.

- Ventilators can have oxygen bled directly into the line if room air is not sufficient for the infant or child.

HOSPITAL DISCHARGE AND TRANSITION TO THE HOME

Coordination of Care

At the time of discharge from the hospital, coordination between the community health nurse and the hospital staff is important. The community health nurse should obtain complete information about the program of home oxygen therapy. This includes the reason for oxygen use, the prescribed concentration and liter flow, hours per day to be used, and type of equipment recommended. The community health nurse may be asked to advise hospital staff on the most appropriate type of oxygen system for home use; factors to consider and information on the options are discussed earlier in this chapter. In this connection, a home care respiratory therapist can also contribute to making an appropriate choice. In choosing an oxygen supplier, a reliable company with 24-hour on-call service is important; other factors to consider are discussed in Chapter 5.

Parental Education

A thorough, well-planned approach to parental education regarding home oxygen therapy can make a substantial difference in parental knowledge, preparedness, and confidence (Brown & Sauve, 1994). Prior to discharge, it is important for the home care nurse to ascertain what parents have been taught about the need for oxygen and its safe and appropriate use; to ascertain parental knowledge of and confidence level in providing all aspects of routine and emergency care; and to determine parental concerns about home use of oxygen for their infant or child. Such information will enable the nurse and family to develop appropriate plans for follow-up teaching and support in the home. (A sample care plan and initial home assessment form are provided in Appendixes 14–A and 14–B, respectively.)

Emergency Preparations

Before hospital discharge, the nurse should ensure that emergency preparations have been made, as discussed in Chapter 12. These include notifying the local rescue squad, electric company, and telephone company of the child's special needs. The electric and telephone companies should be asked to place the home on a priority service list. A list of emergency telephone numbers (see Exhibit 12–1) should be posted near each telephone in the home. Oxygen safety precautions (Exhibit 14–3) should be reviewed.

Transportation Home

Similarly, plans for transporting the infant from hospital to home should be discussed with caregivers prior to discharge. If oxygen is required during transport, the supplier should be notified in advance to ensure that a portable cylinder or liquid oxygen system will be available. Safety measures for transportation include making sure that an adequate amount of portable oxygen is available in case of car breakdown or traffic problems, maintaining the oxygen source in an upright position at all times, securing the oxygen source with a belt or strap in the car to prevent accidental falls, and maintaining adequate ventilation (a window should be slightly open). Oxygen tanks should not be stored in the car trunk. If public transportation is used, a "no smoking" sign should be displayed prominently to warn others of the safety hazard (Sleeper, 1988b).

Exhibit 14–3 Oxygen Safety Precautions

1. Post "no smoking" signs.
2. Avoid smoking, fire, or sparks in the patient's room.
3. Keep oxygen tank and patient's bed at least 5 feet from radiator or heater.
4. Ensure that oxygen tank is secured upright at all times.
5. Avoid use of alcohol, petroleum jelly (Vaseline) or other petroleum-based products, and aerosols.
6. Keep oxygen in a well-ventilated area at all times.
7. If using an oxygen concentrator, do not use an extension cord, and do not plug into outlets being used for other appliances.

ROUTINE HOME VISITS

Assessment of the Infant

On every home visit, the nurse should assess the infant's status, beginning with the pulse and respiratory rate and, if ordered, oxygen saturation. The nurse should also assess the infant's color, noting particularly the presence or absence of pallor or cyanosis, particularly circumorally. The infant should be observed for signs and symptoms of respiratory distress (including nasal flaring, retractions, and labored or rapid respirations). In addition, lung fields should be auscultated and any adventitious sounds or areas of poor air exchange noted. (See Chapter 12 for a complete discussion of auscultation.) Any deviations from the child's normal patterns should be discussed with parents and, if indicated, with the physician.

On each home visit, the nurse should also determine by parental report the frequency and duration of oxygen use. The question of weaning from oxygen is discussed in the final section of this chapter.

Equipment and Safety Concerns

Equipment should be inspected on every home visit. Oxygen and humidity settings should be checked against the recommended settings, and the oxygen source should be inspected for proper functioning and supply level. Of course, ongoing observation for adherence to oxygen safety precautions, as listed in Exhibit 14–3, is critical.

THE FIRST HOME VISIT

Determining and responding to parental concerns and priorities are essential on the first and all home visits. Additionally, the nurse should complete a physical assessment focusing on the respiratory system (see description in routine home visits, above). The nurse should inspect the equipment and supplies and also assess parental preparation for the provision of safe and appropriate care. Of course, if the infant has bronchopulmonary dysplasia (BPD), a tracheostomy, or is on an apnea monitor or a ventilator, the nurse should complete pertinent assessments and teaching on the first home visit. (See Chapters 12, 13, 15, and 16.)

Equipment and Supplies

On the first visit, a careful inspection of equipment and supplies is important. The oxygen source should be examined for proper functioning and for supply level. The source of humidity should be the type recommended and should also be assessed for proper functioning. Whatever source of humidity is used, the vessel should be kept full of sterile, boiled, or distilled water. Extra nebulizer vessels or a cascade and extra tubing should be available in the home to allow regular cleaning and replacement. Finally, the nurse should observe that the nasal cannula, tracheostomy collar, or mask is being used correctly.

Parental Education

On the first home visit, the nurse should also determine parental ability to evaluate the infant's respiratory status. Knowledge and skills should be augmented by the nurse as needed. Parents must be able to assess the infant's color and to observe for signs and symptoms of respiratory distress. Parents may also wish to be taught to count the respiratory rate and pulse and even to auscultate lung fields. Parents should be familiar enough with the infant's baseline respiratory status that deviations can be noted. Of course, if deviations occur, parents should contact the infant's physician for advisement.

In addition, the nurse should assist parents and other caregivers in evaluating their understanding of appropriate use of the oxygen delivery system. Each caregiver should be able to state and demonstrate the prescribed oxygen concentration and liter flow, humidity settings, and the prescribed times for oxygen use. The nurse should advise parents never to change the oxygen settings without consulting the physician. Parents should also be able to assess the amount of oxygen remaining if either cylinder or liquid oxygen is used and should know the level at which to contact the supplier for a new supply.

Parents should be assisted, as necessary, in developing appropriate plans in the event of either equipment malfunction or depletion of the oxygen supply. Depending on the severity of the underlying lung condition, it may be possible to wait for the supply company to repair or replace equipment or to supply additional oxygen. In other cases, it may be necessary to transport the child immediately to the nearest emergency department for supplemental oxygen until the home situation can be remedied. Guidelines for each infant should be developed in conjunction with the physician prior to discharge.

Parents and other caregivers should also be asked to describe and demonstrate cardiopulmonary resuscitation (CPR). CPR guidelines should be posted near the infant's crib for easy reference in an emergency, and CPR techniques should be reviewed regularly.

Safety Precautions

Adherence to oxygen safety precautions, as listed in Exhibit 14–3, should also be assessed during the first home visit. Precautions should be reviewed with parents and other caregivers and a written list provided for reference use.

Although unwarranted fears and misconceptions about having oxygen in the home should be dispelled, a healthy respect for its potential dangers should be encouraged.

SUBSEQUENT HOME VISITS

On each home visit, the nurse should elicit and address any parental concerns. At the same time, the nurse should have a plan in mind for ongoing assessment and teaching. The plan should address those areas described for routine home visits, any teaching initiated or problems addressed on the first visit, and the following aspects of care.

Equipment and Supplies

The nurse should discuss the importance of regular cleaning and maintenance of supplies and equipment to prevent infection; the warm, moist humidification tubing provides a perfect medium for bacterial growth. In this regard, on a regular basis throughout the day, any excess humidity in the oxygen tubing can be drained by gravity or removed (when disconnected from the infant) by a high flow of oxygen through the tubing. The accumulated moisture should not be emptied back into the water source. Guidelines for cleaning respiratory equipment and supplies are provided in the Special Issue, "Cleaning Respiratory Equipment."

Feeding and Development

Feeding is an activity that can be stressful for the infant requiring oxygen. Breastfeeding may be less stressful than bottle feeding. Small, frequent, high-calorie feedings may be helpful if the infant tires easily or shows prolonged cyanosis, flaring, or retractions with feeding. In occasional cases, supplemental tube feeding may be recommended. Chapters 9 through 11 and the Special Issues in Part III discuss nutrition and feeding in greater detail.

The nurse should encourage stimulation and developmentally appropriate activities for the infant on oxygen. Lengthy tubing can facilitate mobility for the infant or toddler using a nasal cannula or tracheostomy mask. If the infant is in an oxygen tent, small, colorful toys can be put inside the tent and pictures hung outside the tent to provide visual and motor stimulation. Parents may need encouragement not to be overcautious in handling of and play with the infant. However, if the infant is stressed by prolonged or intense activity, the following signs and symptoms may be noted: rapid, labored breathing, nasal flaring, retractions, pallor, or cyanosis. If this occurs, the activity should be stopped until the infant returns to normal; playtimes can still be encouraged but for shorter periods. In some cases, the physician may recommend higher oxygen concentrations during activity. (Development is discussed in more detail in Chapters 19 and 20.)

Outings

Parents may wish to take the infant with them during walks outdoors or on other outings. The nurse should encourage this activity unless contraindicated because of severe hyperreactive airways disease. A stroller with a rack or a backpack can be helpful for carrying a portable source of oxygen. (Of course, cylinder oxygen should generally be maintained in an upright position.) If caregivers are uncomfortable about stares or questions related to the oxygen, a blanket over the tank will hide it from view. Of course, parents should avoid exposure to any outdoor sparks or flames, and excursions should be planned according to the time allowed by amount of oxygen in the portable supply.

Family Issues

It is important for the home care nurse to foster independent parental decision-making skills through carefully planned and learner-ready education. Initially, family members may depend on the home care nurse's knowledge to ensure appropriate decisions regarding the care of their child. As parental mastery develops, parents become increasingly expert in their child's care. The home care nurse's role appropriately shifts to one of guidance and support for parental decisions regarding the infant's care.

On home visits, the nurse may note that the affected child's siblings are both curious about and afraid of the oxygen. Both play (e.g., with stethoscopes and tiny cannulas for their dolls made from nasogastric tubes and rubber bands) and active involvement during each home visit may help to reduce their anxieties. Chapter 3 addresses sibling issues in detail.

Since the infant requiring oxygen should only be left with persons familiar with the necessary specialized care, the family may have difficulty in finding a babysitter. At the same time, occasional relief from the infant's care is very important. Some parents prefer only to leave their child with a nurse (Klein-Berndt, 1991). Sometimes friends, relatives, or other parents who have had a child requiring oxygen will be willing to babysit. On subsequent visits, the home care nurse can offer assistance in training a babysitter in the

child's care requirements if the parents wish. Some areas have respite care programs that can provide parents with a break from the demands of the child's care.

ONGOING CONCERNS

Some parents may wish to wean their child from oxygen either for their own convenience or because they have noted that the child "looks fine" and does not "turn blue" when off the oxygen. It is important to stress that even if the child does not become cyanotic, the oxygen level in the circulatory system may be decreased, with adverse effects on all organ systems, including the brain. The nurse should explain that only tests of the blood oxygen levels can determine the infant's need for oxygen.

Discussions with the managing physician should be encouraged if weaning is desired by parents. In infants with bronchopulmonary dysplasia, weaning of oxgyen may be accomplished by decreasing the flow rate (liters per minute) slowly over a period of months. Appropriate weaning follows a series of tests that may include pulse oximetry and blood gas studies both on and off oxygen. Testing should also be done during both sleep and feeding times to assess oxygen requirements fully during these higher demand activities.

REFERENCES

Abman, S.H., & Groothius, J.R. (1994.) Pathophysiology and treatment of bronchopulmonary dysplasia. *Pediatric Clinics of North America, 41,* (2), 277–315.

Brown, K.A., & Sauve, R.S. (1994). Evaluation of a caregiver education program: Home oxygen therapy for infants. *Journal of Obstetric, Gynecologic, and Neonatal Nursing, 23,* (5), 429–435.

Jennings, C. (1982, March/April). An alternative: Nasal cannula oxygen therapy for infants who are oxygen dependent. *MCN: The American Journal of Maternal Child Nursing,* 89, 92.

Klein-Berndt, S. (1991). Bronchopulmonary dysplasia in the family: A longitudinal case study. *Pediatric Nursing, 17*(6), 607–611.

Lucas, J. (1988). Selecting the optimal oxygen system. In J. Lucas, J. Golish, G. Sleeper, & J. O'Ryan (Eds.), *Home respiratory therapy.* Norwalk, CT: Appleton & Lange.

Sleeper, G. (1988a). Home oxygen therapy equipment. In J. Lucas, J. Golish, G. Sleeper, & J. O'Ryan (Eds.), *Home respiratory therapy,* Norwalk, CT: Appleton & Lange.

Sleeper, G. (1988b). Traveling with oxygen. In J. Lucas, J. Golish, G. Sleeper, & J. O'Ryan (Eds.), *Home respiratory therapy,* Norwalk, CT: Appleton & Lange.

Home Care Plan: Respiratory Compromise—Oxygen

Date _____   Case manager _____

Name _____   Hosp # _____   DOB _____

PROBLEM: **RESPIRATORY COMPROMISE: OXYGEN**

GOALS/OBJECTIVES	METHODS	STAFF/REVIEW
Child to be at minimal risk for inadequate oxygenation/respiratory distress	Assess AP, RR. Auscultate lung fields. Assess color, flaring, retractions, level of activity each visit. Assess/teach chest therapy and suctioning if indicated. Contact supplier prn re: concerns related to equipment. Assess oxygen saturation.	
Caregivers will verbalize and use correct oxygen %, flow rate, humidity settings and safety precautions	Assess appropriate use of oxygen (flow rate, tubing and administration set-up, hours/day used) each visit. Teach oxygen safety measures; review prn.	
Caregivers will describe signs/symptoms of respiratory distress and inadequate oxygenation	Assess/teach signs/symptoms of respiratory distress, inadequate oxygenation. Teach auscultation if appropriate.	
Parents will describe interventions for distress/inadequate oxygenation.	Teach when/how to increase O_2 per physician order and when to contact physician.	
Caregivers to verbalize appropriate plan for respiratory distress.	Assess/teach emergency plans. Encourage contacting managing physician. Assess/review CPR regularly.	
Caregivers to verbalize appropriate back-up for equipment malfunction or electric failure.	Assess/assist in developing back-up plans. Arrange for back-up oxygen source. Encourage caretakers to call oxygen supplier, prn.	

GOALS/OBJECTIVES	METHODS	STAFF/REVIEW
Caregivers to have appropriate plans for travel with oxygen.	Ensure that phone and electric companies, rescue squad, and appropriate emergency departments are aware of child's status.	
Child to be at minimal risk for respiratory infection	Assess/assist in developing plans and arranging for portable equipment prn.	
	Teach/assess appropriate plans for oxygen equipment cleaning and maintenance.	
	Encourage avoidance of exposure to people with upper respiratory infections.	
Child to have regular and prn follow-up by managing physician.	Encourage regular and prn appointments.	
	Communicate/coordinate with managing physician on regular and prn basis.	

Source: Courtesy of Children's Hospital National Medical Center, Home Health Care Services, Washington, D.C.

Appendix 14–B

Home Assessment: Oxygen

Name _____ Hosp# _____ DOB _____

Primary caretaker _____ Back-up caretaker _____

Address _____ Address _____

Telephone _____ Telephone _____

Date of hospital discharge _____ Start of service date _____

Diagnoses _____

_____

_____

Reason for oxygen: _____

Physician: _____

Telephone _____ Page _____

Oxygen source _____ liter flow _____

Oxygen hours/day _____

Maintain O_2 sats between _____ and _____

Equipment supply company _____

Telephone _____ 24-hour service telephone _____

Funding for equipment _____

Humidity source and setting _____

EVERY VISIT: Obtain pulse, respirations. Assess respiratory pattern, color; auscultate lung fields; and assess for signs/symptoms of respiratory distress. Check oxygen and humidity settings.

I. Equipment

	Date observed	N/A	Comments
Oxygen source: type			
Humidity source: type			
Nasal cannula			

217

Trach collar _____

Other: _____

Extra tubing/connectors _____

Portable oxygen source type _____

II. Emergency notifications

	Date sent	N/A	Comments
Letter to telephone co.			
Letter to electric co.			
Letter to rescue squad			
Personal contact with squad (opt)			
Letter to nearest emergency room			
Family given ER card			

III. Emergency information posted

	Date observed	N/A	Comments
Rescue squad number			
Physician's number day/evng/wknd (see Vent. Home Assmnt)			
DME number			
Power co. emergency number			
CPR guidelines			
Patient's name & address (opt)			
Directions to the home (so home care nurse can give to EMS personnel)			
Poison control			

IV. Emergency care

	Primary Caretaker Date	Back-up Caretaker Date	Comments
Describes signs/symptoms of respiratory distress			
Describes emergency plan for:			
a. Respiratory distress			
b. Power failure			
Demonstrates CPR:			

V. Routine care

	Primary Caretaker Date	Back-up Caretaker Date	Comments
States reason for oxygen			
Demonstrates how to evaluate:			

a. Respiratory status _____

b. Appropriate intervention for
    deviations from normal _____

States oxygen/liter flow _____

States prescribed amount of
time on oxygen/day _____

Demonstrates and states correct
settings for: _____

a. Oxygen _____

b. Humidity _____

c. Other _____

Demonstrates use of:

a. Oximeter _____

b. Nasal cannula _____

c. Trach collar _____

d. Oxygen mask _____

e. Other _____

Describes how to assess amount
of oxygen remaining_____

Describes or demonstrates use
of portable oxygen _____

Describes cleaning of
supplies and equipment _____

VI. Safety precautions

	Date reviewed	N/A	Comments
Oxygen supports combustion			
No smoking sign posted			
Avoid flames, heat sources, sparks			
Ground all electrical equipment			
Avoid oil, grease, and aerosol sprays			
Keep oxygen in well ventilated areas			
Secure tanks or portable liquid systems			
Fire extinguisher in the home			

Comments: _____

_____

_____

_____

VII. Describe caretaker/child interaction (overall interaction and with respect to oxygen use)

_____
_____
_____
_____

VIII. Describe caretakers' overall confidence and concerns about use of oxygen

_____
_____
_____
_____

IX. Assessment of problems identified

_____
_____
_____
_____

X. Plan to address problems identified

_____
_____
_____
_____

Signature _____Date completed _____

Source: Courtesy of Children's Hospital National Medical Center, Home Health Care Services, Washington, D.C.

Chapter 15

Home Care of the Infant or Child with a Tracheostomy

Revised by Collette Duncliffe Driscoll, RN

The high-risk neonate, with a small airway and a history of multiple or prolonged endotracheal intubations, may develop subglottic stenosis, or narrowing of the tracheal airway. If this occurs, surgical creation of a tracheostomy, through which a tube is inserted, may be necessary to ensure an adequate airway. Use of a tracheostomy tube may also be indicated in some infants if long-term ventilation is required. In addition, tracheostomies may be used for management of other airway disorders or for optimal pulmonary toilet, as in the care of some children with cystic fibrosis.

HOSPITAL DISCHARGE AND TRANSITION TO THE HOME

A successful home discharge for an infant with a tracheostomy should include both intensive predischarge parental training and a plan for a home care program utilizing a multidisciplinary approach (Schlessel, Harper, Rappa, Kenigsberg, & Khanna, 1993). Decisions regarding the scope of home care services should be based on the infant's medical needs and medical stability as well as on parental support needs. At a minimum, all infants should receive the services of a home equipment supplier and some hourly or intermittent home nursing. Social work and speech, occupational, or physical therapy may be additional services that are needed by the child and family.

Discharge Teaching

Discharge teaching with parents should include pathophysiology of the upper airway, care of the tracheostomy, indications and technique for suctioning, management of illnesses or emergencies, use and maintenance of equipment, and daily care and health maintenance (Barnes, 1992). (A predischarge teaching checklist for the child with a tracheostomy is provided in Appendix 5–C.)

Transportation Plans

Similarly, plans for transportation from hospital to home should be discussed with parents prior to discharge. An appropriate carseat is required. When a child has a tracheostomy, two adults should always be in the car so that one can safely drive while the other attends to the infant; both suctioning of the tracheostomy tube and other respiratory care may be needed. A battery-operated suction machine or a mouth suction (DeLee trap) will be necessary in the car. Additionally, the supplies listed in Exhibit 15–1 should be carried with the infant at all times.

Emergency Preparations

Prior to hospital discharge, parents should be assisted in making emergency preparations, including the following:

Exhibit 15–1 Tracheostomy Travel Kit

1. tracheostomy tube of correct size, with ties attached, and obturator in place, labeled "ready to go"
2. tracheostomy tube one size smaller, with ties attached, and obturator in place, labeled "ready to go"
3. blunt-end (bandage) scissors, to cut ties if necessary
4. portable suction machine, tubing, and catheter (optional)
5. DeLee mucous suction trap (needed even with portable suction machine, in case portable machine malfunctions)
6. suction catheter one size smaller (in case of mucous plug)
7. saline vials for instillation
8. small jar with saline to clean suction catheter
9. spare trach ties
10. tissues
11. resuscitation bag
12. tracheostomy humidifying filter

- ensuring the presence of a telephone in the home
- notifying telephone and electric companies of the need to put the family on a priority service list
- notifying the local rescue squad that a child with a tracheostomy is in the community
- posting CPR guidelines (with modifications for a tracheostomy) near the infant's sleeping area
- posting emergency telephone numbers and directions to the home (nearest major intersection) at each telephone.

(Emergency precautions are described in greater detail in Chapter 12.)

Home Nursing Referral

Nursing services required for a child with a tracheostomy may range from intermittent visits to extended hourly or private-duty nursing from 8 to 24 hrs a day. For those infants and their parents who receive extended hourly care, the transition to home may be far less stressful. However, as a practical matter, the availability of funding will often influence the scope of services.

At the time of hospital discharge for any infant with a tracheostomy, coordination between the home health nurse and the hospital staff is important. In order to formulate an effective plan of care, the home care nurse should gather the following information on the infant: diagnosis; medical history; status of parental training; parental response to training; equipment needs, including size and make of the tracheostomy tube; and plans for routine and emergency care.

Predischarge Home Visit

A predischarge home assessment by the home care nurse is valuable for many reasons. For one, families may desire assistance in setting up equipment and supplies. Second, a predischarge home visit offers the family and home care nurse an early opportunity to discuss expectations and concerns regarding home care, laying the groundwork for collaboration. The nurse can help the family assess their needs, strengths, and goals. These form the basis for the plan of care.

ROUTINE HOME VISITS

Assessment

Assessment of the Infant

On each home visit, the nurse should note the infant's pulse and respiratory rate, auscultate the lung fields, and observe the infant's respiratory pattern.

Tracheal Secretions

Assessment of tracheal secretions is another important aspect of routine nursing visits. The quantity, quality, color, viscosity, and odor (if any) of secretions should be observed and documented. Very thick secretions may indicate either insufficient humidity or an infection. Yellow, green, or odiferous secretions may signal an infection. If blood-tinged secretions are noted on a single suctioning, the suctioning technique may be too vigorous, or the humidity may be inadequate. If copious or recurrent bleeding from the tracheostomy is noted, the physician should be notified.

Tracheostomy Site

In addition to regular assessment of tracheal secretions, the nurse should routinely assess for irritation and inflammation at the tracheostomy site. Irritation and inflammation may signal either bacterial or yeast infections or granuloma formation.

Teaching

Care of the Tracheostomy Site

The nurse should review with parents or other caregivers both routine care of the tracheostomy site, including the neck and stoma, and the procedure for changing the ties. The stoma site can be cleaned daily with a cotton swab and either hydrogen peroxide or normal saline alone. The neck may be cleaned with soap and water followed by a saline rinse. Parents should be instructed to observe for signs of irritation and inflammation.

Tracheostomy ties should also be changed daily to prevent irritation to the neck. When changing the ties, caregivers should demonstrate holding the tracheostomy tube carefully in place to prevent it from falling out. Methods for holding the child still and securing the ties are presented later in this chapter.

Tracheal Secretions

While the nurse observes the tracheal secretions, parents can be instructed in what to look for as well (quantity, color, viscosity, and odor). They should also be instructed in appropriate interventions should changes in secretions be noted.

Humidity

Since the tracheostomy tube bypasses the nose and mouth, which normally humidify inspired air, a source of humidity is an essential component of routine tracheostomy care. For this reason, the provision of adequate humidity should be determined on each home visit. Most frequently, a compressor and nebulizer or cascade will be used for humidity, as discussed in Chapter 14. Lengthy tubing can be used to allow the infant or young child freedom to move.

If the child will not be using the regular source of humidity for a prolonged period of time, there are several options for ensuring adequate humidity. First, vaporizers or room humidifiers can assist in maintaining airway humidity. As a second alternative, if the infant begins to sound dry or raspy with breathing, a small amount of preservative-free saline solution (several milliliters) can be instilled into the tracheostomy tube to prevent drying of secretions. Third, a tracheostomy humidifying filter, a small cover for the tube, can assist in keeping secretions moist (see Figure 15–1). It is also useful in preventing aspiration of dust and other particles when the child is either outside or playing on the floor.

THE FIRST HOME VISIT

The first home visit should incorporate all aspects of routine home visits. In addition, the nurse must determine that the needed supplies and equipment are in the home, that equipment is functioning properly, and that parents are prepared to provide safe and appropriate care for the infant.

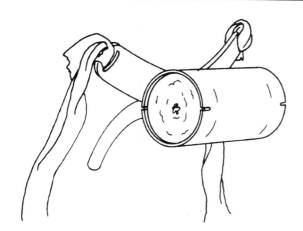

Figure 15–1 Tracheostomy Humidifying Filter

Source: Courtesy of Teresa Ahmann.

Exhibit 15–2 Equipment and Supplies for Tracheostomy Home Care

---

The following equipment should always be at the child's bedside:

1. a *tracheostomy tube of correct size,* with ties attached, and obturator in place, labeled "ready to go"
2. a *tracheostomy tube one size smaller,* with ties attached, and obturator in place, labeled "ready to go"
3. the *obturator* to the tube the child is currently using (taped to the wall near the bed)
4. blunt-end (bandage) *scissors*
5. *saline solution,* including small vials of saline for installation
6. *paper cups*
7. *hydrogen peroxide solution* (in brown bottle) or *white vinegar solution*
8. *cotton swabs* (Q-tips)
9. *gauze pads* or other *small cloths* to clean stoma area
10. *suction catheters* (correct size and one size smaller)
11. *tracheostomy ties*
12. *shoulder roll*
13. *suction machine and tubing*
14. *resuscitation bag*
15. *DeLee suction trap*
16. *source of humidity*

Equipment and Supplies

An evaluation of the equipment and supplies in the home is important on the first visit. All supplies listed in Exhibit 15–2 should be in the home. The nurse should check to ensure that the correct size and correct type (neonatal, pediatric, adult) of tracheostomy tubes and the correct size of suction catheter are available. Although the interior diameter of comparably sized pediatric and neonatal tracheostomy tubes may be the same, the length of the two types of tubes differs. Therefore, it is critical that both the size and the type of tube match that which is prescribed. Table 15–1 indicates the recommended sizes for suction catheters. The suction machine and source of humidity, usually a compressor with a jet nebulizer or cascade, should be assessed for proper functioning.

The nurse should also examine the arrangement of equipment and supplies in the home. The source of humidity, the suction machine, and the apnea monitor, if used, should be arranged at the child's bedside on a set of shelves or a small table. Suction catheters, as well as a tracheostomy tube of the prescribed size and a tube with a lumen one size smaller (both with ties attached, labeled "ready to go") should be at the bedside. Access to these supplies will facilitate suctioning and an emergency tube change, if needed.

Families living in a large house may wish to have these emergency supplies available in several rooms of the house. If a battery-operated, portable suction machine is not available, mouth suction traps (DeLee traps) can be placed in

Table 15–1 Choice of Catheter for Tracheostomy Suctioning

Size of trach tube Shiley	Size of catheter French	Length to insert [a] (cm)	Length to insert [b] (cm)
Neonatal			
00	6.5	5	5¾
0	6.5	5½	6½
1	6.5	5½	6½
Pediatric			
00	6.5	6½	7
0	6.5	6½	7
1	8	6½	7
2	8	6½	7
3	8	6½	7¼
4	8	7	7½

[a]This column indicates the length (in cm) to insert the catheter so that it will extend ¼ inch beyond the end of the trach tube.

[b]This column indicates the length (in cm) to insert the catheter so that it will extend ½ inch beyond the end of the trach tube.

Source: Adapted from *Management of the Child with a Tracheostomy, Protocol #1900A,* with permission of Children's Hospital National Medical Center, Division of Nursing and Patient Services, Washington, D.C., © 1995.

other rooms for easy access. Mouth suction traps should always be available for use in case of either suction machine or power failure. (See Figure 12–2 for an illustration of the mouth suction trap.) Parents and other caregivers should be instructed in their use.

Routine Tracheostomy Care

On the first home visit, the nurse should assist parents and other caregivers in assessing their preparedness to provide competently all aspects of tracheostomy care, including the following:

- suctioning
- removal and insertion of the tube
- the procedure to follow if the tube is difficult to insert
- the procedure to follow if the infant has difficulty breathing.

Anyone who will care for the infant even briefly should be knowledgeable in these procedures and proficient in cardiopulmonary resuscitation (CPR) techniques.

Suctioning

Suctioning on a regular basis is important to maintain an open airway free of secretions and mucus. Suctioning is indicated whenever the following signs occur (Children's National Medical Center, 1988, p. 7):

1. Secretions can be heard bubbling in the airway.
2. Breath sounds are dry and wheezing.
3. Child complains of difficult breathing.
4. Child has fast breathing not caused by activity.
5. Child shows signs of low oxygen such as restlessness, fast heart rate, flaring of the nostrils, blue or dusky color around the mouth or nose.

Several approaches to home suctioning have been recommended: clean (nongloved, washed hands), clean-gloved, and sterile-gloved. As long as the infant is not extremely young and is not prone to frequent infections, the family members may prefer to use the simplest and least expensive method, which is nongloved. If the child has any respiratory infection, clean-gloved or sterile-gloved techniques should be instituted until the infection has cleared. If frequent infections occur, clean-gloved or sterile-gloved technique should become routine. Professional caregivers should always choose a gloved method.

The basic techniques for catheter suctioning are discussed in Chapter 12. Chest therapy (see Chapter 12) may be helpful prior to suctioning, and saline instillation may assist in loosening secretions. In suctioning, the catheter should be inserted into the tracheostomy ¼ to ½ inch beyond the tip of the artificial airway (Runton, 1992) without suction applied; then suction can be applied, and the catheter twirled during its withdrawal from the tube. Withdrawal of the catheter should take no more than 5 sec. Because oxygen desaturation occurs for up to 60 sec after each suctioning attempt, the infant should be allowed to breathe at least a full 30 sec before the catheter is reinserted. During this time, the child who is mechanically ventilated or who does not tolerate suctioning well (e.g., the child who requires oxygen), can be given three or four breaths with the resuscitation bag.

Removing/Inserting the Tracheostomy Tube

On the first home visit, the nurse should also assist parents in assessing their skill and comfort in the procedures for removing and inserting the tracheostomy tube. Supplies for this procedure should always be available at the bedside, labeled "ready to go" in case of the need for an emergency tracheostomy tube change. The tube should be changed regularly, at least once a week. Of course, if the tube has an inner cannula, it should be removed and cleaned daily, as described in the Special Issue, "Cleaning Respiratory Equipment." Thorough hand-washing and careful handling of the tube, by the flanges only, are also important to reduce the risk of contamination.

When removing and inserting a tracheostomy tube, parents can use a shoulder roll (e.g., a small blanket rolled up) to put the infant's neck in the optimal alignment. An active infant should be held by another adult or wrapped snugly in a sheet or blanket.

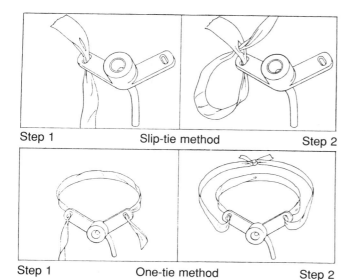

Step 1   Slip-tie method   Step 2

Step 1   One-tie method   Step 2

Figure 15–2 Methods for Securing the Tracheostomy Tube

Source: Reprinted from *Home Care of Your Child with a Tracheostomy: A Parent Handbook* by P. Hennessy (Ed.), p. 12, with permission of Children's Hospital National Medical Center, Washington, D.C., © 1983.

The tracheostomy tube is removed by pulling out and down, along the curve of the tube. The new tube is then placed into the stoma and pushed gently in and down, also along the curve of the tube. The obturator must be removed immediately, and the ties secured snugly. Two methods for securing the tracheostomy tube are illustrated in Figure 15–2.

Emergency Situations

Parents and other caregivers will also need to know the procedure to follow if the tracheostomy tube is difficult to insert—a rare but life-threatening occurrence. In this situation, the infant's head should be repositioned, tipped slightly back; the skin of the stoma spread carefully with the fingers; and the tube inserted as the infant breathes in. If the tube is still difficult to insert, parents should be prepared to use a tube one size smaller. In the event that this smaller tube cannot be inserted, a suction catheter can be placed in the stoma, secretions removed, and breaths given through the catheter. When the infant relaxes, another attempt should be made to insert the tracheostomy tube. If difficulty persists, the rescue squad should be contacted immediately and the infant transported to the hospital. The insertion attempts should continue.

An additional emergency plan that the nurse should review with parents involves appropriate interventions for the infant who either has difficulty breathing or ceases to breathe. In either case, the tracheostomy tube should be suctioned immediately. If respiratory difficulty continues, the tube may be plugged with secretions and should be removed

and replaced immediately. If the infant ceases breathing or the heart stops beating, CPR is necessary, and the rescue squad should be contacted immediately.

However, the nurse should warn parents that not all rescue squad personnel will have experience with tracheostomy care. In an emergency, parents may have to continue the procedures they have learned until the hospital staff takes over.

CPR techniques should be reviewed with parents and other caregivers on the first home visit, as well as on a regular basis on subsequent visits. Each caregiver should describe and demonstrate the correct procedure and timing for CPR, as well as modifications in the CPR procedure for a tracheostomy, as outlined in Exhibit 15–3.

SUBSEQUENT HOME VISITS

On each home visit, the nurse should elicit and address any parental concerns. In addition, the nurse should have a plan in mind for ongoing assessment and teaching that may not be addressed by parental concerns. The plan should address those areas described for routine visits, any teaching initiated or problems addressed on the first visit, and the following aspects of care.

Preventing Infection

Preventing infection is an important aspect of tracheostomy care, and the nurse should review three relevant principles with parents. First, thorough hand-washing prior to tracheostomy care, suctioning, and tube changes is key. Second, proper suctioning technique and regular, thorough cleaning of equipment and supplies are essential. Suction catheters should be rinsed with saline after each use; they then can be stored in a clean towel and reused for up to 6 hr unless the infant either has an infection or is prone to frequent infections. Instructions for cleaning other equipment and supplies can be found in the Special Issue, "Cleaning Respiratory Equipment." Third, if the infant or child does

Exhibit 15–3 CPR Modifications for a Child with a Tracheostomy

- The head should be tilted back so that the chin does not cover the tracheostomy tube.
- In listening for breaths, the ear should be placed at the tube.
- When breaths are given, the infant's nose and mouth should be held closed and breaths given into the tracheostomy tube, using the manual resuscitation device.
- If no breaths go in, the tube should be changed immediately and CPR continued as necessary.
- "If in doubt, change the trach" should be the motto of every person who cares for a child with a tracheostomy (Buzz-Kelly & Gordon, 1993).

acquire an infection with pseudomonas or Serratia, all disposable supplies should be discarded and new supplies used. Fourth, because the child with a tracheostomy may be especially susceptible, protection from exposure to others with upper respiratory infections is an important precaution.

Activities of Daily Living

The effect of the tracheostomy on the activities of daily living for the infant and family is an important area of assessment for the nurse and parents. In regard to feeding, most infants with a tracheostomy tube are able to eat and drink without difficulty. (Special attention may be required when positioning an infant for breastfeeding.) Vomiting may occur when an infant attempts to cough up secretions during or after feedings; suctioning during or after feedings can also stimulate vomiting. To limit the risk of vomiting, the nurse can encourage parents to suction just before feedings and not again until 2 hr afterward. If it is necessary to suction sooner, only gentle, brief suctioning should be used.

Bathing is another aspect of daily care that may concern parents. Although the infant should be carefully attended in the bathtub to avoid getting water into the tracheostomy, there is no reason to avoid bathing the infant or washing the infant's hair. Swimming, however, is contraindicated.

Parents may also have questions about the infant's sleeping arrangements. Because of the potential for respiratory emergencies at night, some parents choose to keep the infant in their room. Other families with extended hourly nursing services choose to have a nurse care for the infant at night. Generally, an infant with a tracheostomy is likely to have an apnea monitor that can alert caregivers of difficulty. The monitor will not alarm for obstructive apnea when there is chest wall movement. However, the tachycardia or bradycardia setting may alert parents to a problem. A pulse oximeter can be used to alert caregivers to hypoxemia, though they have not generally been used with children having tracheostomies. As a further precaution, some parents sew small bells into the infant's clothes so that they will ring as an initial sign of distress if the infant moves restlessly. Some parents purchase inexpensive intercoms so that they can hear the infant at all times. The nurse should assist parents as necessary in determining the arrangements that best meet their own needs for both peace of mind and privacy.

ONGOING CONCERNS

Decannulation

The length of time an infant may require a tracheostomy is variable and is influenced both by the primary reason for the tracheostomy and by any associated conditions. A study by Schlessel and colleagues (1993) found a 2-year mean duration of tracheostomy in young children.

Decannulation may be attempted as the underlying cause for tracheostomy resolves. For infants with mild subglottic stenosis, growth and careful medical management may allow for eventual decannulation. Other infants may require surgical reconstruction of the airway, called *laryngotracheal reconstruction*. The goals of reconstruction are to produce an adequate airway, an acceptable voice, and a larynx competent to avoid aspiration (Zal Zal, 1988).

Communication Development

Communication development is a long-term concern for children with tracheostomies. The ability to vocalize with a tracheostomy in place may be limited, and parents may be concerned about the likelihood of resultant long-term communication disorders. In this regard, Simon, Fowler, and Handler (1983) studied language development in 77 tracheostomized children and found that extensive cooing and babbling was not necessary for later speech development. Children decannulated prelinguistically mastered communication skills appropriate for their developmental level. Children decannulated during linguistic stages did exhibit some speech delays, although with speech or language therapy, nearly all of the decannulated children showed eventual compensation for these delays. Chapter 22 offers a detailed discussion of speech and language development in the child with a tracheostomy; suggestions for intervention to minimize potential problems are included.

Out-of-Home Programs

Conditions, such as prematurity, that led to the infant's need for a tracheostomy may predispose him or her to developmental delay as well. Public Law (P.L.) 99-457 mandates "education and related services" to meet the developmental needs of children requiring special attention. Services include special education, audiology, speech and language therapy, physical therapy, and occupational therapy. Parents may be unaware of the child's entitlement, and nurses should provide them with information about P.L. 99-457 and available programs as appropriate. (See Special Issue, "Early Intervention Services For the High-risk Infant.")

Under P.L. 99-457, a child may receive homebound or school-based services. For a child receiving center-based developmental intervention or attending a day care or school setting, it is essential that someone capable in all aspects of tracheostomy care be available to the child. This may require extensive training of center or school personnel prior to the child's attendance (Dorsey & Diehl, 1992; Haynie, Porter, & Palfrey, 1989). If the child is transported on a school bus, a trained attendant should accompany the child.

Emergency equipment and supplies should accompany the child at all times (see Exhibit 15–1).

Family Concerns

Sibling adjustment is a potential ongoing concern for parents. As with any chronic illness, siblings may experience anxiety, anger, and jealousy related to the child with a tracheostomy. Chapter 3 addresses sibling adjustment issues in detail and provides guidance for the nurse and family.

In addition, providing care to an infant or child with a tracheostomy can shift all family member roles and responsibilities. The extra work that is involved can strain the family's daily schedule. Some families may appreciate the nurse's assistance in evaluating and reorganizing responsibilities and daily schedules. Assisting families to arrange respite care by training babysitters, or by arranging for home nursing care or a respite program, can also be a key factor in making home care more manageable for the family of an infant with a tracheostomy.

For infants receiving extended hourly nursing care rather than intermittent visits, nurses will be providing direct care for a specified number of hours per day. Nurses should evaluate equipment and supplies, review routine and emergency care, and make an initial and then ongoing assessments of the infant's condition. In addition to performing procedures, nurses should provide continuing education and training to parents, assuring that they will be confident and competent caregivers in the absence of nurses. Because private-duty nurses and families share responsibilites in the infant's life, it is essential they have a collaborative relationship. Families must be included in formulating and revising the plan of care. Interventions are more likely to achieve the desired results when the nurse conveys a sense of cooperation and joint responsibility (partnership) with families in implementing the plan of care (Bond, Phillips, & Rollins, 1994). (Chapter 4 discusses these issues in greater detail.)

REFERENCES

Barnes, L. (1992). Tracheostomy care: Preparing parents for discharge. *MCN: American Journal of Maternal/Child Nursing, 17,* 293.

Bond, N., Phillips, P., & Rollins, N. (1994). Family centered care at home for families with children who are technology dependent. *Pediatric Nursing, 20*(2), 123–130.

Buzz-Kelly, L., & Gordon, P. (1993). Teaching CPR to parents of children with tracheostomies. *MCN: American Journal of Maternal/Child Nursing, 18,* 158–163.

Children's National Medical Center. (1988). *Home care of your child with a tracheostomy: A parent handbook.* Washington, DC: Author.

Dorsey, L., & Diehl, B. (1992). An educational program for school nurses caring for the pediatric client with a tracheostomy. *Ostomy/Wound Management, 38*(5), 16–19.

Haynie, M., Porter, S., & Palfrey, J.S. (1989). *Children assisted by medical technology in educational settings: Guidelines for care.* Boston, MA: The Children's Hospital.

Runton, N. (1992). Suctioning artificial airways in children: Appropriate technique. *Pediatric Nursing, 18*(2), 115–118.

Schlessel, J., Harper, R., Rappa, H., Kenigsberg, K., & Khanna, S. (1993). Tracheostomy: Acute and long-term mortality and morbidity in very low birth weight premature infants. *Journal of Pediatric Surgery, 28*(7), 873–876.

Simon, B.M., Fowler, S.M., & Handler, S.D. (1983). Communication development in young children with long term tracheostomies: Preliminary report. *Journal of Pediatric Otorhinolaryngology, 6,* 37–50.

Zal Zal, G. (1988). Use of stents in laryngotracheal reconstruction in children: Indications, technical considerations, and complications. *Laryngoscope, 98*(8), 849–864.

ADDITIONAL RESOURCES

Ahmann, E. (1992). Family centered care: Shifting orientation. *Pediatric Nursing, 20*(2), 113–117.

Ahmann, E. (1994). Family centered care: The time has come. *Pediatric Nursing, 20*(1), 52–53.

Ahmann, E., & Bond, N. (1992). Promoting normal development in school aged children and adolescents who are technology dependent: A family centered model. *Pediatric Nursing, 18*(4), 399–405.

Duncan, B., Howell, L., deLorimer, A., Adzick, N., & Harrison, M. (1992). Tracheostomy in children with emphasis on home care. *Journal of Pediatric Surgery, 27*(4), 432–435.

Fields, A., Rosenblatt, A., Pollack, M., & Kaufman, J. (1991). Home care cost effectiveness for respiratory technology dependent children. *American Journal of Diseases of Children, 145,* 729–733.

Sherman, L., & Rosen, C. (1990). Development of a preschool program for tracheostomy dependent children. *Pediatric Nursing, 16*(4), 357–361.

Warnock, C., & Porpora, K. (1994). A pediatric trach card: Transforming research into practice. *Pediatric Nursing, 20*(2), 186–188.

Zeitouni, A., & Manoukian, J. (1993). Tracheotomy in the first year of life. *Journal of Otolaryngology, 22*(6), 431–434.

Home Care Plan: Tracheostomy

Date _____   Case manager _____

Name _____   Hosp # _____   DOB _____

PROBLEM: **RESPIRATORY COMPROMISE: TRACHEOSTOMY**

GOALS/OBJECTIVES	METHODS	STAFF/REVIEW
Child to be at minimal risk of occluded airway	Assess/teach AP, RR; auscultate lungs; observe for flaring, and retractions. Assess secretions for viscosity, color, odor each visit. Assess/teach appropriate use of humidity, suctioning. Assess/teach correct procedures for trach change. Assess supplies and equipment in the home for appropriateness and safe, easy access.	
Caregivers to have appropriate plans for emergency intervention	Assess/teach appropriate plans for emergency intervention. Assess/teach CPR for trach; review as necessary. Assess plans/assist in planning when to call rescue squad/doctor. Ensure that phone company, power company, appropriate rescue squads and ER notified of child's status.	
Child will be at minimal risk for irritation at trach site	Assess trach site each visit for redness, granuloma. Assess neck for redness, skin breakdown. Assess/teach caregivers appropriate method and schedule for cleaning trach site, changing trach ties.	
Child will be at minimal risk for respiratory/tracheal infection	Assess/teach clean technique for suctioning/trach change.	

GOALS/OBJECTIVES	METHODS	STAFF/REVIEW
	Assess/teach appropriate method and schedule for cleaning equipment and supplies. Teach family to keep child away from persons with URI. Teach caregivers signs and symptoms of infection: 　Elevated temperature 　Change in trach secretions 　　color 　　volume 　　viscosity 　　odor 　Respiratory distress 　　increase in RR 　　retracting, flaring 　　increase in O_2 requirements	
Caregivers to describe appropriate intervention for signs/symptoms of tracheal/respiratory infection	Assess/teach caretakers plans for intervention. If tracheal infection: 　Contact doctor at early signs 　More frequent change of suction catheters 　More thorough cleansing of equipment (or discard disposable equipment if pseudomonas or Serratia) If respiratory infection: 　Contact doctor at early signs 　More frequent change of suction catheters 　Increase chest therapy	
Caregivers to describe/demonstrate appropriate travel plans	Review/assist in planning for safe travel prn. Review/assist in making Travel Kit.	
Child to have regular and prn follow-up by managing physician	Encourage regular and prn appointments. Communicate/coordinate with managing physician on regular and prn basis.	

Source: Courtesy of Children's Hospital National Medical Center, Home Health Care Services, Washington, D.C.

Appendix 15–B

Home Assessment: Tracheostomy

Name _____ Hosp# _____ DOB _____

Primary caretaker _____ Back-up caretaker _____

Address _____ Address _____

Telephone _____ Telephone _____

Date of hospital discharge _____ Start of service date _____

Diagnoses _____

_____

_____

Reason for tracheostomy: _____

Physician managing trach: _____

Telephone _____ Page _____

Type of trach _____ Size of trach _____

Equipment supply company _____

Telephone _____ 24-hour service telephone _____

EVERY VISIT: Assess vital signs, quantity and quality of secretions. Observe respiratory pattern, neck, and stoma site. Auscultate breath sounds, and assess for s/sx respiratory distress.

I. Equipment

	Date observed	N/A	Comments
Humidification System	_____		_____
Vaporizer (opt.)	_____		
Apnea monitor (If yes, refer to Apnea Monitor Assessment in Appendix 13–B)	_____		
Oxygen Source (prn) (If yes, refer to Oxygen Assessment in Appendix 14–B)	_____		

Suction Machine (stationary
and/or portable) _____

Suction Catheters _____

    size # _____, length to insert _____

Portable Suction Catheter
(DeLee) size # _____

Tracheostomy Tubes:
    type & size _____

    prescribed size (min. of 4) _____

    1 size smaller _____

Tracheostomy Ties
(twill tape) _____

Tracheostomy
Humidifying filter _____

Blunt End Scissors _____

Dispose-A-Vial Saline _____

Resuscitation Bag
(size   ) _____

Shoulder Roll _____

White Vinegar _____

Hydrogen Peroxide _____

Q-Tips _____

Paper Cups _____

Wipes (Kleenex,
Handiwipes, etc.) _____

Phone (near patient) _____

Travel Bag:
    prescribe trach tube
    (with ties) "ready to go" _____

    tube one size smaller
    (with ties) "ready to go" _____

    obturator _____

    Addapak saline vials _____

    bandage scissors _____

    Handiwipes or tissues _____

    portable suction catheter _____

    jar-sterile saline _____

II. Emergency notifications

	Date sent	N/A	Comments
Letter to telephone co.			
Letter to electric co.			
Letter to rescue squad			
Personal contact with squad (opt)			
Letter to nearest emergency room			

III. Emergency information posted

	Date observed	N/A	Comments
Rescue squad number			
Physician's number			
Equipment supply co. number			
Power co. emergency number			
CPR guidelines			
Patient's name & address (opt)			

IV. Emergency care

	Primary Caretaker Date	Back-up Caretaker Date	Comments
Demonstrates one-person trach change (pt. or doll)			
Describes procedures when trach tube insertion is difficult			
Describes signs and symptoms of respiratory distress			
Describes emergency plan for:			
a. Respiratory failure			
b. Respiratory distress			
c. Power failure			
Demonstrates CPR:			

V. Routine care

	Primary Caretaker Date	Back-up Caretaker Date	Comments
State reason for tracheostomy			
Describes pulmonary anatomy			
Describes how to evaluate:			
a. Quality & quantity of secretions			
b. Respiratory pattern			
c. Appropriate intervention for deviations from normal			
Demonstrates tracheostomy change			
Demonstrates cleaning of neck and stoma			
Demonstrates changing trach ties			

Demonstrates chest
therapy _____

Demonstrates use of
resuscitation bag _____

Demonstrates operation of
apnea monitor, prn _____

Demonstrates operation of
humidification system _____

Demonstrates operation of
suction equipment _____

Demonstrates safe use
of oxygen, prn _____

Describes cleaning of
supplies & equipment _____

Describes appropriate
arrangement of supplies _____

VI. Safety precautions

	Date reviewed	N/A	Comments
Trach tube, prescribed size, with ties on at bedside			
Trach tube, one size smaller, with ties on, at bedside			
Obturator at bedside			
Scissors & extra trach ties at bedside			
Suction catheters available at bedside			
Travel bag on all trips out of house			
No swimming			
No clothing obstructing trach			
No small beads as toys			

Comments: _____
_____

VII. Describe caretaker/child interaction (overall interaction and with respect to trach care)

_____
_____
_____
_____

VIII. Describe caretakers' overall confidence and concerns about tracheostomy care

_____
_____
_____
_____

IX. Assessment of problems identified

_____

_____

_____

_____

_____

X. Plan to address problems identified

_____

_____

_____

_____

_____

Signature _____ Date completed _____

Source: Courtesy of Children's Hospital National Medical Center, Home Health Care Services, Washington, D.C.

Chapter 16

Home Care of the Infant Requiring Mechanical Ventilation

Revised by Angela Jerome-Ebel, MSN, RN

The use of mechanical ventilation at home has been increasing over the past 15 years. In pediatrics, experience has been gained with young children having spinal cord injuries, congenital and acquired central hypoventilation syndrome, neuromuscular disease, and bronchopulmonary dysplasia (Pilmer, 1994).

DECIDING ON HOME CARE

In considering the feasibility of home ventilation, several factors are important. Of greatest importance is parental participation in the decision-making process. Health care providers must respect the fact that not all families will choose to care for a ventilator-dependent child in the home (Lantos & Kohrman, 1992). In this connection, parents must be thoroughly informed that home ventilation involves a commitment of 24 hours each day. Likewise, they must be advised of its risks and its benefits, as well as other options for the child's ongoing care. The attitude of the parents toward home mechanical ventilation and their motivation and ability to learn the necessary care are important factors in safe, successful management of home ventilation.

Additional considerations regarding the feasibility of home ventilator care include the following:

- the relative stability of the underlying disease process
- the inability to wean from mechanical ventilation over a 3- to 6-month period

- the home environment, especially electrical capability, heat, plumbing, wheelchair accessibility if needed, space for necessary equipment and storage of supplies, and a telephone
- a community support system, including availability of 24-hr servicing for equipment and supplies, reasonable accessibility to both trained rescue squads and an emergency facility, and the availability of appropriately trained home care nurses or other support personnel to provide back-up care
- adequate financial resources, private or public, to support the costs of home care.

PREDISCHARGE PLANNING

Parental Education

If home care is determined to be feasible, the parents and other caregivers must be thoroughly educated regarding the child's condition and care requirements prior to hospital discharge. (See Exhibit 16–1.) Each person who will care for the infant must be involved in discussion, demonstration, and repeat demonstration of all components of the child's care. The teaching should be followed by a 24- to 48-hr period during which two primary caregivers provide the child's complete care in the hospital, with nurses, respiratory therapists, and physicians available only as consultants. (Some institutions require a 12- to 24-hr trial and a 24- to

Exhibit 16–1 Predischarge Teaching for Home Ventilator Care

Underlying disease

Pulmonary hygiene (see Chapter 12)

Ventilator
- operational controls: prescribed settings for rate, tidal volume, pressures, and so on
- procedure and schedule for cleaning and changing circuitry
- source of humidity; use & cleaning
- alarms
- troubleshooting problems
- use of manual resuscitator
- supply inventory
- alternative source of power (duration of charge on internal battery, 12-volt battery)
- cleaning and disinfection of all equipment

Other equipment and care
- apnea monitor
- oxygen
- tracheostomy care
- oximetry

Emergency care and precautions
- prenotification of rescue squads, nearest emergency facility, electric and telephone companies, and road commission (in rural areas)
- troubleshooting alarms (see Figure 16–1)
- signs and symptoms of respiratory distress or failure
- criteria for calling equipment supplier, rescue squad, and physician
- CPR
- hurricane/flood plan if appropriate

Medications: dosages, frequency, actions, and side effects

Health maintenance plan, including location of source of primary care and arrangement of follow-up appointments

Developmental program including arrangement for occupational, physical, and/or speech therapy, if necessary

Travel and transportation plans

Daily care plan

Supply inventory and source of 24-hour supply and service

48-hr trial at home or in a nearby hotel before discharge.) Even with such practice, written instructions for all aspects of routine and emergency care, including equipment inventory and daily schedules or checklists, may be necessary to assist the family in providing appropriate care at home.

Financial Arrangements

The financial support for home care must also be thoroughly investigated before a decision to discharge can be made. Private insurers and Medicaid vary in the amount and extent of coverage provided for home care (Kaufman,

1991a, 1991b). Coverage and caps for medical equipment, supplies, prescriptions (including oxygen), home nursing care, and other necessary services should be explored. Creative approaches to financing home care may be necessary.

Home Nursing Support

The first several weeks of home care are a critical time period as the family is still in the process of learning the care of their child. Readmission to the hospital is a significant risk during this period. To minimize this risk, the family should consider, and the discharge planning team should assist in arranging, 24 hr per day of home nursing care for at least 3 weeks. If financial restrictions necessitate it, care can gradually be transitioned down to 8 hr of nursing care per day after the initial adjustment period. Careful evaluation of medical needs must be assessed before reducing home nursing coverage.

CHOICE OF A VENTILATOR

A ventilator is a device that moves air into the lungs. Ventilators can move air into the lungs using either positive or negative pressure. Ventilators vary in design, and it is possible to select a specific model and settings that can best meet the needs of the infant or child.

Choice of a home ventilator depends on several factors:

- the child's underlying disease process
- the mode of ventilation required
- the need for positive end-expiratory pressure (PEEP)
- the need for oxygen
- ventilator capabilities, including ease of operation, portability, reliability, and functioning alarm system
- community experience with a particular type of ventilator.

Whatever type of ventilator is selected, certain services should be expected to be provided in conjunction with its purchase or lease. (See Chapter 5.) The family, and any nurses providing care for the child at home, should be assisted in becoming thoroughly familiar with the operation of the chosen ventilator before it is used in the home. Use of the home ventilator for 24 to 48 hr in the hospital before discharge will enable the family to become familiar with its use. A troubleshooting manual should be provided with the ventilator. However, it is also important to have 24-hr servicing and 24-hr respiratory therapy assistance available in case of equipment malfunction. It is further advisable to have a back-up suction, humidifier, and ventilator readily available (though not necessarily in the home) in case of malfunction.

Positive Pressure Ventilation

Positive pressure ventilation supports the infant by pushing air into the lungs, holding it there for a predetermined amount of time, and letting it return to baseline (Dupuis, 1986). During a ventilator breath, the chest will rise. Positive pressure ventilation can be provided through a tracheostomy tube or by a face/nose mask. There are several ways that positive pressure ventilation can be provided: volume controlled, pressure controlled, or bilevel positive airway pressure (BiPab® Respironics).

Volume Ventilator

The Aequitron LP-6, LP-6 plus, or LP-10, Lifecare PLV102, BEAR 33, and Puritan-Bennett Companion 2801 (no longer manufactured) are common volume ventilators used in the home. Volume ventilators provide a preset tidal volume or "breath size" to the infant while the pressure needed to deliver the volume may vary. It is common in infants to use a volume ventilator with a pressure limit control device to provide "pressure-limited" ventilation.

Pressure Ventilator

Pressure ventilation is used primarily in the acute care setting and only occasionally in home care. The most common pressure ventilators for use in the home include the BEAR Cub infant ventilator, the Sechrist, and The Newport E100i, but most of the volume ventilators (noted above) can also provide pressure ventilation (though without continuous flow). With pressure ventilation, air is moved into the lungs at a prescribed pressure, while the tidal volume that the lung receives may vary (Dupuis, 1986). Pressure ventilation requires a continuous air source that can be difficult to maintain in the home care setting, especially during transport of the child.

BiPAP (Bilevel Positive Airway Pressure)

BiPAP® by Respironic, Inc., is a low-pressure ventilatory support system that provides pressurized air to the infant through a face/nose mask or a tracheostomy tube (Respironics Inc., 1990a, 1990b). Although Respironics does not endorse trach tube application, use this way is gaining widespread acceptance. During inspiration (IPAP), a breath is delivered at a prescribed level. The device then senses expiration, bringing the pressured air down to a lower level (EPAP) to allow for exhalation. BiPAP can be set in several modes that meet the specific needs of the infant or child, including continuous positive airway pressure (CPAP). It can be set up with or without a back-up rate. Although this device was not intended to be used as a life-support ventilator, it often is.

Negative Pressure Ventilation

Negative pressure ventilation moves air into the lungs by using devices to apply subatmospheric pressure around the chest (Dupuis, 1986; Hill, 1994). Inhalation occurs when the chest cavity is expanded periodically; exhalation occurs by passive relaxation of the chest wall and lungs. Intermittent ventilation improves gas exchange and allows fatigued muscles to rest. The efficiency of negative pressure ventilation is based on lung and chest wall compliance and the quality of the seal of the chest device.

There are two components of a negative pressure ventilation system. The first component is the ventilator that creates the negative pressure. Common negative pressure ventilators used in the home care setting include Lifecare's NEV-100 and the Thompson Maxivent, Emerson, and other positive pressure ventilators with a negative pressure capability. The second component of the system is the body device that attaches to the negative pressure ventilator. Common body devices include the Lifecare "shell" or cuirass, "Pulmo-Wrap," "Nu-Mo" garments, and "Poncho." Another device that is used in the home care setting is the Port-a-lung, which is an adaptation of the Emerson tank ventilator or "iron lung" (McNichol-Dougherty, 1990).

HOSPITAL DISCHARGE AND TRANSITION TO THE HOME

In the past, infants being discharged to home on a ventilator remained in the acute care hospital prior to discharge to home. Recently, skilled nursing facilities that provide transitional care for infants requiring long-term mechanical ventilation are becoming increasingly available. Therefore, the trend may be to discharge to home from the skilled nursing facility instead of the acute care hospital. Regardless of the institution from which the infant or child is discharged, discharge planning must be a collaborative process involving parents, hospital nurses, respiratory therapists, physicians, other health care personnel, and home care personnel, including a case manager or nursing supervisor, and representatives of the durable medical equipment (DME) or home medical equipment (HME) company. (See Chapter 5.)

Selection of Home Nurses

The family should be provided information to assist in selection of a qualified nursing agency and DME provider. Occasionally, a "back-up" agency may be necessary to ensure the full coverage the family needs. It will be particularly important for both companies to provide the family with information regarding their overall experience with other ventilator-assisted children. Nurses can be located through nursing agencies or through newspaper advertisements. Of course, nurses with both pediatric and ventilator experience are preferable, and any nurses recruited should be trained in the specifics of care for the infant or child prior to hospital discharge. When possible, setting up a schedule for nurses in advance will help minimize gaps in coverage.

Home Care Referral

As discharge approaches, the community health nurse should obtain a thorough history of the child's course and information about the underlying disease process leading to the need for continued mechanical ventilation. The nurse should also obtain, in writing, the physician's instructions for ventilator settings. (See Exhibit 16–2.) Prescriptions, including oxygen, if required, should be listed by the physician. Additionally, individualized guidelines for responding to respiratory distress in the infant should be worked out with the physician, nurse, and parents before hospital discharge.

The home care nurse will be better able to address issues and problems arising in home care if familiar both with the ventilator to be used in the home and with the daily care of the infant or child prior to hospital discharge. An awareness of the parents' skill with the infant's special care, their understanding of the infant's condition, and their general level of acceptance of the home care plan will form the basis for initial support and teaching at home. Both parents and the home care nurse(s) will find it helpful if hospital nurses prepare a list of the infant's daily schedule of medications, treatments, and other care requirements. While the infant's

Exhibit 16–2 Ventilator Settings and Respiratory Parameters

Mode (Control, intermittent mechanical ventilation [IMV] or
    CPAP)
Pressure limit
PEEP (positive end-expiratory pressure)
Rate
Flow rate
Inspiratory time
Expiratory time
Volume (when applicable)
Heater temperature ranges
Low-pressure alarm
High-pressure alarm
Breathing effort
FiO_2 (when and how to titrate O_2 according to SpO_2)
Exhaled volume, normal ranges
Own breath volume ranges
Weaning schedule

Note: These settings may apply to some, but not all, ventilators and some, but not all, modes of ventilation. The settings may vary significantly depending on the child's size, age, underlying condition, and the size of the trach tube.

schedule may be rearranged at home, the hospital schedule will provide material with which to work.

Predischarge Home Visit

It may be useful for the home care nursing supervisor or case manager to make a home visit prior to discharge to assist the family in assessing the electrical capability of the home, accessibility, and adequacy of space in the home for the necessary equipment and supplies. During the visit, the nurse can also assist parents, as needed, to determine optimal locations for equipment and supplies in the home. In this regard, ease of care and ready access in case of emergencies are primary considerations.

Emergency Preparations

Prior to discharge, it is important to ensure that emergency preparations, as discussed in Chapter 12, have been addressed (Steele & Morgan, 1989). Emergency preparations include the following:

- ensuring that there is a telephone in the home
- notifying telephone and electric companies and the road commission that the family needs to be on a priority service list
- informing rescue squad and emergency department personnel of the child's presence in the home and special requirements
- posting cardiopulmonary resuscitation (CPR) guidelines
- posting a list of important telephone numbers (see Exhibit 12–1).

Transportation

The nurse should also discuss with parents plans for safe transportation of the child. (See also Chapter 5.) Arrangements should be made for ventilation during transport. Options include running the ventilator on a 12-volt battery; plugging it into an automobile cigarette lighter electrical adapter; or, alternatively, the use of a portable ventilator. Age-appropriate carseat or tie-downs for a wheelchair are needed. Transport by ambulance can be arranged when no other alternatives are available or in case of emergency. Two adults should always be in the vehicle when the child is transported; this permits at least one adult to respond to respiratory emergencies.

In addition, transportation to and from visits to the physician or clinic will need careful planning. Some families may already have or may be able to purchase a van or a station wagon; others may need to use ambulance services. Families using their own vehicles can be advised to obtain a handicapped permit or license plates to facilitate parking.

ROUTINE HOME VISITS

The plan of care should be negotiated with the family, and the concerns and priorities of family members should receive attention on each home visit. (A sample care plan is provided in Appendix 16–A.) Additionally, the nurse should complete a thorough assessment of the infant or child; assist family members in assessing their ability to provide safe and appropriate care; and provide teaching, support, and referrals as neccessary.

Assessment of the Infant or Child

On all home visits, vital signs of the infant or child should be obtained and the observed respiratory rate should be checked against the rate of the ventilator. In addition, it is important to assess regularly both the infant or child and the ventilator to identify actual or potential problems during mechanical ventilation.

For assessment, the nurse should note skin color and respiratory patterns and should observe the chest for regular rise and fall with each breath. Lung fields should be auscultated for the presence of adventitious sounds, and the infant or child should be assessed for signs and symptoms of respiratory distress or failure, including dyspnea, restlessness, pallor, fatigue, and periorbital edema. Additionally, the pulse oximeter will generally be used in assessment. Deviations from the individual's normal condition should be brought to the attention of both the parents and the physician.

Assessment of the Ventilator

For assessment of the ventilator, all settings should be checked against those recommended. The ventilator should also routinely be observed for the following:

- Chest wall moves with ventilator breath.
- Low-pressure alarm goes off with tubing disconnection.
- Dial goes up to patient's norm with each ventilator cycle.
- Dial returns to zero or the recommended PEEP.
- High-pressure alarm goes off with circuit occlusion.
- Circuit temperature is at recommended range.
- Exhaled volumes, using a respirometer, are within recommended range.
- SpO_2 levels are appropriate.
- O_2 concentration is accurate.

Any problems should be brought to the attention of the parents and, as appropriate, the physician, the supply company representative, and/or the respiratory therapist.

Parental Education

The care plan for a mechanically ventilated child should address the risks of barotrauma (e.g., pneumothorax or pneumomediastinum), decreased cardiac output, and fluid imbalance. Although these particular risks are low when a child has stabilized on mechanical ventilation, it is nevertheless important to assess for these problems on each home visit. Parents should be taught to observe their child for the signs and symptoms of cardiorespiratory problems: dyspnea, restlessness, pallor, fatigue, and periorbital edema. If such changes are noted, the physician should be contacted promptly. Growth and energy levels should also be monitored.

Atelectasis is also a potential problem for the mechanically ventilated child, particularly if mobility is limited. The nurse should review with parents instructions for frequent position changes, regular and vigorous chest therapy (see Chapter 12), and periodic hyperinflation as preventive measures. Suctioning as needed can assist in the removal of copious secretions, which may otherwise contribute to the risk of atelectasis as well as inadequate ventilation. (Suctioning is discussed in more detail in Chapters 12 and 15). Hyperinflation and hyperoxygenation before and after suctioning are sometimes recommended, particularly in infants because of their small lung volumes. It is also important while suctioning to ventilate the infant, mechanically or manually, between each pass of the catheter.

THE FIRST HOME VISIT

Establishing rapport with the family is an important aspect of the first home visit. Parental concerns and questions should be solicited and addressed, and parents should play a central role in the development of the plan for home care of the infant or child.

The nurse should have a plan in mind to address all aspects of routine home visits, as previously detailed, on the first home visit. In addition, the nurse must determine that needed supplies and equipment are available in the home, that equipment is functioning properly, and that parents are well prepared to provide safe and appropriate care.

Equipment and Supplies

Essential equipment and supplies for respiratory care should be available in the home, both at the infant's bedside and at any other location at which care may be provided. (A list of supplies is part of Appendix 16–B.) Some families find shelved carts with wheels very useful for storing supplies.

Essential bedside supplies include an extra tracheostomy tube with ties attached, a tube one to two sizes smaller, suction equipment, and a manual resuscitator. All tracheostomy supplies, apnea monitor supplies, oximeter and supplies, and oxygen equipment, if needed, should be arranged for safety and ready access. An extra set of tubing (including PEEP valve, etc.) should be kept "ready to go" to use if necessary to resolve a continuous low-pressure (or other) alarm problem. The new tubing can be put in place and the old tubing then examined piece by piece for small leak holes.

A back-up power source for the ventilator should be available for use in an electrical "brown-out" or "black-out"; 12-volt batteries are often used for this purpose. Some families may need an electrical generator for the house to ensure adequate power. If a back-up power source is an impractical expense, parents must be instructed in ventilation using an oxygen cylinder and a manual resuscitator in case of power loss.

If a cardiorespiratory monitor or oxygen is being used, the essential equipment knowledge, and skills for their safe and appropriate use should likewise be reviewed. (Apnea monitoring and home oxygen therapy are discussed in Chapters 13 and 14, respectively.)

Review Ventilator Settings

On the first home visit, the nurse and/or the respiratory therapist should review with parents their knowledge of the prescribed ventilator settings. It can be helpful to post prescribed settings on or near the ventilator for quick reference. (See Exhibit 16–2.) The settings should be checked every 4 hours if the infant is on the ventilator continuously and before use if mechanical ventilation is needed only at night. Parents should also have an understanding both of the meaning of each setting and of how the ventilator functions. In this regard, they can be asked to describe the ventilator circuitry, including the source of humidification.

Safety Concerns

If there are curious siblings in the family, or if the ventilated child is ambulatory, it is important to childproof the ventilator dials and switches. Putting the ventilator out of reach and using childproof plastic panels to cover control knobs will help ensure that the settings are not mistakenly changed by curious hands. (Such panels can be obtained from the manufacturer or supplier.)

Parental Education

Respiratory Distress

On the initial visit, the nurse should also assess parental knowledge of signs and symptoms of respiratory distress, inadequate ventilation, and respiratory failure as well as appropriate interventions. Respiratory distress (described in Chapter 12) may result from partial or complete occlusion of the tracheostomy tube, from hyperreactive airways disease, from a pulmonary infection, or from other cardiopulmonary disorders. Basic guidelines for intervention in the event of respiratory distress, which must take into consideration the child's underlying lung condition, should be developed in conjunction with the physician prior to discharge. Parental familiarity with these guidelines is essential. Parents should be encouraged to contact the physician as necessary should questions or concerns arise. Parents should also be instructed in steps to follow if the trach tube comes out and cannot be reinserted. (See Chapter 15.)

Troubleshooting Ventilator Alarms

Both inadequate ventilation and respiratory failure may have various causes. Of primary importance is the ability to differentiate between ventilator problems and problems originating in the infant or child, as indicated in Figure 16–1. Caregivers should be familiar with methods of troubleshooting ventilator alarms. In this regard, they should know that the first step upon hearing an alarm sound is to

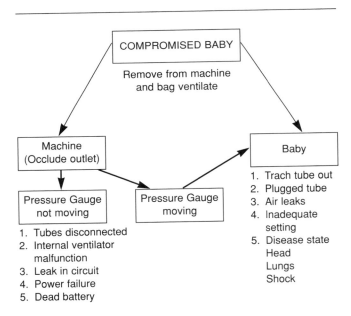

Figure 16–1 Troubleshooting Mechanical Ventilation Alarms

Source: Adapted from "Basic Concepts in Positive Pressure Ventilation of the Newborn" by S.K. Gottschalk, B. King, and C.R. Schuth, *Perinatology/Neonatology,* Vol. 4, with permission of Brentwood Publishing Corporation, © March-April, 1980.

assess the infant. Then the ventilator circuitry should be examined for disconnections (Witham-Wilson, 1991). If the alarm is not merely signaling a disconnection of circuitry, the infant should be removed from the ventilator and manually ventilated with the manual resuscitator until the reason for the alarm is identified and corrected. Causes may include the following: the need for suctioning, an air leak around the trach tube, the need for a nebulizer treatment, an empty oxygen tank, and so forth.

A manual or set of written instructions detailing troubleshooting methods, generally supplied by the manufacturer, should always be kept near the ventilator. Additionally, the 24-hr number for the equipment supplier should be posted near the telephone. (See Exhibit 12–1.) Guidelines for when to contact the equipment supplier, the physician, and the rescue squad are an important element of planning for potential emergencies. They should be developed in conjunction with the physician prior to discharge and reviewed with caregivers at home both initially and again at intervals as necessary.

Emergency Interventions

In order to manage ventilatory insufficiency and possible respiratory failure, it is essential that caregivers be able to clear an obstructed airway and to provide CPR, if indicated. These crucial skills should be reviewed on the first home visit and subsequently at regular intervals. (Chapters 12 and 15 are useful in this regard.)

SUBSEQUENT HOME VISITS

Home visits should generally begin by addressing any problems or concerns identified by caregivers. At the same time, the nurse should have a plan in mind for ongoing assessment and teaching. The plan should address those areas described for routine home visits, any teaching initiated or problems addressed on the first visit, and the following aspects of care.

Preventing Infection

The prevention of infection is one important aspect of the care plan for a child on a ventilator. The nurse should stress thorough hand-washing and should caution parents to avoid exposing the infant to persons with upper respiratory infections.

Another potential source of infection is water that accumulates in the ventilator tubing. As it accumulates, the water should be emptied from the circuit. It can be disposed of into a plastic-lined garbage can placed nearby; it should not be emptied back into the humidifier.

The methods and schedules for cleaning and disinfection of ventilator circuitry are also important. Although there is debate over how often, if ever, tubing and connections can reasonably be reused, financial constraints will sometimes necessitate the reuse of at least some of the equipment. If portions of the ventilator circuitry are to be reused, regular cleaning is essential. (See Special Issue, "Cleaning Respiratory Equipment.") If problems occur with frequent tracheitis, unusually frequent upper respiratory infections, or pneumonia, both a more stringent cleaning and disinfection schedule and sterile technique for tracheostomy care are recommended, as well as more frequent filter changes on the respiratory equipment.

Health Maintenance

Health maintenance needs must also be addressed. (See Chapter 8.) In the midst of the many demands of caring for a ventilated child, they easily can be neglected. The family may need assistance in locating a pediatrician or nurse practitioner who will make home visits. Alternatively, the nurse can assist in arranging health maintenance visits at the medical center in conjunction with any visits to other specialists. Visits should be coordinated in order to limit the number of trips the family must make to the medical center. Examination rooms must, of course, be arranged to accommodate the ventilator, suction machine, and oxygen if required.

Nutrition and Feeding

A thorough nutrition and feeding assessment should be conducted by the nurse. For many children with respiratory compromise, obtaining adequate nutrition can be challenging. (See Chapter 9.) Additionally, for many ventilator-dependent infants, early lack of oral experience or developing orally aversive behaviors may interfere with optimal oral intake, and special intervention by an occupational or speech therapist may be helpful.

Development

Developmental issues and assessment are discussed in Chapters 19 and 20. Many infants and young children who are ventilator-dependent will benefit from developmental intervention because of consequences of prematurity, chronic illness, and technology dependence. Initially, it may be necessary to provide early intervention or school services in the home-based setting. When appropriate, however, the child can be transitioned to the mainstreamed setting. The community health nurse can assist the school nurse, therapists, and educators by providing information regarding the child's equipment and care in order to plan for the special needs in the school setting.

ONGOING CONCERNS

Many of the ongoing concerns families face can be ameliorated with effective case management. An effective case manager will be knowledgeable of local community resources, strategies for working with insurance companies, other funding possibilities, and financial management.

Organizing Time

Care of an infant requiring mechanical ventilation at home can be very complex and time consuming. Caregivers may benefit from assistance in organizing their daily or weekly care plans or checklists. (See Exhibit 16–3.)

Respite

Furthermore, although parents will often be reluctant to leave the infant with anyone else, over the long term, some form of respite from the demands of care will likely be important for the family. The nurse can assist family members to strategize options based on their finances and a knowledge of community resources and local programs.

Long-term Coping

A major stressor for families is the ongoing responsibility for the care of the child (Scharer & Dixon, 1989). Weaning from the ventilator is a slow process that may take months to years, if it is at all possible. Some children may have a severe developmental delay with limited improvement becoming apparent over time. Furthermore, nursing care in the home can be stressful even in the best of situations. At the same time, the reality of the long-term nature of the underlying disease process and the care intensity can be difficult to accept.

Families can be assisted to identify their coping mechanisms and to draw on their support mechanisms as they face these challenges. Some families may additionally want a referral for counseling to help them develop healthy coping skills to adjust to difficult changes throughout the family lifespan.

Financial Pressure

Another major strain of home care for many families is financial pressure (Fields et al., 1991). Supplies and equipment are costly, utility bills increase, transportation costs may be burdensome, and both physician visits and occasional rehospitalization are costly. At the same time, some insurance plans and health maintenance organizations offer limited home care benefits (Kaufman, 1991a, 1991b). Piecing funds together from programs such as Supplemental Security Income (SSI) and Medicaid, as well as various community organizations, may be necessary to ensure financial stability for the family of a ventilator-dependent child. (See Chapter 7.) Consultation with a nurse or social worker (e.g., a case manager) who is aware of available community resources, coupled with a creative and assertive approach, may be helpful. Case management is an important service to offer this population (Lewis et al., 1992).

Exhibit 16–3 Sample Weekly Schedule for the Care of a Mechanically Ventilated Child[a]

To Do	Sun	Mon	Tues	Wed	Thurs	Fri	Sat
Tracheostomy care, change ties	X	X	X	X	X	X	X
Tube change						X	
Check ventilator settings	X	X	X	X	X	X	X
Chest therapy	X	X	X	X	X	X	X
Rinse and wash suction container	X	X	X	X	X	X	X
Make fresh saline		X		X		X	
Soak parts of suction machine		X				X	
Soak parts of resuscitation bag and valve						X	
Empty and refill cascade on ventilator		X		X		X	
Change ventilator tubing and soak all parts						X	
Check oxygen level in all tanks	X	X	X	X	X	X	
Check contents of travel bag	X	X	X	X	X	X	X
Inventory all supplies		X					

[a]For children with increased secretions or those prone to infection, some of this care and cleaning may need to be more frequent.

REFERENCES

Dupuis, Y. (1986). Ventilators: Theory and application. St. Louis, MO: Mosby.

Fields, A.I., Rosenblatt, A., Pollack, M.M., et al. (1991). Home care cost-effectiveness for respiratory technology-dependent children, *American Journal of Diseases of Children*, *145*, 729–733.

Hill, N. (1994). Use of negative pressure ventilation, rocking beds, and pneumobelts. *Respiratory Care, 39*(5), 532–543.

Kaufman, J. (1991a). An overview of financing for pediatric home care: Part 1. *Pediatric Nursing, 19*(3), 280–281.

Kaufman, J. (1991b). An overview of financing for pediatric home care: Part 2. *Pediatric Nursing, 19*(4), 380–381, 422.

Lantos, J.D., & Kohrman, A.F. (1992). Ethical aspects of pediatric home care. *Pediatrics, 89*(5), 920–924.

Lewis, C.C., Alford-Winston, A., Billy-Kornas, M., McCaustland, M.D., & Tachman, C.P. (1992). Case management for children who are medically fragile/technology-dependent. *Issues in Comprehensive Pediatric Nursing, 15*(2), 73–92.

McNichol-Dougherty, J. (1990). Negative pressure devices in pediatric practice. *Pediatric Nursing, 16*(2), 135–138.

Pilmer, S. (1994). Prolonged mechanical ventilation in children. *Pediatric Clinics of North America, 41*(3), 473–510.

Respironics Inc. (1990a). *BiPAP S/T ventilatory support system: Patient pamphlet.* Murrysville, PA: Author.

Respironics Inc. (1990b). *Patient accessory guide.* Murrysville, PA: Author.

Scharer, K., & Dixon, D. (1989). Managing chronic illness: Parents with a ventilator-dependent child. *Journal of Pediatric Nursing, 4*(4), 236–247.

Steele, N., & Morgan, J. (1989). Emergency planning for technology-assisted children. *Journal of Pediatric Nursing, 4*(2), 81–87.

Witham-Wilson, M. (1991). Accidental breathing circuit disconnections in the neonatal or pediatric critical care setting. *Pediatric Nursing, 17*(3), 283–286.

ADDITIONAL RESOURCES

Aequitron Medical, Inc. (1991). *LP-10 Volume ventilator with pressure limit: User's manual.* Minneapolis, MN: Author.

American Thoracic Society. (1990). Position paper: Home mechanical ventilation of pediatric patients. *American Review of Respiratory Disease, 141*(1), 258–259.

Edwards Hazlett, D. (1989). A study of pediatric home ventilator management: Medical, psychosocial, and financial aspects. *Journal of Pediatric Nursing, 4*(4), 284–294.

Goldberg, A. (1991). Your role in pediatric home ventilation. *The Journal of Respiratory Diseases, 12*(5), 471–480.

Grossman Nissim, L., & Sten, M. (1991). The ventilator-assisted child: A case for empowerment. *Pediatric Nursing, 17*(5), 507–511.

Kacmarek, R. (1994). Home mechanical ventilatory assistance for infants. *Respiratory Care, 39*(5), 550–560.

Lucas, J., Golish, J., Sleeper, G., & O'Ryan, J. (1988). *Home respiratory care.* Norwalk, CT: Appleton & Lange.

Mallory, G., & Stillwell, P. (1991). The ventilator-dependent child: Issues in diagnosis and management. *Archives of Physical Medicine and Rehabilitation, 72,* 43–55.

Youngblut, J., Brennan, P., & Swegart, L. (1994). Families with medically fragile children: An exploratory study. *Pediatric Nursing, 20*(5), 463–468.

Home Care Plan: Mechanical Ventilation

Date _____   Case manager _____

Name _____   Hosp # _____   DOB _____

PROBLEM: **VENTILATOR**

GOALS/OBJECTIVES	METHODS	STAFF/REVIEW
Child will be at minimal risk of respiratory failure	Obtain AP and RR each visit; check vent settings each visit; assess for spontaneous respirations; assess color, respiratory pattern; auscultate lung fields for signs/symptoms of respiratory distress or failure each visit.	
Caregivers will state correct settings for ventilator and will demonstrate correct/safe operation of ventilator and humidifier	Assess knowledge and observe use of equipment; teach/reinforce as necessary. Observe arrangement of equipment and supplies for safety and accessibility.	
Caregivers will describe signs/symptoms of respiratory distress and inadequate ventilation	Assess knowledge; teach/reinforce as necessary.	
Caregivers will develop appropriate plans for emergency intervention	Ensure that phone and electric companies, rescue squads, and emergency departments are aware of child's status. Assess knowledge of when intervention is necessary. Teach/review as needed. Assess knowledge of how to troubleshoot ventilator alarms. Teach/review as needed. Assess plans for emergency intervention and assist in developing as needed.	

GOALS/OBJECTIVES	METHODS	STAFF/REVIEW
	Assess caregivers' ability to provide CPR competently; teach/review regularly. Review with caregivers the indications for calling doctor/equipment supplier/rescue squad/home care nurse.	
The child will be at minimal risk of infection or atelectasis	Assess for signs of infection or atelectasis. Review preventive measures each visit.	
Child to have age and condition appropriate developmental stimulation and motor activity	Assess appropriateness of developmental stimulation and motor activity; offer recommendations prn. Consult with OT/PT/speech therapist as necessary in planning.	
Caregivers to adjust to activities of daily living to allow for hearing vent alarms at all times	Assess effect of home ventilation on caregivers' daily schedules. Assist in developing new patterns of family member responsibilities and/or developing clear daily schedules for the child's care if needed. Assist in developing safe travel plans if needed.	
Caregivers to have all needed supplies and to clean reusable supplies appropriately	Assess regularly for adequate stock of needed supplies. Assist caregivers in developing inventory list, schedule for ordering supplies. Communicate with supplier(s) prn re: concerns. Assess caregivers' schedule, and techniques for cleaning reusable supplies and equipment; teach prn.	
Child to have regular and prn follow-up by managing physician	Encourage regular and prn visits with managing physician. Assist in arranging plans for safe visits to physician or home visits by physician. Communicate/coordinate with managing physician(s) on a regular basis and as needed for problems.	

Source: Courtesy of Children's Hospital National Medical Center, Home Health Care Services, Washington, D.C.

Appendix 16–B

Home Assessment: Mechanical Ventilation

Name _____ Hosp# _____ DOB _____

Primary caretaker _____ Back-up caretaker _____

Address _____ Address _____

Telephone _____ Telephone _____

Date of hospital discharge _____ Start of service date _____

Diagnoses _____
_____
_____

Reason for ventilator: _____

Physician managing ventilator: _____

Telephone _____ Page _____

Type of ventilator _____ Humidity source _____

Prescribed settings _____

Prescribed time on ventilator _____

Equipment supply company _____

Telephone _____ 24-hour service telephone _____

Funding for equipment _____

Trach type: _____ Size: _____ Suction catheter size: _____

EVERY VISIT: Assess vital signs, observe respiratory pattern and color. Auscultate breath sounds, assess for signs/symptoms of respiratory distress. Check ventilator settings for accuracy.

I. Equipment

	Date observed	N/A	Comments
Ventilator (type)			
Portability changes			
Humidity (source)			
Compressor			
Ventilator tubing			
Extra exhalation valve			

Manual resuscitator _____

Sterile water and
  normal saline _____

Suction machine &
  catheters (refer also
  to Trach 15 Assessment,
  Appendix 15–B) _____

Apnea monitor ____
  (If yes, refer to Apnea
  Monitor 13 Assessment,
  Appendix 13–B) _____

Oxygen source ____
  (If yes, refer to
  Oxygen Assessment, 14
  Appendix 14–B) _____

Oximeter _____

II. Emergency notifications

	Date sent	N/A	Comments
Letter to telephone co.			
Letter to electric co.			
Letter to rescue squad			
Personal contact with squad (opt)			
Letter to nearest emergency room			
Family given ER card			

III. Emergency information posted

	Date observed	N/A	Comments
Rescue squad number			
Physician's number (day, evng, wknd)			
Equipment supply co. number			
Power co. emergency number			
CPR guidelines			
Patient's name & address (opt) with directions to home			
Home health care agency			

IV. Emergency care

(See also Tracheostomy Assessment)

	Primary Caretaker Date	Back-up Caretaker Date	Comments
Describes signs and symptoms of respiratory distress:			
Describes signs and symptoms of inadequate ventilation:			
Describes emergency plan for: a. Respiratory distress			

   b. Respiratory failure _____

   c. Ventilator alarm _____

   d. Power failure _____

Demonstrates CPR _____

Demonstrates use of manual resuscitator _____

V. Routine care (see also Tracheostomy Assessment, Appendix 15–B)

	Primary Caretaker *Date*	*Back-up Caretaker* *Date*	*Comments*
States reason for ventilator			
Describes pulmonary anatomy			
Describes how to evaluate respiratory pattern/ breath sounds			
Describes appropriate interventions for deviations from normal			
States ventilator settings			
Demonstrates operation of ventilator & humidification			
Demonstrates use of oximeter			
Demonstrates trouble-shooting techniques			
Demonstrates operation of apnea monitor			
Demonstrates operation of suction equipment			
Demonstrates safe use of oxygen			
Demonstrates cleaning of supplies & equipment			
Demonstrates appropriate arrangement of supplies			
Demonstrates vent. circuit change			
Describes travel plan			

VI. Safety precautions (see also Trach Assessment, Appendix 15–B)

	Date reviewed	*N/A*	*Comments*
Can hear ventilator alarms at all times			
Transport with two adults			
Check ventilator settings regularly/post near vent.			

Check ventilator circuit
  connections regularly _____

Shake excess water out of
  tubing regularly _____

Child-proof equipment
  settings prn _____

Charge car battery for power
  back-up_____

Phone near child's bedroom_____

Ventilator manual in home _____

Comments: _____

_____

_____

_____

Caretaker description of planning daily tasks to enable hearing ventilator (e.g., vacuuming)

Primary caretaker: _____

_____

_____

Back-up caretaker: _____

_____

_____

VII. Describe caretaker/child interaction (overall interaction and with respect to ventilator)

_____

_____

_____

_____

VIII. Describe caretakers' overall confidence and concerns about ventilator

_____

_____

_____

_____

IX. Assessment of problems identified

_____

_____

_____

_____

X. Plan to address problems identified

_____

_____

_____

_____

Signature _____Date completed _____

Source: Courtesy of Children's Hospital National Medical Center, Home Health Care Services, Washington, D.C.

Part V

Neurological Concerns

A Parent's Perspective on Hydrocephalus

Brenda Bird, RN, MSN

It was our worst nightmare. I will never forget the day we were told that our son James had suffered a grade IV IVH (intraventricular hemorrhage). My husband, Jim, and I were visiting the neonatal intensive care unit (NICU). James was in his isolette on a ventilator. He was only a week old, born at 28½ weeks gestation. The neonatal nurse practitioner (NNP) was at the bedside, and I asked her what the results of the head ultrasound done 2 days earlier were. She searched through the chart, at first unable to find the report. I insisted it was there since radiology had informed me the report had been delivered. (I worked as a nurse at the hospital.) The NNP then found the report, took a few moments to scan it and said to us, "It's bad. It's a grade IV bleed." She explained that they would be closely monitoring James for hydrocephalus and referred us to one of the neonatologists if we wanted to go over the ultrasound reports with someone.

We were devastated. My husband and I were unable to speak, cry, or move. We both looked at our tiny infant son and thought, "No, it can't be." James, of course, looked no different, and it wasn't until we were alone, away from the hospital that we fell apart, crushed by grief. I'm not sure that one ever comes to terms with the grief, but you learn to live with it. It was important to us not to let it consume us and adversely affect James.

When we were able to discuss the ultrasound with the neonatologist, it helped us gain some perspective on the future for James. The neonatologist explained that with brain injury of this type, there was no way to predict exactly what the deficits might be. He did state that James would have right-sided hemiparesis since the bleed occurred on the left, but he could not estimate the level of functioning. His feeling was that James' development would be mildly affected and that he had great potential. We left the discussion feeling even more devastated as the enormity of the problem became more real.

We had hoped, by some miracle, that James would not develop hydrocephalus. That was not to be the case. At less than 4 weeks of age, it was obvious that James would undergo a ventriculoperitoneal (VP) shunt insertion. We had been given the option of first attempting serial spinal taps to clear the exudate from the bleed that was thought to be the cause of the hydrocephalus. After weighing the possible risks and the fact that James probably would need a shunt eventually, we opted for the shunt. Within a month of shunt placement, James required a revision to remove the exudate that had obstructed the shunt tube distally.

Each surgery was a frightening experience, and we worried that each would delay James' homecoming. James did very well with the surgeries. I will never forget the OR (operating room) nurse bringing us the first hair shaved from his head for us to save. It meant so much. We were so fragile then.

The first year was a blur. We did our share of crying but a lot of the time were able to use denial as a means of coping. We had the support of family from a distance and friends who were wonderful. One friend gave me a number of books to read that were very helpful. The book that I found invaluable was Helen Featherstone's *A Difference in the Family*. It was very touching and helped me to recognize and deal with many emotions that I had buried in order to survive.

Everyone's grieving is different, but I feel very strongly that it lasts a lifetime. The pain never goes away. It seems you just find a place for it so that you can focus on life and enjoy your child. If you dwell on it, the grief can consume you. Sadness does creep in when you are most vulnerable, but then you must gather your resources and go on.

Guilt can be overwhelming for the family. I blamed myself for James' early delivery even though intellectually I knew I had done nothing wrong. I had sought prenatal care and trusted in my obstetricians but later felt cheated when I looked back to see they failed to pick up cues that something was not right. I was large for the gestational age of the baby, the baby never moved to the left side, I had contractions from 20 weeks on, and a month earlier a band or "synechiae" had been discovered on ultrasound. I had been to the doctor's office the morning before my water broke and everything was fine. I was angry at the physician group that had followed me but also at myself for not being more concerned about these different things. I carry this guilt with me to this day.

We were so eager to have James home yet very anxious too. Even though I am a pediatric nurse, I was afraid of leaving the safety of round-the-clock nursing care. My husband and I didn't sleep much the first few weeks but gradually grew into our roles as parents. We enrolled James in an early intervention program as soon as we could. He qualified for physical therapy (PT), occupational therapy (OT), and speech. It was a homebound program, so the therapists came to the house. My husband, Jim, was the primary caretaker and worked with James a great deal. James flourished. We were greatly encouraged by his progress but always worried what the future might bring.

We have the support of quite a number of doctors, between the pediatrician and the many specialists. But the question we continue to struggle with when James does not seem well is: "Is James sick or does he have a shunt malfunction?" There have been a number of times when James was vomiting that we brought him to the pediatrician worried it might be the shunt. Since there is no way to tell for sure, even the pediatrician will admit he's not certain. It can be very frustrating, but we have learned that, as parents, we are the experts on our child and have to trust our instincts.

James went to school at the age of 2 years in a handicapped preschool class of eight children. He received his therapies there and continued to follow up with many specialists. He was doing well, although we had hoped he would progress more rapidly.

James was having some difficulty breathing at night and naptime. He often had colds that we assumed were the problem. Since the problem persisted, we had a sleep study done. He was diagnosed with obstructive apnea and scheduled for a tonsillectomy, adenoidectomy, and myringotomy tubes. I spoke to the neurosurgeon about the possibility of having his shunt revision done at the same time as the other surgeries. A computed tomography (CT) scan and abdominal X-ray were ordered and confirmed the need for shunt revision for tube lengthening and valve change. James was over shunted

and had slit ventricles. We were very anxious about yet another surgery, but at least he would only have anesthesia once. One of the nurses in the postanesthesia recovery unit (PACU) asked if he had come in for his 10,000 mile check!

James did very well following the surgery and made remarkable gains in his development. His speech flourished, and he began walking at 34 months of age. He has just completed his second year in the handicapped preschool program and loves to tease his younger sister, Victoria. His developmental quotient was recently assessed at 95! We couldn't be happier. He talks in full sentences, walks, runs, and seems to charm everyone. His future looks bright.

We recognize that we have been extremely lucky. James has not had any shunt infections or serious malfunctions. Although his IVH was a grade IV, the sequelae have been minimal. He continues to wear bilateral ankle-foot orthoses, uses a right soft hand brace, and has some difficulty with stuttering. He still has a long way to go, and we realize it will always be a struggle for him. We have not yet had to deal with possible learning disabilities but recognize that we might. Every day I put him on the bus with the blue handicapped sign on it, I am reminded that he has special needs. And no matter what anyone says, it still hurts.

I think the most important thing for home care nurses to remember about caring for a high-risk infant is that the family is in crisis. It is so devastating and overwhelming to everyone concerned that not only the infant, but also the family, need care. Nurses should empower parents/caregivers by giving them the education and support necessary to take care of the infant. Make sure the family is aware of resources and support groups in the community. The family often doesn't have the energy to seek those out initially, but they can prove to be invaluable in the future. If the family seems to be in denial, remember that it may be their only means of dealing with the situation. Be aware of how you present things. Be empathetic, not sympathetic. Acknowledge grief if it is presented to you, but do not try to minimize it and cheer up the person. Remember that you may have to repeat instructions and answer the same questions over and over regardless of the parent's/caregivers's level of education. Respect the parents/caregivers as people with their own needs. When you nurture the family, you will inevitably improve the quality of care the infant will receive at home.

I know that becoming the parent of a neurologically impaired child has changed my nursing practice when dealing with other parents/caregivers. Parents appreciate being listened to, not talked at. You don't have to be a social worker and counselor, but some of their listening skills are useful. A family may be very angry and feeling: "Why our child? Why us?" They need your guidance and support. In these times of managed care, you may see infants going home much earlier with many more needs to address. The families may not have the resources to deal with the infant's needs prior to discharge. More of the responsibility will be yours, and you will be asked to do more with less. As a nurse and a parent, I urge you to take care of yourself so you can be better prepared to handle the stress of dealing with families in crisis.

Chapter 17

Home Care of the Infant with Seizures

Revised by Marian J. Kolodgie, MSN, CPNP

Seizures are the clinical manifestations of excessive and/or hypersynchronous abnormal activity of neurons in the cerebral cortex (Engel, 1992). A seizure is not a disease in itself but a symptom, the cause of which must be sought and treated if possible. Epilepsy is the recurrence of chronic, unprovoked seizures. Somewhat over 4% of all children experience one or more seizures between infancy and childhood. Roughly 1% of all neonates will have a seizure, and the incidence among premature infants in the modern neonatal intensive care unit is approximately 20% (Painter, 1988). This chapter reviews the evaluation and treatment of neonatal seizures and home nursing care, including family support and education.

RECOGNITION OF NEONATAL SEIZURES

Infants exhibit various behavioral phenomena, described below, that may at times be difficult to distinguish from seizures. For this reason, an electroencephalogram (EEG) should be performed on infants at risk or those who present with seizure-like behaviors before starting anticonvulsant therapy. In the absence of a conclusive EEG, prolonged video monitoring may confirm the diagnosis. Abnormal nonepileptic behaviors should not be treated with anticonvulsants.

Distinguishing Nonseizure Behaviors

Infants exhibit a variety of behavioral phenomena. Twitching, posturing, head turning, sucking, and eye devia-

tion may appear during certain phases of the sleep–wake cycle in the normal neonate (Clancy, Legido, & Lewis, 1988). In sick neonates, bradycardia, apnea, color changes, eye deviation, and posturing may be confused with seizure activity. These behaviors may arise from cortical or subcortical structures whose electrical discharges are not easily transmitted to the scalp (Clancy, 1988). It may be difficult to distinguish seizures from normal or pathological nonepileptic behaviors.

It can be helpful to be aware of certain distinctions. Neonates rarely present with generalized tonic-clonic seizures. Apneic spells, especially in the premature infant, are usually related to pathologic mechanisms other than seizures (Legido, Clancy, & Berman, 1988; Mizrahi, 1990). "Jitteriness" is nonspecific and lacks the stereotypical quality of seizure behaviors: it can be provoked by tactile stimulation and is sensitive to restraint (gentle holding) (see Table 17–1).

Neonatal Seizures

It was previously thought that an immature nervous system was the cause for neonatal seizures. On the contrary, the neonatal brain has a very high threshold for seizure activity. However, incomplete neuronal structure and immature cellular migration mechanisms prevent seizure activity from generalizing in the way it does in older individuals (Legido et al., 1988). Neonatal seizures have unique clinical and electrographic qualities not found in older children and

Table 17–1 Distinguishing Seizure Activity from Tremor/Jitteriness

Tremor/Jitteriness	Focal Clonic Seizure
Intermittent, irregular	Rhythmic, regular
Fast, 5–6 jerks/sec	Slow, 2–3 jerks/sec
Provoked by tactile stimulation or repositioning	Not affected by repositioning
Stops with passive restraint	Not affected by restraint
No abnormal eye movements	Eye deviations common

adults. Neonatal seizures are not included in the International Classification of Epileptic Seizures (Exhibit 17–1). In fact, there is controversy regarding the categorization of neonatal seizures. However, research using EEG and simultaneous video monitoring has made it possible to distinguish neonatal seizures from other types of neonatal behavior (Mizrahi, 1990; Mizrahi & Kellaway, 1987).

Categories of Neonatal Seizures

Mizrahi (1990; Mizrahi & Kellaway, 1987) categorized neonatal seizures into three major types according to the absence/presence of an electrocortical signature and clinical correlates (Exhibit 17–2). These include clinical seizures accompanied by an electrocortical signature, clinical seizures not accompanied by an electrocortical signature, and electrical seizures without clinical correlates.

Clinical Seizures Accompanied by an Electrocortical Signature

Clinical events accompanied by an electrocortical signature are subcategorized according to the appearance of specific behavioral phenomena (Exhibit 17–3) and are described below.

Focal Clonic Seizures. Focal clonic seizures present as rhythmical, slow, jerking affecting one (unifocal) or more

Exhibit 17–1 International Classification of Epilepsy

Generalized Seizures
  Absence
  Tonic
  Clonic
  Myoclonic
  Tonic-clonic
  Atonic/drop
  Status epilepticus

Partial Seizures
  Simple partial (no impairment of consciousness)
  Complex partial (consciousness impaired)
  Complex partial with secondary generalization

Exhibit 17–2 Classification of Neonatal Seizures

SEIZURE TYPES

1. Clinical seizures with a consistent electrocortical signature
2. Clinical seizures without a consistent electrocortical signature
3. Electrical seizures without clinical seizures

Source: Courtesy of E. Mizrahi, Associate Professor of Neurology and Pediatrics, Baylor College of Medicine, The Methodist Hospital, and Texas Children's Hospital, Houston, Texas.

(multifocal) muscle groups. They may be confined to one side of the body (hemiconvulsive) or the trunk/midline (axial). The movements may alternate among muscle groups or migrate from one area to another, depending on whether the electrical discharge is localized or generalized. The typical progression from one muscle group to another (jacksonian march) does not occur in infants. Focal clonic seizures may be accompanied by facial twitching, tongue thrusting, and twitching of the neck and trunk, and should be differentiated from tremor or clonus, which subsides with passive restraint of the affected extremity.

Exhibit 17–3 Categorization of Clinical Seizures with and without Consistent Electrocortical Signatures

---
CLINICAL SEIZURES WITH A CONSISTENT ELECTROCORTICAL SIGNATURE

I.   Focal clonic
     A. Unifocal
     B. Multi-focal
        1. alternating
        2. migrating
     C. Hemiconvulsive
     D. Axial

II. Focal Tonic
     A. Asymmetric truncal
     B. Eye deviation

III. Myoclonic
     A. Generalized
     B. Focal

CLINICAL SEIZURES WITHOUT A CONSISTENT ELECTROCORTICAL SIGNATURE

I.   Myoclonic
     A. Generalized
     B. Focal
     C. Fragmentary

II. Generalized Tonic
     A. Extensor
     B. Flexor
     C. Mixed extensor/flexor

III. Motor Automatisms
     A. Oral/buccal/lingual
     B. Ocular signs
     C. Progression movements
        1. pedaling
        2. stepping
        3. rotary arm movements
     D. Complex purposeless movements

Source: Courtesy of E. Mizrahi, Associate Professor of Neurology and Pediatrics, Baylor College of Medicine, The Methodist Hospital, and Texas Children's Hospital, Houston, Texas.

Focal Tonic Seizures. Focal tonic seizures appear as asymmetric flexion or stiffening of the trunk or extremities. They are often accompanied by apnea, grunting, changes in heart rate, repetitive eye opening, nystagmus, or pupillary dilatation/constriction. They can also appear as sustained eye deviation or dystonic posturing.

Myoclonic Seizures. Myoclonic seizures are rapid, isolated muscle jerks that may be generalized or confined to a specific muscle group. Some myoclonic seizures are accompanied by an electrocortical signature, and others are not.

Clinical Seizures without an Electrocortical Correlate

Clinical seizures without an electrocortical correlate (see Exhibit 17–3) include myoclonic (some), generalized tonic, numerous motor automatisms (sucking, pedaling, rotary arm movements), and posturing. These behaviors can be suppressed with restraint or repositioning, or provoked by tactile stimulation. Infants exhibiting these types of seizures have usually experienced some degree of hypoxic-ischemic encephalopathy and have a poor prognosis (Mizrahi, 1990).

Electrical Seizures without Clinical Behaviors

Electrical seizures (those having an electrocorticographic signature) may be present in the absence of observed clinical behaviors. This seizure type is most commonly observed in infants with severe encephalopathy, those who are pharmacologically paralyzed, and those who are already being treated with anticonvulsants (Mizrahi, 1990).

ETIOLOGY AND TREATMENT OF SEIZURE DISORDERS

Seizures arise from many different causes, including the following:

- hypoxic ischemic encephalopathy
- central nervous system (CNS) infection
- intracerebral hemorrhage
- infarction/malformation
- inborn errors of metabolism
- subarachnoid hemorrhage
- metabolic disturbances.

Approximately 60% of neonatal seizures result from severe brain insult (Mizrahi, 1990).

Prompt identification of seizures is essential since prolonged seizure activity can inhibit neurocognitive functioning and may lead to subsequent neuronal injury. Treatment should be aimed at the underlying pathophysiology. The diagnostic workup for an infant includes EEG, magnetic resonance imaging (MRI), septic workup with lumbar puncture, and metabolic studies (Painter, 1988). In the presence of a structural or metabolic abnormality, a genetics consultation may be warranted. The developmental specialist should also evaluate those infants at risk for neurocognitive delay.

When the diagnosis of seizures is confirmed, antiepileptic drug (AED) therapy will be instituted. (See Appendix 17–B.)

Phenobarbital, depakote, tegretol, and phenytoin are the first-line drugs used to treat infants. Phenobarbital is the drug of choice; however, the sedative side effects may inhibit important neurocognitive functioning. Depakote should be used cautiously in infants under 2 years of age due to its effect on hepatic enzymes. However, it can be a very useful AED when accompanied by careful monitoring of blood levels. Monotherapy (the use of a single AED) is preferred; however, if the seizures are refractory to treatment, second-line drugs may be added.

HOSPITAL DISCHARGE AND TRANSITION TO THE HOME

Preparation for hospital discharge includes ensuring both that the home care nurse has complete information regarding the infant's condition and care and that the parents or other caregivers are well prepared to manage the infant's care at home.

Coordination with the Home Care Nurse

Prior to the infant's discharge from the hospital, the home care nurse should obtain complete information on the infant's condition, including the following:

- seizure type
- clinical behaviors
- duration and frequency
- parts of the body affected
- associated automatisms (chewing, sucking, eye blinking, fumbling)
- precipitating factors
- postictal state
- prescribed medications
- response to AEDs
- presence and nature of developmental delay.

The nurse should determine the parents' understanding of the diagnosis and prognosis and clarify any misconceptions.

Parental Education

Recognition and Documentation of Seizure Activity

Parents should be taught to recognize seizure activity and to document activity during and after the seizure. (See Exhibit 17–4.) Parents should be instructed to record seizure

Exhibit 17–4 Documentation of Seizure Activity

• precipitating factors	• progression of seizure
• typical onset	• duration
• description of specific behaviors	• frequency

appearance, duration, and frequency in a brief diary for future reference. They should be instructed to describe seizure-related behaviors observed in their child and can be taught to look for eye deviation, facial twitching, tongue thrusting, or other behaviors that may assist in describing the evolution of the seizure. In the presence of automatisms and stereotyped behaviors, it may be helpful for the parent to see if the activity stops when passive restraint is applied. Parents should also note the presence of asymmetric movements or muscle weakness following a seizure. Careful observation and documentation are important, as appropriate management varies depending on the type of seizure.

Seizure Management

Seizure management involves several steps, with the overall goal of care being to ensure the safety of the infant. Parents and other caregivers should be taught each step. In general, the infant should be placed on the side to maintain the airway. Nothing should be placed in the mouth, as it may further occlude the airway and can cause injury. Parents should be informed that irregular respirations and/or mild color changes may accompany seizure activity. While CPR is not indicated for acute seizure management, parents should be instructed both in how to assess respirations and to call 911 in the event of respiratory distress or a prolonged seizure (usually over 5 min). Parents can be encouraged to caress and talk to the infant in a soft tone during the seizure, as it enables them to use familiar skills and helps to determine the return to responsiveness.

Guidelines for Medical Follow-up

Parents should be instructed to seek medical attention if they notice changes in seizure activity or signs of medication reactions. These include the following:

- prolonged seizure greater than 5 min
- significant change in seizure number or frequency
- occurrence of new seizure behaviors
- sudden change in behavior
- loss of developmental skills
- vomiting
- rash
- lethargy
- any other changes that seem suspicious.

Providing parents with specific guidelines can ease anxiety and prevent complications. Parents will make frequent telephone calls immediately following discharge but become more confident as their expertise increases. Initial concerns can be useful teaching opportunities to aid parents in becoming adjusted to their child's seizures.

Plans for medical follow-up should be determined prior to discharge. All disciplines involved in managing the infant's care should be identified and appropriate follow-up visits scheduled. The first neurology visit is usually 2 to 4 weeks after hospital discharge. If the seizures are under good control, subsequent neurology visits may be scheduled every 3 to 6 months. If the seizures are poorly controlled, the infant may be seen more frequently. Infants receiving steroids should be seen weekly or biweekly for the first 4 to 6 weeks of treatment. Routine primary care visits should also be scheduled. Parents should be provided with specific telephone numbers for physicians' offices, the neurology on-call system, and the local emergency department.

Prescriptions

Prescriptions should be obtained and filled prior to discharge so medication will be available when the infant arrives home. Additionally, parents should be encouraged to obtain refills of prescribed medication before running out. Interruptions in AED therapy related to unavailability of the medication is unsafe.

ROUTINE HOME VISITS

On each home visit, the nurse should assess the infant's overall health and neurological status, obtain an interim seizure history (see Exhibit 17–4), review medication dosage and schedule with the parents, and observe for medication side effects. Any parental questions and concerns should be addressed. Exhibit 17–5 outlines other duties of the home care nurse in the care of the infant with seizures.

THE FIRST HOME VISIT

On the first home visit, the nurse should address any parental questions and concerns. The nurse should both obtain a health history and perform a physical and neurological assessment, including evaluation of muscle tone, posture, observation for asymmetry, reflexes, suck/swallow abilities, reflexive eye movements, and general activity.

Review Seizure Recognition and Management

The nurse should review seizure recognition and management to ensure that caregivers understand the clinical pre-

Exhibit 17–5 Role of the Home Care Nurse When an Infant Has Seizures

Assess infant's response to treatment progress.
Review medication dosage, administration, side effects.
Obtain interim seizure history.
Evaluate parent's level of skill performance.
Validate parent's observations of infant's progress.
Provide anticipatory guidance:
• reinforcement of information provided to parents;
• effect of diagnosis on family/relationships;
• emotional support;
• prognosis/planning for future.
Assist parents with problem solving:
• obtain equipment, medication;
• organize appointments, follow-up care;
• manage behavioral changes.
Identify available resources:
• Epilepsy Foundation referral;
• counseling;
• infant developmental programs/placement.
Communicate with primary health care providers.

Source: Adapted from *Pediatric Nursing,* Vol. 20, No. 6, May-June, p. 272, with permission of Janetti Publications, Inc., Pitman, New Jersey, © 1994.

sentation of their child's seizures and are aware of appropriate first-aid measures. Witnessing a seizure can be very frightening for parents, and they may need both continued support and ongoing reinforcement of skills.

Address Medication Regimen

The dosage, administration, and side effects of prescribed AEDs should be reviewed. The nurse should check the medication label against the prescription for any discrepancies. Each parent should be observed measuring the prescribed dose. Accurate dosage of medications is essential in providing effective seizure control and avoiding hazardous toxic doses. If a medication is in suspension, parents should be reminded to shake the bottle vigorously before each use. The nurse should review the medication schedule and assist the parents to adjust administration times according to their family's schedule. For example, medication may be given before, during, or after feeding times. Parents should be reminded that dosage times can be spread throughout the infant's waking hours, and it is not necessary to awaken the infant to give medications.

Observe for Medication Side Effects

The infant should be evaluated for the presence of side effects related to the medication. (See Appendix 17–B.)

Many side effects are listed for the AEDs; however, each infant's response may vary due to individual metabolic rates and pharmacodynamic drug properties. Side effects most commonly observed in infants include the following:

• sleep disturbances
• nausea/vomiting/constipation
• sedation
• lethargy/irritability
• hyperactivity
• altered blood studies
• rash
• tremor
• increased secretions
• increase or change in seizure pattern.

It is most practical to instruct parents to observe their infant for *any* changes resulting from AED therapy. Should changes occur, they are probably due to the medication. Some of the side effects observed following initiation or alteration of AED therapy are expected and should resolve within 2 to 3 days. If this does not occur, therapy may need to be revised.

Particular attention should be given to the possibility of Stevens-Johnson syndrome, which can occur with almost all anticonvulsants. The initial sign of this syndrome is development of a rash, which may erupt into a systemic infection and is potentially fatal. The syndrome is associated with conjunctivitis, iritis, stomatitis, fever, and arthralgia. Parents should be instructed to contact the neurologist immediately if any signs of rash develop, as the medication in use must be discontinued immediately and another drug substituted.

SUBSEQUENT HOME VISITS

Each home visit should include a general physical examination and neurological assessment of the infant as described above. An interim seizure history should be obtained, including a review of both the seizure diary and postictal symptoms. If there has been a significant change in frequency or type of seizures, the physician or nurse practitioner should be contacted. A change in the medication may be necessary in order to obtain improved seizure control. Medication, dosage, administration, and side effects should be reviewed with parents periodically. The nurse should also review the infant's developmental progress and assist parents as necessary in communicating with the therapists involved in the child's care.

Medication Renewal

The importance of medication renewal should be impressed on the family. Abrupt cessation of medication can precipitate seizure breakthrough or status epilepticus (a prolonged seizure greater than 30 min). Parents should be encouraged to call in prescriptions at least 10 to 14 days before they expect to run out of medication. This will allow plenty of time in the event there is a delay in obtaining a refill.

Appointments and Labwork

The nurse should also encourage parents to keep their follow-up appointments and obtain labwork as directed by the health care provider. AED blood levels should be recorded in the seizure diary. Therapeutic levels may vary from child to child. The given ranges should be used as guidelines only. For example, most drugs start at the lowest dose and are increased until the seizures are controlled or side effects appear. Some patients require only minimum medication doses to achieve good seizure control with mildly subtherapeutic levels. Other patients may require high doses and run very high blood levels. In the absence of side effects, this may be acceptable. Parents need to be aware of this so they do not panic if their child's level is not within a given range. Other parameters, such as a complete blood count, platelet count, and liver function tests, may be indicated to rule out the presence of side effects. As the infant grows, medication dosages will need to be readjusted to coincide with the child's weight gain.

Managing Precipitating Factors

As parents become more sophisticated in managing their infant's seizures, they may notice that certain factors influence seizure activity. Anticipatory guidance can be provided regarding common precipitating factors in infants, including the following: illness, fever, drowsiness, and natural evolution or cycling of seizure activity. Parents should seek early treatment of any suspected illness to prevent seizure breakthrough. In the event additional medications (including over-the-counter) are prescribed, parents must remind the physician and pharmacist that their child is receiving AEDs so that other contraindicated medications can be avoided. Drugs containing antihistamines are not often prescribed, as they can precipitate seizure breakthrough.

Obtaining Routine Health Care

It is important that the infant's general health is periodically evaluated. The child should have regularly scheduled visits with the primary care provider. Immunizations should be kept up to date. Some physicians prefer not to administer the pertussis vaccine to infants with epilepsy. (See Chapter 8.) Parents should discuss the risk factors with their individual providers.

Safety Precautions

The family should adhere to common child safety measures. If the older infant is prone to loss of muscle tone or falling over during a seizure, it may be necessary to restrict some activities or have the child wear a helmet to prevent head injury. The child should never be left alone in the bath or near a pool. Seatbelts and infant carseats must be used as required by law. The nurse may want to review appropriate use of these measures because mistakes are common and can be serious. Babysitters and other caregivers should be instructed in seizure first aid and management. Every parent should know CPR regardless of his or her child's health status. The nurse should clarify that CPR is not indicated in seizure management but should be initiated if cardiorespiratory compromise is suspected.

ONGOING CONCERNS

Since seizures are symptoms of an underlying problem, the long-term prognosis is dependent on the nature and severity of the causative disorder and the promptness of treatment (Legido, Clancy, & Berman, 1991; Temple, Dennis, Carney, & Sharich, 1995). Infants with normal development in whom no causative factor can be identified generally have a better prognosis. Developmental delay and seizures that are refractory to treatment are poor prognostic indicators. Although the prognosis may be guarded, maximal effort should be made to assist the infant in achieving his or her developmental potential.

Ongoing assessment of the child's growth and development should be performed. The Denver II developmental assessment (Frankenberg & Dobbs, 1990) is a useful screening instrument and can be applied as major milestones are anticipated. Specific attention should be paid to language, cognitive development, and motor activity. The child should be referred to the appropriate discipline for a thorough evaluation if there are any concerns about developmental progress. Early intervention plays a significant role in developmental outcome. Promoting optimal development is important not only to meet the needs of the child but also to impart a sense of hope for the parents.

Neonatal seizures are often an ominous sign to parents. Parents may find it very difficult to cope with the diagnosis and will grieve over the loss of the child they had hoped for. They may need continued reassurance and support as they deal with their infant's uncertain prognosis. The factor most predictive of how well a child eventually copes with having seizures is how the parents respond to this diagnosis. Thus, early support and counseling can be critical factors in helping the entire family adjust to this disorder.

If there are other children in the family, it is important to clarify each sibling's understanding of epilepsy. The parents may need assistance explaining epilepsy to siblings, other family members, or friends.

Families whose child has a chronic illness often find themselves isolated from their social network. Parents may be reluctant to leave their infant for fear that a seizure may occur. The nurse can suggest resources to parents for planning activities and obtaining appropriate child/respite care. Understandably, parents may have difficulty separating from their child for even short periods of time. Some families may need assistance from the nurse or a referral for counseling both to cope with the sense of loss or guilt associated with the diagnosis and to restructure their lives.

Parents may need additional support in developing discipline and parenting skills for the young child with a seizure disorder. Because of their concern about the seizures, some families may be overprotective, placing unnecessary restrictions on the child's activities. When this occurs, the child may become manipulative and resentful. Education and support at the time of diagnosis will help parents to be more comfortable with the increased independence that is a normal part of growing up. Families can also be referred for counseling or parenting classes to address these issues.

When the child enters school, the family will need to make a decision regarding whether or not to inform school personnel about the seizure disorder. This is a very personal decision. Consideration should be given to the frequency and type of seizure. If the child is at risk for having a seizure in school, the diagnosis of epilepsy should be reported on the school health form. This prepares the teachers and school staff to administer appropriate first aid as well as to manage the classroom of students in a calm, reassuring manner during a seizure. The child's self-perception and adjustment to epilepsy will in large part be affected by how those around him or her react to the epilepsy. Both parents and nurses can affect the attitudes of school personnel.

The Epilepsy Foundation of America (4351 Garden City Drive, Landover, MD 20785) is an excellent resource providing education, written materials, counseling, and other services to persons coping with epilepsy. It also has a film library addressing different issues related to seizure disorders. Tertiary centers with epilepsy programs may also provide counseling, education, or support groups to serve this population.

REFERENCES

Engel, J. (1992). *Seizures and epilepsy.* Philadelphia, PA: F.A. Davis.

Frankenberg, W.K., & Dodds, J.B. (1990). *Denver II.* Denver, CO: Denver Developmental Materials, Inc.

Legido, A., Clancy, R., & Berman, P. (1988). Recent advances in the diagnosis, treatment, and prognosis of neonatal seizures. *Pediatric Neurology, 4,* 79–86.

Legido, A., Clancy, R., & Berman, P. (1991). Neurologic outcome after electroencephalographically proven neonatal seizures. *Pediatrics, 88*(3), 583–596.

Mizrahi, E. (1990). Analysis of neonatal seizures. In Wasterlain, C., Vert, P., (Eds.), *Neonatal seizures,* New York, NY: Raven Press.

Mizrahi, E., & Kellaway, P. (1987). Characterization and classification of neonatal seizures. *Neurology, 37,* 1,837–1,844.

Painter, M. (1988). Neonatal seizures. *International Pediatrics, 3*(2), 97–103.

Temple, C., Dennis, J., Carney, R., & Sharich, J. (1995). Neonatal seizures: Long term outcome and cognitive development among normal survivors. *Developmental Medicine and Child Neurology, 37,* 109–118.

ADDITIONAL RESOURCES

Akiko, M., Kazayoshi, W., & Midori, S. (1985). Predictors of long term outcome of convulsive disorders in the first year of life: Clinical use of five risk factors. *European Neurology, 24,* 62–68.

Reynolds, E., Ring, I., Farr, A., Heller, R., & Elwes, R. (1991). Open double-blinded and long term study of vigabatrin in chronic epilepsy. *Epilepsia, 32*(4), 530–538.

The U.S. Gabapentin Study Group. (1994). The long term safety and efficacy of gabapentin (Neurontin) as add-on therapy in drug resistant partial epilepsy. *Epilepsy Research, 18,* 67–73.

Home Care Plan: The Infant with Seizures

Date _____   Case manager _____

Name _____   Hosp # _____   DOB _____

PROBLEM: **SEIZURES**

GOALS/OBJECTIVES	METHODS	STAFF/REVIEW
Caregivers will demonstrate appropriate seizure management	Assess caregivers' knowledge regarding: seizure recognition and observation seizure first aid (acute seizure management) precipitating factors.	
Infant will demonstrate minimal AED side effects	Assess caregivers' knowledge of dosage, side effects, and administration of AED. Evaluate caregivers' knowledge of drug levels.	
Caregivers state when to call physician	Instruct regarding criteria of concern: Prolonged seizure greater than 5 min Breakthrough seizures Evidence of possible medication side effects Sudden change in seizures or child's condition as described in discharge instructions	
Infant will function at highest level of developmental abilities	Provide resources for developmental/cognitive assessment. Assess family's level of knowledge and compliance with developmental treatment plan. Evaluate infant's progress or decline of milestones.	
Child will receive comprehensive care	Communicate with physician and neurologist as necessary. Educate family regarding potential risks of immunizations, if applicable.	

GOALS/OBJECTIVES	METHODS	STAFF/REVIEW
	Assist family to coordinate follow-up care including blood levels, EEG, and other diagnostic testing. Provide anticipatory guidance for potential childhood illnesses/health problems.	
Caregivers/parents will be able to identify appropriate coping strategies	Evaluate family for stressors related to caring for child with long-term illness. Provide community resources/ referrals. Assess compliance with follow-through on recommendations.	

Source: Courtesy of Children's Hospital National Medical Center, Home Health Care Services, Washington, D.C.

Medications Used in the Management of Seizures

Medication	Common Indications	Dosage	Optimal Serum Level (therapeutic range)	Side Effects and Nursing Considerations
Phenytoin (Dilantin)	Generalized psycho-motor, and focal seizures	5–8 mg/kg/day	10–20 µg/mL	Nystagmus, ataxia, slurred speech, mental confusion, dizziness, insomnia, transient nervousness, motor twitching, hirsutism
				Nausea, vomiting, constipation; may decrease if given after meals
				Rashes: scarletiniform, bulbous, exfoliative purpura, dermatitis, lupus; also Stevens-Johnson syndrome, which *can be fatal* (first signs usually appear 7–10 days after beginning medication). *If rash develops, contact physician immediately*
				Gingival hyperplasia; encourage gum brushing, gum massage and good dental care
				Available as suspension, but must be shaken well
				Contraindicated in hepatic damage
Phenobarbital	Generalized	4–6 mg/kg/day	15–40 µg/mL	Sedation (frequently decreases after the first few days); excitability with increased motor activity, short attention span, distractibility and hyperactivity; sleep disturbances (especially in toddlers); depression; potentiation of existing behavior problems
				Dizziness, headache, "hangover," exacerbation of preexisting pain

Medication	Common Indications	Dosage	Optimal Serum Level *(therapeutic range)*	Side Effects and Nursing Considerations
				Diplopia, nystagmus, nausea and vomiting, epigastric pain
				Hypotension, facial edema, skin rash, purpura, erythema multiforme, exfoliative dermatitis (severe rash may indicate degenerative changes in liver)
				Megaloblastic anemia, agranulocytosis, thrombocytopenia
				Abrupt cessation (missed dose) may cause tremulousness, weakness, insomnia, convulsions, delirium
				Contraindicated in severe renal or hepatic dysfunction or in patients with hypersensitivity to barbiturates
Clonazepam (Clonapin)	Absence, complex partial, akinetic, and myoclonic seizures	0.1–0.2 mg/kg/day	20–60 ng/mL	Changes may be dosage-related and can be exaggerated.
				Drowsiness, tremor, ataxia, nausea, bradycardia, hypotonicity, rash, personality changes (such as hyperactivity, irritability, depression, sedation, aggression)
				May cause increase in nasopharyngeal secretions
				Diplopia, nystagmus, constipation, gastritis, nausea, dysuria, enuresis, urinary retention
				Contraindicated in hepatic disease with benzodiazepan sensitivity; use with caution in chronic respiratory disease; never withdraw drug suddenly
Valproic acid (Depekane)	Generalized, absence, complex partial, and focal seizures	10–40 mg/kg/day	50–11 µg/mL	Nausea, vomiting, and indigestion (may be transient), diarrhea, abdominal cramps and constipation
				Sedative effects (mostly if combined with other drugs), ataxia, headache, nystagmus, diplopia, "spots before eyes," tremor, dysarthria, dizziness, incoordination

Medication	Common Indications	Dosage	Optimal Serum Level (therapeutic range)	Side Effects and Nursing Considerations
				Transient hair loss, emotional upset, depression, psychosis, aggression, hyperactivity, behavioral deterioration
				Altered bleeding time, thrombocytopenia
				Advise patients to take with meals
				Obtain liver function studies, platelet count, and prothrombin time initially and on regular basis
				Contraindicated in patients who have any hepatic condition; may cause acute hepatic necrosis
Carbamazepine (Tegretol)	Psychomotor and temporal lobe or generalized tonic-clonic seizures Mixed seizures of above or complex partial seizures that secondarily generalize	7–20 mg/kg/day	8–12 µg/mL	Dizziness, vertigo, drowsiness, fatigue, ataxia, congestive heart failure, hypotension, conjunctivitis, dry mouth and pharynx, blurred vision, diplopia, nystagmus, nausea, vomiting, diarrhea, anorexia, urinary frequency, glycosuria, water intoxication, skin rash
				Diplopia may be first sign that dose is too high; potentially serious side effects include aplastic anemia; get pretreatment blood counts to rule out abnormalities and repeat frequently; stop drug with bone marrow depression: monitor status with CBC, platelet and reticulocyte counts, serum iron determinations, liver function studies
				NOTIFY DOCTOR if symptoms of fever, sore throat, ulcers in mouth, easy bruising petechiae, purpura (early toxic signs) appear
				Eye changes; baseline and periodic eye examinations are essential
				Renal dysfunction; baseline and periodic determinations of urine and BUN are essential
				Contraindicated in patients with bone marrow depression

Medication	Common Indications	Dosage	Optimal Serum Level (therapeutic range)	Side Effects and Nursing Considerations
Ethosuximide (Zarontin)	Absence, akinetic, and myoclonic seizures	20–30 mg/kg/day	40–100 µg/mL	Nausea, vomiting, leukopenia, eosinophilia, agranulocytosis, pancytopenia, aplastic anemia, drowsiness, headache, dizziness, ataxia, irritability, hiccups, euphoria, lethargy, myopia
				Diarrhea, weight loss, cramps, anorexia, epigastric and abdominal pain, vaginal bleeding, urticaria, pruritic erythematous rashes
				Use with caution in hepatic or renal disease
				Obtain frequent CBC
Adrenocorticotropic hormone (ACTH)	Infantile spasms	Dosage varies; must be given by injection; often given on a daily basis		Edema with weight gain, sodium and potassium retention, muscle weakness and loss of muscle mass, irritability, petechiae, acne, hirsutism, hypertension, headache, thrush, vertigo, negative nitrogen balance, allergic response to proteins, dizziness, nausea, vomiting, diarrhea
				Will need to monitor blood pressure
Vigabatrin (not approved for use in United States)	Complex partial epilepsy	40 mg/kg/d	Unknown	Drowsiness, ataxia, headache, aggressive behavior in mentally retarded children
Gabapentin	Add-on medication for partial refractory seizures	300 mg qd, titrate to 600–1,800 qd	4–16 µg/mL	Drowsiness, fatigue, weight gain, 5% ataxia, diplopia, headache, nausea
Lamotrigine	Add-on medication for partial refractory seizures	Starting dose 2 mg/kg/d Maintenance dose 5–15 mg/kg/d If patient is receiving sodium valproate: initial dose 0.5 mg/kg/d; maintenance dose 1–5 mg/kg/d	2–20 µg/mL	Skin rash (especially if used with depakote), lethargy, drowsiness

Abbreviations: µg = micrograms; ng = nanograms; CBC = complete blood count; BUN = blood urea nitrogen.

Chapter 18

Home Care of the Infant and Young Child with Hydrocephalus

Revised by Brenda Bird, RN, MSN, and Elizabeth Ahmann, ScD, RN

Hydrocephalus means "water head" and is defined as an abnormal accumulation of cerebrospinal fluid (CSF) within the ventricles of the brain. Hydrocephalus may occur as frequently as 1 in every 500 children born (Jackson, 1990). It results from a congenital or an acquired alteration in the normal absorption or production of CSF, resulting in an enlargement of the ventricular system and an increase in CSF pressure. In some cases, the specific cause may be unknown; in other cases, the causative factor may be any of the following:

- congenital problems (e.g., spina bifida, arachnoid cysts, Dandy-Walker syndrome)
- infections (e.g., meningitis)
- trauma (including intraventricular hemorrhage)
- tumors.

Among premature infants, hydrocephalus is one of the more common neurologic sequelae.

Generally, hydrocephalus is a lifelong condition. The prognosis depends on the specific cause of the hydrocephalus, episodes of infection, and the response of the individual's brain tissue to both infection and increased pressure. Nursing care should be directed toward promoting optimal outcomes by providing appropriate assessment of the infant, ensuring early intervention, and providing family education. This chapter discusses the pathophysiology of hydrocephalus, treatment approaches, and issues relevant to home care of the infant with hydrocephalus.

PATHOPHYSIOLOGY OF HYDROCEPHALUS

CSF is formed continuously by the choroid plexus in the lining of the ventricles. The function of the CSF is thought to be essentially mechanical: it protects the central nervous system (CNS) by acting as a shock absorber, thereby reducing the force of impact on the brain. CSF also carries nutrients into and waste products away from the brain.

CSF circulates from the two lateral ventricles through the foramen of Monro to the third ventricle, which communicates posteriorly through the aqueduct of Sylvius, to the fourth ventricle. (See Figure 18–1.) The CSF then passes into the subarachnoid space to be reabsorbed eventually into the venous system of the brain.

Types of Hydrocephalus

Two major types of hydrocephalus are defined by the point of obstruction of the CSF. *Noncommunicating hydrocephalus* is the result of obstruction of the normal flow at some point within the ventricular system. *Communicating hydrocephalus* results from obstruction distal to the outlets of the fourth ventricle in the subarachnoid space. (See Figure 18–1.) In this case, there is no obstruction of the normal flow between ventricles, but CSF flow becomes backed up because of slow or poor reabsorption.

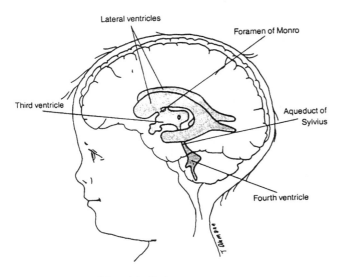

Figure 18–1 Ventricles of the Brain

Source: Courtesy of Teresa Ahmann.

Intraventricular Hemorrhage

Intraventricular hemorrhage (IVH) is a potential cause of hydrocephalus in premature infants, particularly those less than 32 weeks gestation or 1,500 g at birth. The immature brain of the premature infant contains richly vascular areas that are poorly supported by tissue mass; it is in these areas that hemorrhage occurs. The amount of hemorrhage can vary and is generally graded, by findings on computed tomography (CT) scans, as follows:

- Grade I: subependymal hemorrhage (bleeding in lining over ventricles)
- Grade II: IVH without ventricular dilatation (blood in the ventricles)
- Grade III: IVH with ventricular dilatation (blood in enlarged ventricles)
- Grade IV: IVH with parenchymal hemorrhage (bleeding in the tissues of the brain).

IVH can result in either acute obstructive hydrocephalus or secondary communicating hydrocephalus. Hydrocephalus occurs in approximately 10% of infants with mild IVH and as many as 65% to 100% of those who survive Grade IV IVH (Minarcik & Beachy, 1989).

DIAGNOSTIC TESTS

Families should be counseled about the importance of routine follow-up neuroradiographic diagnostic tests to evaluate the status of the child's hydrocephalus. While there

may be no obvious symptoms of a problem, diagnostic tests are the only way ventricular size can be determined, and ventricular size reflects the status of the hydrocephalus.

For infants with an open fontanel, the head ultrasound or craniosector scan (CSS) is the preferred method used to assess ventricular size. However, CT scan is the method of choice for diagnosing and assisting management of hydrocephalus after fontanel closure. When a CT scan is required, families often benefit from anticipatory guidance regarding the length of the test (approximately 15 min); the need for sedation so that the young child will lie still; prescan procedures, including NPO and sleep deprivation; and the size of the scanner, which can be quite intimidating.

Magnetic resonance imaging (MRI) is less frequently used for diagnostic purposes because of its longer duration (approximately 30 min) and its far greater cost. When it is the method of choice, anticipatory guidance is useful regarding the length of the test; the need for sedation; and the importance of compliance with preprocedure instructions, which vary among institutions.

TREATMENT

The goal of neurosurgical care for the infant with hydrocephalus is removal of the obstruction or, if this is not possible, diversion of the CSF produced into another body cavity. Occasionally, medications are used to reduce the production of CSF. However, standard treatment involves the surgical placement of a shunt system. A shunt system diverts the CSF from the ventricles either to the peritoneal cavity (ventriculoperitoneal shunt) or to the atrial cavity of the heart (ventriculoatrial). In infants, placement of a ventriculoperitoneal shunt, a relatively simple surgical procedure, is the method of choice (see Figure 18–2). An extra length of catheter is generally coiled in the peritoneum to extend as the infant grows. Ventriculoperitoneal shunts are generally safer than ventriculoatrial shunts (Shiminski-Maher & Disabato, 1994).

A variety of shunts is manufactured. Each type consists of three basic components: (1) the ventricular catheter (proximal end), (2) the bubble or reservoir (a pump with or without a valve), and (3) the peritoneal or atrial drainage end (distal catheter). The shunt tube, made of soft, pliable plastic, is approximately 1/8 inch in diameter. Shunts are designed to permit only unidirectional flow of CSF, away from the ventricles.

HOSPITAL DISCHARGE AND TRANSITION TO THE HOME

In preparing parents for home care of an infant with hydrocephalus, instructions should be given regarding shunt

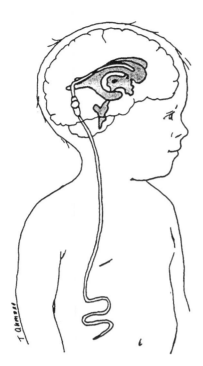

Figure 18–2 Ventriculoperitoneal Shunt

Source: Courtesy of Teresa Ahmann.

function, signs and symptoms of shunt malfunction and infection, how and when to contact the physician, and the infant's general care. Plans for safe transportation should be reviewed. Any parental concerns should also be addressed.

The community health nurse should obtain information from the hospital staff regarding the infant's particular history, including the following:

- previous symptoms of increased intracranial pressure (ICP)
- the location of the shunt
- the type and pressure of the shunt
- a record of serial measurements of the infant's head circumference
- a history of the infant's overall neurologic status
- prognosis as explained to the parents
- parental understanding of the infant's problem
- the need for follow-up care.

This information will assist the nurse in developing an appropriate home care plan with the family (see Appendix 18–A).

Safe transportation for the infant with hydrocephalus includes the use of an appropriate carseat. Some infants may require additional support for an enlarged head (Bull, Stout, Stroup, & Rust, 1991).

ROUTINE HOME VISITS

On each home visit, parental questions and concerns should be addressed. The nurse should also assess the infant's status relative to hydrocephalus.

Assessment of the Infant

Important elements of the history and physical examination include the following:

- level of orientation
- alertness
- behavior
- sleep patterns
- head circumference
- fontanels
- suture lines
- shunt insertion site
- eye movements
- bowel elimination pattern
- abdominal incision site
- shunt tract.

Examination of the head is critical and begins with measurement of the head circumference. If the infant's head circumference is increasing more rapidly than is normal, indicated by the normal curve on a growth chart, or more than 1.75 cm per week (Gardner & Hagedorn, 1992), the physician should be notified.

The character of the anterior fontanel should also be noted: on a quiet infant in the sitting position, the site should be soft and flat. On palpation, suture lines (coronal, sagittal, lambdoidal) should not be appreciably split or overlapping. The shunt insertion site, usually located above and slightly behind the ear, should be gently palpated and checked for redness, edema, or drainage. Ability to pump the reservoir does not indicate functioning; this maneuver can, in fact, lead to problems and should not be done unless the parent has special instructions from the neurosurgeon.

As part of the physical examination, the nurse should observe the infant's eye movements:

- Does the infant follow an object in all visual fields?
- Is there nystagmus (rapid, involuntary eye movement)?
- Can the infant look above midline without tilting his or her head?
- Can the infant visually converge on an object?

These findings should be compared to discharge data.

Assessment of Potential Complications

On each routine home visit, the nurse should also assess for symptoms of shunt malfunction, including shunt obstruction and infection. The shunt can become partially or completely blocked, for various reasons. The resulting obstruction will lead to increased intracranial pressure (ICP). Symptoms of shunt obstruction are somewhat different for infants and toddlers and are listed in Exhibit 18–1.

Infection is another potential complication. With an infection, the infant or toddler may exhibit the signs of shunt obstruction. In addition, fever, redness, and tenderness or puffiness along the shunt tract may be noted. Abdominal distension and tenderness may also be indicative of a shunt infection.

Other complications include disengagement of the shunt components, valve failure, and overdrainage. Most complications requiring shunt revision occur within the first 6 to 12 months after surgical placement of the shunt system.

Rare complications related to the use of a shunt include the following:

- *subdural hematoma (bleeding over the brain):* signs include increasing head circumference, full anterior fontanel, sunset eyes, and other signs of hydrocephalus.
- *paralytic ileus (abnormal bowel blockage):* signs include enlarged abdomen, vomiting, and absence of bowel sounds.

Exhibit 18–1 Signs and Symptoms of Increased Intracranial Pressure in Infants and Toddlers

In infants (before closure of sutures), symptoms of concern include the following:
- a tense, bulging fontanel when infant is upright and quiet
- increased head circumference
- prominent scalp veins
- split sutures
- vomiting
- change in appetite
- irritability
- increased sleepiness or lethargy
- "sunset" eyes (intermittent or continuous downward deviation of the eyes)
- seizures

In toddlers (after closure of sutures), symptoms of concern include the following:
- head enlargement
- vomiting, abdominal pain
- headache
- irritability
- sleepiness or lethargy
- behavior changes
- loss of previous abilities (e.g., sensory or motor function)
- seizures

- *cranial stenosis (early closure of cranial sutures):* signs include a change in head contour, particularly overlapping or ridges along the suture lines.

THE FIRST HOME VISIT

On the initial home visit, the nurse should elicit and address family concerns and needs. Additionally, the nurse should complete a thorough history and a detailed physical examination of the infant, for the purpose of establishing a baseline assessment. Assessment should also include all the elements of a routine visit, discussed in the previous section.

Parent Education

On the first home visit, it is generally helpful to review with parents the pattern of CSF flow and, if known, the specific cause of the hydrocephalus in their infant. Pictures such as those in Figures 18–1 and 18–2 can be used to help the parents understand the problem. The functioning of the shunt should also be reviewed. The nurse should assess parental knowledge of the signs and symptoms of potential shunt malfunction, particularly obstruction and infection.

Although parents need not regularly measure the head circumference, they should be instructed to regularly check the infant's fontanel. This should be done when the infant is upright and quiet. The nurse can demonstrate this procedure, and parents should be asked to provide a return demonstration.

In regard to the care of the infant with a shunt, the nurse should review with parents guidelines for contacting the primary care provider. These guidelines should be developed for each infant prior to hospital discharge and should include the signs of increased ICP listed in Exhibit 18–1. A fever of 101.5 °F (38.5 °C) is usually also a reason to contact the primary care provider (Gardner & Hagedorn, 1992). In general, concern is not for one episode of vomiting but rather for an overall pattern indicative of increasing ICP, including several of the signs and symptoms. However, some infants may have no symptoms of problems with the shunt except for a rapidly increasing head circumference. Therefore, if this is noted, it is a sufficient reason to contact the primary care provider. Of course, the parents should know how to contact the primary care provider and neurosurgeon around-the-clock.

Because a child with hydrocephalus is at an increased risk of seizure activity, parents should be taught both how to recognize seizures and how to observe and care for an infant or child during a seizure. (See Chapter 17.) Any seizure activity should be reported promptly to the primary care provider and neurosurgeon.

Primary Care

It is important for the family to have a source of regular pediatric care for the infant. The pediatrician or nurse practitioner can assist the family in answering general care questions and in assessing whether any symptoms the infant presents may be cranial in nature. Additionally, the primary care provider will evaluate the appropriateness of the standard immunization schedule in relation to the neurological status of the infant or young child. (See also Chapter 8.) Antibiotic prophylaxis is recommended for dental work and surgical procedures. Regular vision and hearing screenings will be important because of the increased risk of visual problems associated with hydrocephalus and the risk of hearing impairment associated with shunt malfunction and CNS infection.

SUBSEQUENT HOME VISITS

On subsequent home visits, parental concerns and questions should be elicited and addressed. At the same time, the nurse should have a plan in mind for ongoing assessment and intervention. This plan should address all elements of routine home visits and of the first home visit previously discussed in this chapter. In addition, the following areas should be addressed.

Assessment of the Infant

A developmental screening evaluation should be completed by the nurse to determine the infant's baseline development status. (See also Chapters 19 and 20.) If the assessment indicates a delay, the nurse should contact the physician to request a formal evaluation. If deficits are confirmed, the nurse can then assist the parents to obtain physical or occupational therapy and to enroll the infant in a developmental program. The nurse should also provide guidance and support to families regarding normal developmental activities.

On subsequent home visits, it is also important for the nurse to assess the infant's nutritional intake and growth pattern. Some neurologically involved infants feed poorly and have erratic growth patterns. Constipation should also be avoided since it can potentially cause problems with the distal end of the shunt tubing. The nurse can provide guidance regarding recommended intake, feeding patterns, methods to supplement the infant's caloric intake as necessary, and bowel elimination patterns. Chapter 9 provides an in-depth discussion of assessment and intervention related to nutrition and feeding.

Common Parental Concerns

Some parents will be concerned about the physical appearance of the infant with a shunt. In an infant, the shunt site and the tubing will be noticeable. The nurse can reassure parents, however, that as the child grows and develops more subcutaneous fat and thicker hair, the shunt will no longer be visible (although it can usually still be felt under the skin).

Parents may also be concerned about the shape of the infant's head after the shunt insertion and resulting ventricular decompression. The sutures may overlap and create the appearance of ridges. Parents can be reassured that most of these ridges will disappear as the infant grows. Additionally, parents can be instructed in frequent position changes to assist in uniform molding of the infant's head.

Activities of Daily Living

Because of the presence of the shunt, children with hydrocephalus may be at greater risk of CNS infection than their peers. The risk of shunt infection is greatest in infants. For this reason, when day care is necessary, care at home or in a small family day care setting is optimal to minimize exposure to common pathogens (Jackson, 1990).

Parents should be informed that toilet readiness can be delayed in children with neurological impairments. Guidance can be provided individually, as necessary.

As the child grows, parents are often concerned about the safety of play and other daily activities in the child with a shunt. The nurse should reassure them that it is very difficult to injure the shunt tubing and that the shunt will not become dislodged during normal activities. As children get older, activities should be limited as little as possible. However, some practitioners discourage direct-contact sports such as football. The use of helmets is often recommended when the older child engages in activities frequently resulting in falls (e.g., bicycle and skateboard riding; Jackson, 1990).

ONGOING CONCERNS

Shunt Revisions

Parents commonly fear future shunt revisions. However, it is typical for infants to require two to three revisions to accommodate for growth and, when necessary, to correct shunt malfunctions. Parents can be reassured that the surgery is relatively common.

The use of a shunt controls, but does not cure, hydrocephalus. Except in rare cases, hydrocephalus is a lifelong illness requiring consistent care and ongoing follow-up. Parents must remain alert to signs and symptoms of shunt malfunction or infection and should be encouraged to report suspicious changes promptly to avoid complications.

Ophthalmologic Follow-up

Children with hydrocephalus commonly have visual problems, even with proper shunt function and control of intracranial pressure. Problems may include disorders of gaze and eye movement as well as errors of refraction and accommodation. For this reason regular ophthalmologic evaluation, with an initial complete examination at approximately 6 months is warranted (Jackson, 1990).

Developmental Prognosis

The developmental prognosis for the infant with hydrocephalus often concerns parents. The nurse can encourage parents to express fears and concerns. Parents can also be counseled that each child will develop differently. Eventual intellectual function is difficult to predict early in the disease process and relates in part to associated brain injury (Jackson, 1990). Motor disabilities are fairly common, varying from mild weakness to more severe disability. The severity is generally diagnosis-related; children with conditions such as meningomyelocele or Dandy-Walker malformation have more serious impairments than those with uncomplicated hydrocephalus. In premature infants, other factors also affect developmental prognosis. (See Chapters 12 and 20.)

Information about local developmental resources can be provided to the family. Useful resources include the following: neurodevelopmental pediatrician, pediatric psychologist, physical therapist, occupational therapist, speech therapist, and neuro-ophthalmologist. Parents can be encouraged to advocate for the needs of their child in both the health care and, eventually, the educational systems.

REFERENCES

Bull, M.J., Stout, J., Stroup, K.B., & Rust, J. (1991). Safe transportation home for infants with severe hydrocephalus. *Journal of Neuroscience Nursing, 23*(6), 369–373.

Gardner, S.L., & Hagedorn, M.I. (1992). Physiologic sequelae of prematurity: The nurse practitioner's roles. Part VII. Neurologic conditions. *Journal of Pediatric Health Care, 6*(5), 263–270.

Jackson, P.L. (1990). Primary care needs of children with hydrocephalus. *Journal of Pediatric Health Care, 4*(2), 59–71.

Minarcik, C.J., & Beachy, P. (1989). Neurologic disorders. In G.B. Merenstein & S.L. Gardner (Eds.), *Handbook of neonatal intensive care* (2nd ed.). St. Louis, MO: Mosby.

Shiminski-Maher, T.S., & Disabato, J. (1994). Current trends in the diagnosis and management of hydrocephalus in children. *Journal of Pediatric Nursing, 9*(2), 74–82.

Home Care Plan: The Infant with Hydrocephalus

Date _____   Case manager _____

Name _____   Hosp # _____   DOB _____

PROBLEM: **HYDROCEPHALUS**

GOALS/OBJECTIVES	METHODS	STAFF/REVIEW
Child will maintain adequate drainage of CSF	Measure head circumference at each home visit. Assess for symptoms of increased ICP: bulging fontanel, sunset eyes, vomiting, lethargy, irritability, headache, change in level of consciousness, failure to thrive.	
Child will receive prompt treatment for signs and symptoms of increased ICP or infection	Assess caregivers' knowledge of signs and symptoms of increased ICP or infection; teach/review as needed. Assist caregivers in planning how to contact physician when problems are noted (including nights, weekends).	
Child will be at low risk of infection	Assess for swelling or redness along shunt track. Review signs and symptoms of infection with caregivers.	
Child will receive well-coordinated care	Communicate with primary physician or neurosurgeon as indicated.	
Child will be able to function with minimal restrictions	Discuss with family the effects of hydrocephalus on lifestyle of child and family: babysitters, vacations, activity. Provide information as needed.	

Source: Courtesy of Children's Hospital National Medical Center, Home Health Care Services, Washington, D.C.

Part VI

Developmental and Sensory Concerns

Early Intervention Services for the High-risk Infant

Jennifer Smith Stepanek

In recent years, there has been a complex evolution of laws, regulations, and policies supporting children with illnesses or disabilities and the families and professionals caring for them. In the arena of education and child development, the passage of Public Law 99-457 (Amendments to the Education of the Handicapped Act) mandated a rigorous national agenda to increase and improve services for infants and young children needing specialized care and their families. This agenda, "fueled by the needs of children and families and by the documented benefits of early intervention and preschool services" (Trohanis, 1995, p. 1), has been strengthened and renewed in subsequent reauthorizations of the law, the most recent being Part H of Public Law 103-382, amendments to the Individuals with Disabilities Education Act (IDEA) in 1993.

The passage of these regulations supports numerous initiatives related to early childhood development including research, training, educational technology, demonstration, outreach, and technical assistance (Trohanis, 1995). Equally important, however, is the fact that Part H regulations also mark an initiative to develop and implement family-centered practices in early intervention programs serving eligible children aged birth to 3 years. This legislation legally recognizes parents and family members as an integral part of the interdisciplinary educational and therapeutic teams caring for their young children needing specialized services (Poyadue, 1988).

Although the legislation is a decade old, the field of early intervention will continue to define itself based on the growing body of information documenting the specific needs of infants and young children. So, too, will ensuing regulations and the renewal of legislation persist in their evolution, as more and more policymakers are convinced of the benefits of early intervention and of family-centered approaches to working with children. However, it is important to have a fundamental understanding of current early intervention legislation—its intent, its components, and its implementation—to continue both supporting children with illnesses and disabling conditions and empowering the families and multidisciplinary professionals caring for them.

To help families and professionals better understand the collaborative process and the roles of various team members in the early intervention system, numerous publications have been developed by individuals and advocacy organizations supporting children's health and developmental care (e.g., Beckman & Boyes, 1993; Bishop, Woll, & Arango, 1993; Consortium of Family Organizations, 1994; McGonigel, Kaufman, & Johnson, 1991; Shelton & Stepanek, 1994; Trohanis, 1995; Von Rembow & Sciarillo, 1993). Exhibit 1 lists organizations providing information, resources, or technical assistance related to early intervention services. This Special Issue will provide a summarized overview of this literature and of basic information related to Part H services for infants and toddlers.

THE INTENT AND COMPONENTS OF PART H

The federally mandated Part H Infants and Toddlers Program (ITP) is a nationwide effort to assist states and juris-

Exhibit 1 Organizations Providing Information, Resources, or Technical Assistance Related to Early Intervention Services

Association for the Care of Children's Health (ACCH)
7910 Woodmont Avenue, Suite 300
Bethesda, MD 20814
301-654-6549

National Association of Protection & Advocacy Systems (NAPAS)
900 2nd Street, Suite 211
Washington, DC 20002
202-408-9514

National Early Childhood Technical Assistance System (NEC*TAS)
137 East Franklin Street, Suite 500
Chapel Hill, NC 27514
919-962-2001

National Information Center for Children and Youth with Disabilities (NICHCY)
PO Box 1492
Washington, DC 20013
1-800-659-0285

National Information Clearinghouse for Infants with Disabilities and Life-Threatening Conditions (NIC)
Center for Developmental Disabilities
University of South Carolina
Columbia, SC 29208
1-800-922-9234

Technical Assistance for Parents Programs (TAPP)
95 Berkely Street, Suite 104
Boston, MA 02116
617-482-2915

dictions with funding to plan, develop, and implement comprehensive, coordinated, community-based services for all eligible young children with disabilities from birth to age 3 years. Each state or jurisdiction is responsible for designating a lead agency that will ensure the availability of family-centered, responsive, collaborative, culturally competent, and high-quality early intervention services that are multidisciplinary and interagency in nature and that are (with certain exceptions) provided at no cost to the family.

These voluntary ITPs are to be offered to children and families in natural settings (e.g., homes, day care centers, libraries) whenever possible to enhance the integration of children with and without disabilities within communities. An Interagency Coordinating Council (consisting of agency, service provider, university, and family member representatives) is also to be appointed within each state and jurisdiction, to advise and assist the lead agency (Trohanis, 1995; Von Rembow & Sciarillo, 1993).

While specific policies and practices related to the implementation of Part H may vary from state to state, several ITP

components are nationally mandated. These include eligibility criteria, timelines for assessment and intervention, providers of early intervention services, and the range of entitlement and linkage services available. Federal guidelines also call for the development of an Individualized Family Service Plan (IFSP) for each eligible child and family.

All evaluation and intervention information is confidential, and procedural safeguards exist to protect certain parental rights (e.g., confidentiality, timely mediation, and conflict resolution). Furthermore, because participation in ITP is voluntary, parental consent must be obtained prior to all evaluations and/or program changes, and parents are entitled to have access to all information in their child's early intervention file.

PART H SERVICES

Any parent, professional, or relevant individual (e.g., day care provider, grandparent) can refer an infant or toddler to the local lead agency for evaluation. (For information regarding system contacts for early intervention services in each state, refer to Von Rembow and Sciarillo [1993] or to a local Child Find office, listed in most telephone books.) In collaboration with the family, the individual needs and developmental levels of the referred child will be assessed by a multidisciplinary team of two or more professionals to determine eligibility.

Eligibility

According to federal regulations, infants and toddlers from birth until the age of 3 years qualify for early intervention services if they fall into one of three eligibility categories:

1. *developmental delay* in one or more areas (i.e., cognitive, gross motor, fine motor, vision or hearing, expressive or receptive communication/language, social/emotional, and/or adaptive/self-help skills);
2. *high probability condition* (e.g., Down syndrome, cerebral palsy); or,
3. *at-risk or atypical development* as defined by each state (e.g., prematurity).

Timelines

Under Part H, evaluation of any referred child must be completed within 45 days from the date of referral. If the child is determined to be eligible for ITP services, an IFSP or Interim IFSP must also be developed within this timeline. The IFSP must then be implemented within 30 days of its development and signing. Because ITP services are only provided through age 2 years, a transition plan for toddlers must be initiated 6 months prior to a toddler's third birthday. If a child no longer requires intervention, community referrals such as Head Start, library programs, or play groups will be recommended. If a child meets eligibility requirements, he or she will be transitioned into Part B of IDEA, serving children ages 3 to 21 years, and an Individualized Education Plan (IEP) will be developed.

Services and Service Providers

ITP services must be provided by qualified personnel in collaboration with families. The types of "entitlement" services offered include assistive technology; audiology; family counseling/training; certain health, nursing, and diagnostic medical services; nutrition services; occupational, physical, speech/language, and/or vision therapies; psychological services; social work; special instruction; and transportation. A number of "linkage" services may also be needed by the family, such as information about local and national resources.

Part H also mandates the provision of a service coordinator who may be a direct service provider, a professional or paraprofessional service coordinator, or another individual chosen by the family. In addition to helping the family coordinate any evaluations and services the child may require, the service coordinator is responsible for making sure that the child and family have been informed of procedural safeguards, that the IFSP document is completed appropriately and implemented in a timely manner, that transition plans are initiated, and that the family is aware of relevant and available local and national resources.

The IFSP

The IFSP is the name for both the process and the document through which free and appropriate early intervention services are provided to children and their families. Developed collaboratively with family members and professionals, the IFSP contains important information about family-identified concerns, priorities, and resources/strengths related to the child's development; the child's current levels of functioning across developmental domains; specific goals and objectives for the child's development; providers and locations of intervention services; funding sources; timelines; and criteria for evaluation. The IFSP is reviewed by families and professionals at least twice a year, and a new IFSP is developed annually.

CONCLUSION

In our rapidly changing society with its complex health care situation, we must ensure that children's developmental needs are adequately and responsibly met. Part H of IDEA represents one of many recent legislative acts and amendments relating to mental health, maternal and child health, education, and developmental disabilities, each strengthening the commitment to family-centered policies and practices for children needing specialized health and developmental services and their families. In addition to providing valuable and comprehensive early intervention services to young children and their families, Part H demonstrates a recognition of the central role that the family plays in a child's life, and of the critical need to understand and incorporate the psychosocial needs of children into the service delivery system. Awareness of the intent, components, and implementation of these services benefits infants and toddlers with illnesses and disabling conditions and the families and professionals who care for them.

REFERENCES

Beckman, P.J., & Boyes, G.B. (1993). *Deciphering the system: A guide for families of young children with disabilities.* Cambridge, MA: Brookline Books.

Bishop, K.K., Woll, J., & Arango, P. (1993). *Family/professional collaboration for children with special health needs and their families.* Burlington, VT: Family/Professional Collaboration Project.

Consortium of Family Organizations. (1994). Principles of family-centered health care: A health care reform white paper (family policy report). *The ACCH Advocate, 1*(2), 11–20.

McGonigel, M.J., Kaufman, R.K., & Johnson, B.H. (1991). *Guidelines and recommendations for the individualized service plan.* Bethesda, MD: Association for the Care of Children's Health.

Poyadue, F.S. (1988). Parents as teachers of health care professionals. *Children's Health Care, 17*(2), 82–84.

Shelton, T.L., & Stepanek, J.S. (1994). *Family-centered care for children needing specialized health and developmental services.* Bethesda, MD: Association for the Care of Children's Health.

Trohanis, P.L. (1995). Progress in providing services to young children with special needs and their families: An overview to and update on implementing the Individuals with Disabilities Education Act (IDEA). NEC*TAS NOTES, (7).

Von Rembow, D., & Sciarillo, W. (1993). *Nurses, physicians, psychologists, and social workers within statewide early intervention systems: Clarifying roles under Part H of the Individuals with Disabilities Education Act.* Bethesda, MD: Association for the Care of Children's Health.

Normalization: A Guide for Parents

Belinda Ledbetter, BA

Being the parent of a child who is medically fragile is a challenging, emotionally draining, exhausting job. Being a child who is medically fragile is a tough job, too. Developmental tasks that happen so easily and naturally for other children can be a major struggle. Yet, there are many things you, as a parent, can do to help your child cope with obstacles created by high-technology medical care and the underlying medical limitations.

What is your underlying view of your child? Your child probably started life as a high-risk infant. Is your child as vulnerable as he or she once was? Are you still worrying about medical concerns that have been resolved? The health care system must, of necessity, focus much of its attention on what is wrong with your child. Are you able to see and appreciate the facets of your child that are normal and healthy? Can you see and appreciate that which is unique and special about your child? You are the mirror for your child and will have much to do with how your child views himself or herself. Will that picture of self be one of a confident, active explorer? Will your child make needs known and get a response? Will your child express a full range of feelings and know that all are acceptable? Can you transfer your child's trust in you to other caregivers, helping him or her understand they are helping even if what they do does not always feel good?

HELPING YOUR CHILD COPE WITH
MEDICAL CARE

Receiving medical treatments is difficult at any age, but the younger the child, the more difficult the treatments are because of the child's inability to understand. When a child approaches about 10 months developmentally, and sometimes even younger, if health care has been frequent or traumatic, he or she starts to benefit from using medical play to express feelings about what is being done. This also gives the child an opportunity to be the one who is the "doer" for a change, rather than the one having things done to him or her. Medical play also allows your child to become more familiar with medical equipment and how it works.

Allowing your child to suction a tracheostomy on a doll, practice a central line or gastrostomy tube dressing change on a doll, or give a nebulizer treatment to a teddy bear offers the opportunity for learning, being the "doer" and expressing feelings. When a young child starts to pull at his or her own tubes or other equipment or to interfere with dressing changes, this is often an expression of a developmentally appropriate need to explore the world—a world that happens to include medical equipment. Providing opportunities for medical play on a doll will help meet the child's need for exploration, often with the additional benefits of increased cooperation with care requirements. Of course, if the child's procedure is painful or creates discomfort, your child will need to express these feelings. To express feelings in proportion to the child's experience is a healthy goal.

HOME ENVIRONMENT

Ideally, home should be a safe haven from the world. Providing medical care in your home can interfere with a child's feelings of protection and relaxation. To help home feel safer and nurturing, two seemingly opposite plans can be used; the choice usually depends on the nature of your child's medical needs.

Care that is painful, difficult for your child, or expected to be of short duration often is best isolated from the child's home life. Consider creating a treatment area in the home, preferably where a child will not need to go for any other purpose. If possible, store medical supplies and all possible medical equipment in this area. This leaves the remainder of your home to be your child's safe haven from the world.

For treatments that your child does not find stressful, especially those that will be continued for a long time, incorporating the treatments into everyday life may be most appropriate for your child. For example, you can turn an intravenous (IV) pole used for night feedings into a stuffed animal rack or make a nebulizer treatment as much a part of the day's routine as changing a diaper.

When a child must receive many types of care at home, a combination of isolating some aspects of care and incorporating others into the daily routine may work best. Whatever you do, it is important to keep a child's bed safe by doing no medical care there. This will allow your child to relax, feel safe, and sleep more soundly.

PASSIVITY VERSUS ACTIVE PARTICIPATION

Most medical care promotes passivity in patients of any age. This is particularly true for infants. Your child benefits from your responsiveness to his or her cues. Getting the appropriate response encourages more cues. A cycle thus begins of communication and a self-image of being an active participant in one's own world. Cues like avoiding eye contact, turning his or her head away, yawning, or hiccuping often mean, "Give me a little space, I've had enough for now." Attentiveness and eye contact say, "Come on, let's continue." The more often caregivers respond to the infant's cue, the stronger the infant's reinforcement to continue actively communicating.

EXPRESSION OF FEELINGS

An emotionally healthy child can express a full range of feelings. The child can let you know when he or she is excited, frustrated, contented, angry, or confused, and you can understand the message. Medical care can complicate the process. When painful medical procedures are performed, the adult often feels upset and subconsciously wants the child to help him or her feel better. This is understandable but unfair. While it is desirable for the child to understand over time that the health care provider is a helper, in the immediate time, your child needs the freedom to express the pain and anger that may be felt when, for example, a blood test is done. If necessary, you may need to remind some health care providers of your child's needs.

When a child has a long and complex medical history, there has inevitably been much discomfort. This child especially needs to be allowed to express whatever he or she is feeling. Hearing your child moan because he or she is uncomfortable is painful for you as a parent, but your child needs to learn that all physical and emotional feelings are acceptable and can be expressed. If the child learns early in life that anger or pain should be suppressed or ignored, this suppression will often become a lifelong habit, and he or she will later have to work hard to unlearn it.

EATING AS A NORMAL ACTIVITY

Many children requiring high-technology home care will have received food through nasogastric (NG) or gastrostomy (G) tubes or by total parenteral nutrition (TPN). The quantity of food taken in will often have been a source of concern. When oral feedings are started, several steps may help. (See also Chapters 9, 10, and 11.)

As far in advance as possible, encourage sucking on a pacifier the same shape as the nipple that will be used. Ideally, no other pacifier should have been used. With your physician's permission, start introducing a taste of formula on the pacifier or your finger for a few days before oral feedings will be started so the child can become accustomed to the taste.

If medically permitted, when oral feedings are started, stop other feedings several hours in advance to allow the child time to become hungry. Be prepared to continue the previous feeding method while your child becomes accustomed to oral feedings. For at least several days, often much longer, oral feedings should only be a learning experience, and the amount of food taken should not matter. When a child has never taken in food through his or her mouth, the experience is strange, and it takes some time for it to become familiar.

Remember that eating is not another medical procedure but a normal life activity that should be a pleasure. Also keep in mind that you want your child to eat—an active taking of food by the child—not simply to be fed, which is a passive process of being given food.

If getting your child to eat or to eat a sufficient quantity is a struggle, several things may help. One possibility is that when a young child feels out of control, controlling food intake may be one of the few opportunities to take charge. Giving your child age-appropriate choices, such as choosing which clothes to wear or which cup to drink from, will start to create an appropriate arena for control and may decrease the need for control at meal time. Another possibility is that food has become a source of fear or anger, particularly if oral feedings were started and stopped on several occasions or if pain or discomfort was associated with eating at some time. Talking about past problems and reassurance that the previous problem has been fixed may be helpful, depending on the age of the child. Acknowledging how scary eating must be because of past experience will often help more than coaxing or threatening. Temporarily allowing eating while being distracted, perhaps by a favorite video movie or while receiving a great deal of attention from Mom or Dad, may help break down a barrier. Sometimes many small snacks through the day, even if eaten while up and playing rather than at the table, will provide the necessary calories. A third possibility is that eating has become a control struggle between you and your child. Try giving up as much control as you can tolerate, and see if eating becomes less of a struggle. Eating mashed potatoes with the fingers is not harmful, whereas stuffing them in an ear could be a problem. Can you give your child food and then ignore him or her for awhile? Excessive praise does not usually work well because a child then learns to expect praise for a normal process that should be self-rewarding.

Keep in mind that struggles over food are a normal developmental occurrence for a toddler. This "problem" may be a result of the normal struggle for independence rather than a result of your child's medical history. Read about eating behaviors of toddlers in a parenting book, and see if they sound familiar. As frustrating as the battles may be, this may be a reason to rejoice. Also, check with your physician about the necessary number of calories. There is a usual point at which the calorie requirements drop due to slowing down of growth, but this may depend on your child's medical requirements.

MOBILITY

If your child's mobility is limited, what degree of limitation is actually necessary? Is a walker, safely supervised, a possibility? Is a toy or padded board on wheels a possible way for the child to move himself or herself around the house by hand? Learn exactly what is required, then be creative in using whatever mobility is possible. For example, can a child in a body cast safely be propped in an upright position to allow increased arm movements through space? If your child must stay in a confined space, such as a wheelchair fitted with a ventilator, how creative can you be with enhancing that space for your child? For example, if your child can watch construction work out your living room window and is fascinated by it, is it possible to take your child out to see some of the work up close or to meet the workers? Can you pull out toys that can be used to imitate the work that he or she is watching? Can books be read about the work? Can your child draw "pictures" about the scene or activity?

Another way to help increase a limited experience of mobility is to provide ways for your child to move objects through space. Throwing a ball, operating a remote-controlled toy, or rolling cars down a ramp and into a pan several feet away are examples of this type of play. Also, with supervision, can a stuffed animal on a leash be "walked across the room"? Can wind chimes hung from the ceiling across the room be activated by pulling a rope, again with supervision? If your child cannot go to the object, then help find a way to allow moving the object from where he or she must stay.

GIVE YOUR CHILD A VOICE

If your child is unable to make sounds due to medical equipment, he or she still needs to develop a self-image as a communicator with the world, starting when other children are making early sounds. (See also Chapter 22.) At about 4 months of age or when your child begins to bat at toys, frequently hang bells, rattles, tambourines, and other noisemakers where your infant can use them and be rewarded by creating sound. When possible, respond to these sounds as if they were your child's own early sounds.

As your child develops, include more sound-producing toys that will encourage self-expression. A drum, xylophone, or cymbals can be used most expressively. Of course, you may need to choose soundmakers that you can live with, and attention to safety is paramount. While you would probably remove a xylophone from your healthy 9-month-old child's crib during a nap, a child who cannot make sounds needs the toy to stay in the crib so he or she can "speak up" when naptime is over or signal to let you know he or she is not sleepy yet. While you may not always be thrilled to hear these sounds, they are the sounds of your infant communicating with you. You may be surprised at the variety of messages that can be communicated through a xylophone.

As your child becomes ready to communicate more precisely, when other children are saying their first words, you can start teaching standard sign language. Begin by choosing a few signs that visually resemble the word. Pictures taken of your child forming words in his or her growing vocabulary can be in an album or on a poster to facilitate communication with babysitters, home nurses, visitors, and playmates. A source of sound still needs to be provided to enhance communication, particularly strong feelings common for children at this age. Some excellent children's books on sign language are available.

CONCLUSION

High-technology medical care will almost certainly have an impact on your child's development, but much can be done to reduce the limitations your child must experience. (See also Chapters 19 and 20.) Some examples of ways to normalize your child's life have been offered here. If you need more suggestions, talk to your home care nurse, ask for help from clinic staff, or call a child-life specialist who can be found working in children's hospitals, most hospitals with large pediatric units, and some community hospitals.

Chapter 19

Overview of Developmental Issues

Revised by Penny Glass, PhD, and Rachel Blinkoff, MA

Medical and technological advances in perinatal care have led to an increase in the survival rate of extremely small and premature infants (Hack et al., 1994). As late as 1970, fewer than 50% of infants born weighing 1,500 g or less survived, whereas today, almost 90% born weighing 1,500 g and 50% born weighing 700 g or less are discharged from the hospital (Batshaw & Perret, 1992; Glass, 1994). This increase in survival rates of infants with complex medical problems poses many challenges for the parents and professionals caring for them. Preterm infants develop differently from others and are at a greater risk for developmental problems throughout infancy and into early childhood (Hack et al., 1994). The immaturity of their organ systems also places them at greater risk for dependence on medical assistive technology, which interferes with the normal developmental process (Batshaw & Perret, 1992). As the lives of increasingly immature infants are being sustained, efforts must be undertaken to optimize the developmental aspects of their care.

A home care nurse is in a unique position to expand his or her traditional role by addressing the developmental needs of this high-risk population. This chapter presents a framework for understanding developmental issues related to caring for the high-risk infant at home. More specifically, this chapter provides the following:

- developmental principles and characteristics related to normal infant development
- the spectrum of developmental problems associated with the premature infant

- a general overview of assessment strategies and techniques to monitor the development of the high-risk infant
- specific intervention issues relevant to working with families of high-risk infants.

The reader is cautioned, however, that this chapter is only an overview. The education and training of each practitioner will determine the depth of knowledge and level of skill that are brought to working with the unique developmental needs of high-risk infants and their families (Ichord, 1986).

BASIC CONCEPTS OF NORMAL INFANT DEVELOPMENT

Principles of Early Development

In order to understand what places an infant at risk for developmental problems, one must first understand the natural progression of early development in healthy, full-term infants. Although there is no one specific theory of early development, a number of general principles exist. As suggested by Kopp (1994), Meisels and Provence (1989), and Hanson (1984), these principles provide a foundation for understanding early development:

- Early development is complex and is determined by multiple factors that are interdependent.

- Physiological characteristics of the infant at birth are subject to environmental influences, and the interaction between the two must be considered.
- Early development unfolds in orderly, predictable patterns; the differentiation of the infant's skills and abilities occurs over time.
- Early development is an active process that occurs through the infant's direct actions and the external responses received as a result of these actions.
- The family plays a unique role in the early development of the infant.

Subsumed within these general principles are four domains that comprise an infant's early development. Table 19–1 lists the four major developmental domains and some of the skills acquired during early development. These domains—social, language, cognitive, and motor development—are most easily described as part of the sensorimotor period (Coling, 1991). The sensorimotor period, between birth and approximately 2 years of age, was first described by Jean Piaget in the 1950s. According to Piaget, normal development occurs through the infant's active exploration of his or her environment. Although this is the optimal con-

dition, it is not necessarily essential. This is an important consideration for medically compromised infants: normal cognitive development can occur in the presence of sensory deficits as well as motor impairment.

Sensory Development

Each of the six sensory systems is equipped with specific receptors that respond to immediate information that is then filtered, organized, and integrated by the brain. The onset and rate of maturation of each sensory system varies and contributes differently to the infant's early development. However, all of the senses are functional at birth. Medically fragile infants are frequently described as either overreactive or underreactive to standard levels of sensory input. Even in healthy infants, the level of sensory stimulation in one modality may adversely affect the infant's response to stimulation in another modality. For example, an infant may respond aversively to voice under conditions of bright light and yet respond positively to the same level of voice under lower illumination (Haith, 1980).

Tactile System

The tactile system consists of touch receptors that are located in the skin and includes sensations relating to pressure, pain, and temperature. This system is believed to develop early in fetal life with most of the body becoming sensitive to touch by 15 weeks conceptual age (Glass, 1994). Infants are extremely responsive to touch and may react to tactile stimuli in one of two ways: either (1) in a defensive, protective way or (2) as a means for perceptual or discriminatory learning (Coling, 1991).

Vestibular System

The vestibular system is responsive to movement and directional changes in gravity. Receptors of the vestibular system are located in the inner ear and are believed to reach full size by 20 weeks (Glass, 1994). Infants use the information processed through the vestibular system to maintain balance and normalize muscle tone (Coling, 1991).

Gustatory-olfactory System

The gustatory-olfactory systems relate to the chemical senses of taste and smell. Taste receptors are located in the taste buds, which are found on the tongue, soft palate, and epiglottis. Taste receptors are functional before birth and develop with associated changes in preference and sensitivity (Glass, 1994). Even newborn infants demonstrate characteristic different facial expressions to samples that are sweet, sour, salty, and bitter. Thus, it should not be surprising when infants respond negatively to administration of certain oral medication. Olfactory receptors are located in

Table 19–1 Domains of Early Development

Area of Development	Related Skills
Social	Interpersonal skills Personal relationships and attachments Development of trust and independence
Language	Ability to express oneself through words and gestures Ability to understand what others are communicating
Cognitive	Imitation skills Problem-solving skills Ability to integrate (interpret) information obtained through the senses
Motor	Ability to control and coordinate muscles
Gross motor	Overall posturing and mobility Activities that require the use of large muscles, such as sitting, crawling, walking
Fine motor	Smaller muscle groups controlling hand movements and oral functions Activities such as grasping, manipulating, and chewing Visual tracking sometimes considered a fine motor skill

the nasal passage and are believed to be functional prenatally (Glass, 1994). Although smell in newborns is not well differentiated, infants are known to recognize the odor of their mother's milk within the first few days of life (Smolack, 1986). Both the gustatory and olfactory systems affect oral motor and feeding development.

Auditory System

The auditory system, which is composed of both peripheral and central components, is structurally in place by 25 weeks. Glass (1994) has shown that healthy full-term neonates demonstrate a preference for sound that they were exposed to in utero. Infants will localize sounds very early in life and show a preference for their mother's voice. Even in the newborn period, the two hemispheres of the brain respond differentially to speech (left hemisphere) compared to nonspeech sounds (right hemisphere). Auditory responses to information continue to develop postnatally and play a significant role in the development of language and communication.

Visual System

The visual system is the least mature sensory system at birth, with extensive maturation and differentiation during the third trimester and up to around 4 months postterm (Glass, 1993). Newborn infants are able to attend to form, object, and face, and visual development includes selective attention to specific features and discrimination of patterns. Visual motor integration assumes an intact visual as well as motor system. Information processed through the visual system significantly affects development. Motor milestones and exploratory behavior are dependent on visual responses, as are communicative and social behavior.

Infants learn about their world through each of the sensory systems. The perceptual capabilities embedded in the infant's sensory systems are instrumental in the later development of more complex social and cognitive skills (Smolack, 1986).

Motor Development

Motor development involves the ability to gain control of and coordinate muscles for movement; it is heavily dependent on the functioning of the central nervous system. Motor development may be more specifically defined as gross motor or fine motor development. Gross motor skills involve controlling and coordinating the large muscles used for activities such as sitting, crawling, and walking. Fine motor skills involve the smaller muscles and are used during activities such as grasping, manipulation, chewing, and visual tracking.

In general, motor development progresses in a cephalocaudal pattern in which maturation or motor control proceeds from head to toe. For example, the infant must first develop head control before being able to control his or her trunk. Motor development also progresses in a proximal-distal pattern in which growth and control begin at the center of the body and move outward. For example, the infant must develop arm control before being able to use his or her hands. The acquisition of gross motor skills generally precedes the refinement of fine motor skills. In the medically fragile infant, the problem of energy expenditure during gross motor activity may necessitate a different approach. Stabilization or support of the infant's arm, for example, may allow for refinement of hand usage even without normal gross motor development.

Motor development is generally described in terms of reflexive behavior, muscle tone, and postural control. Reflexes are stereotypical movements or postures produced in response to a specific stimulus and are present at birth. In normally developing infants, these reflexes eventually become integrated into more directed and purposeful behavior. Muscle tone is defined as the amount of tension in the body's muscles, and postural control varies according to a particular muscle group and the type of activity being employed. Muscle tone may fluctuate between the extremes of increased (hypertonic) and decreased (hypotonic). In the healthy, full-term infant, a balance exists between the two extremes, allowing for controlled movements of flexion and extension.

Within the realm of normal development, there is much variation in the maturational patterns associated with motor and sensory skills. Some infants develop quickly and reach expected milestones early, whereas others develop more slowly. The infant brain seems to be "programmed" toward normal development, even when circumstances are not optimal. Resolution of medical complications is often followed by a spurt in progress toward milestones.

DEVELOPMENTAL CONSIDERATIONS FOR THE PRETERM INFANT

Developmental Patterns of the Preterm Infant

Healthy, term infants are equipped with the sensory and motor capacities that are necessary to develop the social, perceptual, and cognitive skills that help them learn about and function in their environment (Ichord, 1986). Premature infants, who are born before being physically ready to enter the world, have poor neurological maturation. Als (1982) has documented the differences between the premature and healthy, full-term infant in the autonomic, motoric, state, attention, and regulatory systems. In the healthy, full-term infant, these systems function smoothly and support and enhance one another. Conversely, the premature infant's systems do not develop simultaneously and are often characterized by signs of stress (Als, 1982).

Premature infants tend to be less alert and therefore have less time for optimal interaction with their caretaker and environment. They also tend to have poor sleep-wake cycles and have difficulty making the transition from one state of consciousness to another. When awake, premature infants often react defensively when touched or moved and may be extremely irritable. Their own ability to self-calm is compromised, and both their irritability and their defensiveness make it difficult to console and calm them. Premature infants tend to have irregular breathing patterns and immature sucking patterns, which make it difficult and time-consuming to feed them. They also tend to display irregular, jerky movements, often in the form of extensor patterns. These infants tend to show a higher number of asymmetrical movements, due to their lack of muscle power and control. Unlike the term infant who has maintained a flexed position as a result of the boundaries in utero, the premature infant has difficulty maintaining the normal flexed position in part due to limited exposure to those natural boundaries.

Environmental Influences

Premature infants who have medical problems that require some dependence on technology tend to display additional characteristics that interfere with normal development. Mechanical ventilation, oxygen use, and apnea monitoring can restrict the infant's mobility (Ahmann & Lipsi, 1992). Prolonged ventilation—specifically, the presence of a tracheostomy—can interfere with the development of speech production. Premature infants who have little energy and require the use of technology may have an even more difficult time communicating their needs. Feeding may be more challenging in this population. In addition to the premature infant's immature suck and swallow, infants who require tube feeding and ventilation may become extremely sensitive to normal oral stimulation.

The responses evident in premature and technologically dependent infants make it difficult for them to adapt to their environment. These response patterns are not only stressful for the infant but also tend to be difficult for the parent and the home care nurse. The caregiver may experience feelings of inadequacy and helplessness because of the infant's inability to respond. Moreover, the infant's irregular sleeping and feeding patterns may cause parents to be deprived of sleep and may result in their being both physically and emotionally exhausted. In addition, the infant's prolonged hospitalization at birth often interferes with and delays the normal maternal–infant bonding process. The end result is that the parents of a preterm or technology-dependent infant may not have had adequate opportunities to become comfortable caring for the infant and instead may feel scared or overwhelmed. This in turn can have a negative impact on the interaction between the parent and infant. The home care nurse, on the other hand, may respond competently to the medical needs of the child but may remain emotionally detached. Neither approach is optimal for the child's development.

Risk Factors and Developmental Outcomes

In addition to immature body systems, there are several medical complications that may contribute to the way a premature infant develops. Many learning problems found in school-age children who were premature infants are often attributable either to overt brain damage or a generalized disturbance in brain organization (Glass, 1994).

Intraventricular Hemorrhage

A medical complication highly predictive of developmental outcome in premature infants is the presence of severe intracranial hemorrhage (Volpe, 1989). Intraventricular hemorrhage (IVH) is actual bleeding into the fluid-filled chambers of the brain. When limited, IVH is not strongly associated with adverse effects on developmental outcomes. However, when the brain parenchyma itself is damaged, either from an extension of an IVH or from an ischemic injury such as periventricular leukomalacia (PVL), the outcome is most often motor handicap, such as cerebral palsy. The severity of the motor handicap is correlated with the extent of injury to the brain parenchyma. Mental retardation usually accompanies the more extensive lesions (Batshaw & Perret, 1992).

Seizures and Hydrocephalus

Other dysfunctions of the brain that frequently lead to developmental problems include seizures and hydrocephalus. The functional impact of both complications is highly variable and relates directly to the degree of underlying brain injury (Ichord, 1986). While the vast majority of seizures are adequately controlled by medication, they continue to place the infant at risk for a range of developmental problems (Ichord, 1986). Hydrocephalus may require the surgical placement of a shunt. Both seizures and hydrocephalus should be recognized as indications of brain dysfunction, requiring consistent monitoring for associated perceptual, learning, and motor problems (Ichord, 1986).

Respiratory Problems

In addition to neurological complications, many premature infants experience respiratory problems. Bronchopulmonary dysplasia (BPD) results from the changes in the lungs associated with long-term respiratory support. Infants with moderate to severe BPD often have poorer developmental outcomes, including language deficits, feeding, and behavioral problems (Batshaw & Perret, 1992; Bernbaum, Friedman, Hoffman-Williamson, Agostino, & Farran, 1989). Infants who require prolonged ventilation utilize most of their energy for breathing, leaving little strength for developmental activities (Ahmann & Lipsi, 1992). Technology associated with ventilatory support imposes many restrictions on the child's ability to move about and explore his or her environment. The technology may also interfere with the child's ability to use expressive language and produce speech. Young children who are ventilator-dependent may become extremely frustrated with their inability to communicate, resulting in aggressive or difficult behavior (Batshaw & Perret, 1992). (Chapter 22 addresses communication issues in detail.)

Sensory Impairment

Additional medical complications associated with prematurity include vision and hearing problems. (See Chapters 21 and 23.) Retinopathy of prematurity (ROP) is a proliferative vascular disease of the retina most strongly associated with extreme prematurity (< 28 weeks gestation; Glass, 1993). Only the most severe ROP leads to the detachment of the retina and subsequent blindness. Severe ROP is reported to affect as many as 4% of infants weighing less than 1,000 g at birth (Glass, 1993). Whether or not the infant had ROP, the preterm child is more likely to develop squint (crossed eye), lazy eye, or extreme nearsightedness. Premature infants are also at risk for hearing problems, with as many as 3% reported as having sensorineural hearing loss at hospital discharge (Bernbaum et al., 1989). Children with chronic respiratory problems are also at increased risk for hearing problems. Unidentified hearing problems significantly affect the child's language and communication skills.

Birth Weight

The extensive medical risks faced by premature infants also make them highly susceptible to developmental problems in early childhood and in school. Recent research shows that 20% to 50% of children born at extremely low birth weight (< 750 g) who survive have some neurodevelopmental impairment during early childhood, and as many as one half of school-age children born at extremely low birth weight display some type of learning problem (Hack & Fanaroff, 1989; Hack et al., 1994). While the spectrum of learning problems is vast, it may include children of low average or otherwise normal intelligence who have deficits in language, visual perception, or visuomotor integration; deficiencies in attention span; hyperactivity; or social immaturity (Glass, 1994).

Environmental Factors

Understandably, extremely fragile neonates are more vulnerable to developmental problems than healthy term infants. However, not all infants born at the same gestational age are prone to the same vulnerabilities (Hanson, 1984). The number of medical complications, as well as factors such as socioeconomic status and quality of parent–infant interaction, can significantly affect the infant's development.

Extensive research has shown that premature infants born to families without adequate economic resources and those who are deprived of quality interaction are more at risk for later health problems and lingering vulnerability (Hanson, 1984).

ASSESSING DEVELOPMENT IN THE PRETERM INFANT

Neonatal Assessment

Because of the extensive array of risk factors involved in the development of the premature infant, it is imperative that the infant be monitored during the first few years of life. Monitoring can occur through informal screening procedures or formal assessment. Developmental assessment should begin well before discharge from the nursery. Initial screening of the infant's risk status can begin as soon as the infant's condition is sufficiently stable. A more formal neurodevelopmental examination of the infant's capabilities should be done close to the time of discharge.

Neonatal assessment of the high-risk infant is important for a number of reasons. First of all, it is critical for the needs of the infant and family to be identified early to ensure optimal developmental progression and parent–infant interaction. Furthermore, through neonatal assessment, state and local governments can obtain an estimated figure of the number of children who may require special education services. Increased public awareness of high-risk infants has enabled many hospitals to institute tracking systems through their state governments to follow any infant weighing less than 1,500 g. These systems have been established in an effort to provide more accessible and better quality services for high-risk neonates and their families.

High-risk Follow-Up

Following discharge from the hospital, the premature infant should continue to be monitored. This is often accomplished by a home health nurse or an established neonatal follow-up clinic. If the infant returns to the hospital for developmental follow-up, visits should be coordinated with other clinic appointments. The assessment of a premature infant is generally a multidisciplinary process and involves a team of professionals working with the family. Members of the assessment team may include a developmental pediatrician, psychologist, developmental specialist, neonatologist, nutritionist or dietitian, speech pathologist, and occupational or physical therapist. Other fundamental members of the team include pediatric nurses and the parents. The nurse is often the initial point of contact and assists in coordinating services for the family (Ahmann & Lipsi, 1992). The parents are in a position to provide invaluable information to the team about the infant's behavior and the general needs of the family.

The premature infant who has not suffered any brain injury will generally follow the same sequence of development as a term infant (Ichord, 1986). However, the degree of prematurity can significantly affect the interpretation of a child's developmental status. Thus, when assessing the premature infant, the general practice is to adjust the infant's age according to the degree of prematurity. (Chapters 9 and 20 contain a description of the process of age adjustment.) The concept of corrected age is generally useful even until the child is 3 years of age.

Before the development of the infant is assessed, it is necessary to obtain a detailed medical and social history. Feeding and sleep patterns should also be reviewed, providing insight into the adaptive behavior of the infant.

The development of the infant is assessed by comparing his or her skills to the normal sequence of developmental skills. (See Chapter 20.) Particular areas of development that should be assessed include motor, language, social, cognitive, and behavioral domains. The assessment of the infant includes observation of spontaneous play as well as the administration of structured tasks. Throughout the assessment, parental reports of the infant's behavior and any family concerns, priorities, and resources should be considered. Table 19–2 provides examples of accessible screening tools and methods.

Table 19–2 Options for Developmental Screening of the High-risk Infant

Process	Description
Child Find	The single point of entry within the public school systems for children ages birth to 21 years suspected of having developmental delays.
Early and Periodic Screening, Diagnosis, and Treatment (EPSDT)	A child-specific component of the Medicaid program that provides periodic screenings, diagnostic services, and health care treatment to children identified with health care needs.
Developmental checklists	A listing of developmental milestones to assist the professional in screening particular areas of development.
Denver Developmental Screening Test II	A frequently used screening instrument for children from 0–6 years, covering the areas of gross motor, language, fine motor/adaptive, and personal/social. Easy to administer and interpret.

Once the developmental status of the infant and the needs of the family have been assessed, impressions and recommendations should be shared with the family and other professionals involved. The most important aspects of the infant's evaluation to focus on while talking with parents include the current functional level of each domain, the long-term priority, what the medically fragile child is most capable of learning, and ways that the therapeutic experience can be "normalized." (Chapter 20 provides additional detail on the assessment process; see also Special Issue, "Normalization: A Guide for Parents.")

INTERVENTION AND THE PRETERM INFANT

A primary purpose in assessing the infant's abilities is to guide the interaction of parents and professionals with the child. Secondary purposes include planning for appropriate intervention strategies. After the needs of the infant and family have been determined, a developmental plan is constructed with the family. In some cases, specific suggestions can be provided to the family for appropriate interaction and play. In other cases, specific developmental needs may be identified warranting more formal intervention strategies.

Criteria for Referral

As suggested by Bernbaum and colleagues (1989), referral for more formal assessment should occur if any of following circumstances are noted:

- Questions or concerns arise about a specific aspect of the infant's development.
- After correcting for prematurity, an overall delay in the child's development is evident.
- Development appears uneven or abnormal.
- The parents have questions about behavior that the screening professional is not able to address directly.

Public Law 99-457

Early intervention services for developmentally vulnerable children and their families have evolved over the last decade through the implementation of Part H of the Individuals with Disabilities Education Act (IDEA), Public Law (P.L.) 99-457 and (P.L.) 103-382. (See also Special Issue "Early Intervention Services for the High-risk Infant.") Through this legislation, states have received federal funds to assist in the provision of early intervention services. As written in the law, early intervention services are intended to enhance the development of at-risk and vulnerable children and provide support and assistance to the family.

Part H requires the development of an individualized family service plan (IFSP) for each infant and family. This plan must include, at a minimum, the following components:

- a statement of the child's present level of development
- the family's statement of its strengths and needs related to enhancing the child's development
- the family's statement of major outcomes expected to be achieved by the child and family
- criteria, timelines, and procedures for determining progress
- specific early intervention services necessary to meet the needs of the child and family
- projected dates for initiation of services and expected duration
- name of service coordinator
- procedure for transitioning from early intervention into preschool.

Specific early intervention services covered by the law may include but are not limited to audiology, speech and language pathology, special education, physical and occupational therapy, psychological services, parent/family training and counseling, transition to preschool, diagnostic medical services; and health services that allow the child to benefit from other intervention services.

Although each state provides services somewhat differently under the federal law, all early intervention programs are based on the same premises. One major principle of all early intervention services is that services are provided as a means to help children achieve particular developmental gains. They are based on individual goals the family and professionals have for the child and are outcome oriented. A second principle is that all programs are designed to be family-focused, meaning that the child is not viewed as an isolated entity (Meisels & Shonkoff, 1992). Families are encouraged to be involved in all aspects of intervention, including assessment, planning, and implementation of services.

Initiating a Referral

Nurses working with families need to be aware of the types of services available to vulnerable infants and the policies that influence these services. (See Special Issue, "Early Intervention Services for the High-risk Infant.") Although each state varies in its systematic arrangements, there are generally a number of entry points to the service network for infants in the local community. The public school system, local health departments, and Child Find programs are common agencies involved in providing early intervention services. While parents may initiate referrals, it is not uncommon to feel frustrated and overwhelmed by the process. Thus, the nurse may frequently take the initiative in sug-

gesting referrals to early intervention programs and supporting the parent's efforts at advocating for their child. Exhibit 19–1 lists the essential steps involved in referring a child to an early intervention program.

THE ROLE OF THE NURSE

The nurse's role in developmental assessment and intervention will vary depending on the individual needs of the child and family as well as the nurse's own level of training. However, all nurses must have an understanding of the screening and assessment processes necessary to monitor the high-risk infant. Furthermore, while the nurses who spe-

Exhibit 19–1 Steps for Referring a Child to an Early Intervention Program

1. Determine the medical and developmental needs of the infant or young child.
   - Assess the abilities of the infant or young child in the areas of cognition, speech and language, fine and gross motor skills, and social interaction.
   - Note any behavioral concerns.
   - Include the strengths and weaknesses of the infant or young child.
   - Note any equipment, medication, and medical needs.

2. Determine the family's needs.
   - Assess particular needs, including mention of other children, number of caretakers, available resources, transportation.
   - Note family concerns and priorities.

3. Discuss the possibility of an early intervention program with the family.
   - Allow the parent to make the ultimate decision in the placement.
   - Offer to initiate the referral.
   - Provide the parent with any program names and numbers.

4. Determine the family's preference for services.
   - Do they prefer home-based or center-based services?
   - Do they prefer individualized therapy or group therapy?
   - What types of services are needed (physical therapy, occupational therapy, speech and language therapy, parent education, case management, social services)?

5. Contact the local early intervention program or the single point of entry for the particular area.
   - Provide the agency with basic information (names, address, child's date of birth, telephone number).
   - Offer to provide pertinent medical, developmental, and social information.
   - Additional information may include the physician's name and number and insurance policy.

6. Follow up with the agency and parent to confirm placement.

cialize in the problems of premature infants obviously need to be aware of critical developmental issues faced by high-risk infants, they also need a basic awareness of normal developmental progression. A nurse who understands normal developmental patterns and progression will be better able to identify abnormal or deviant behaviors or patterns (Ichord, 1986). When concerns arise, the nurse should consult with a developmental specialist prior to formal referral.

If a referral to an early intervention program is necessary, the nurse can assist the family in the enrollment process. After a child is referred for early intervention services, the nurse should collaborate closely with any professionals involved in the family's case. The nurse should continue to monitor the child's tolerance for the intervention strategies (see Chapter 20) and should communicate observations and concerns to parents and to the specialists involved. The nurse can also assist in implementing recommended activities, emphasizing the importance of applying techniques and suggestions to the home environment (Ichord, 1986). Throughout the entire assessment and intervention process, the nurse will remain a consistent support and advocate to the family. In this regard, the nurse's role is critical.

CONCLUSION

Premature infants are born before being physically ready to enter the world; thus, they have a difficult time adjusting to the postnatal environment. They typically display different developmental patterns than healthy, full-term infants. These infants are also at a greater risk for developmental problems in infancy and early childhood than other children. Developmental progress is further complicated for those infants who are technology-dependent.

Home care nurses are in a unique position to support the development of medically fragile or high-risk infants. When working with infants and young children, it is important to maintain a balanced approach, focusing on all areas of development. Of particular importance, nurses must recognize the social–emotional impact medical intervention and technology may have on a developing child. During infants' early years, their sense of trust and independence is developing. The necessary hospitalizations and medical intervention required by high-risk infants make it more difficult for them to develop such competencies. Being separated from parents and exposed to strangers, painful procedures, and noxious medication can be confusing and difficult for a young child. Technology that restricts movement, the ability to communicate, and overall independence can be frustrating and difficult for a child who is attempting to learn about the world. Home care nurses are in a position to alleviate the impact of chronic medical conditions on the growing child and, in turn, the family.

REFERENCES

Ahmann, E., & Lipsi, K. (1992). Developmental assessment of technology-dependent infants and young children. *Pediatric Nursing, 18*(3), 299–305.

Als, H. (1982). Towards a syntactic theory of development: Promise for the assessment of infant individuality. *Infant Mental Health Journal, 3,* 229–243.

Batshaw, M.L., & Perret, Y.M. (1992). *Children with disabilities: A medical primer.* Baltimore, MD: Paul H. Brookes Publishing.

Bernbaum, J.C., Friedman, S., Hoffman-Williamson, M., Agostino, J.D., & Farran, A. (1989). Preterm infant care after hospital discharge. *Pediatrics in Review, 10*(7), 195–206.

Coling, M. (1991). *Developing integrated programs: A transdisciplinary approach to early intervention.* Tucson, AZ: Therapy Skills Builders.

Glass, P. (1993). Development of visual function in preterm infants: Implications for early intervention. *Infants and Young Children, 6*(1), 11–20.

Glass, P. (1994). The vulnerable neonate and the neonatal intensive care environment. In G. Avery (Ed.), *Neonatology: Pathophysiology and management of the newborn* (4th ed.). Philadelphia, PA: J.B. Lippincott.

Hack, M., & Fanaroff, A.A. (1989). Outcome of extremely-low-birth-weight infants between 1982 and 1988. *New England Journal of Medicine, 321,* 1,642–1,647.

Hack, M., Taylor, H.G., Klein, N., Eiben, R., Schatschneider, C., & Mercuri-Minich, N. (1994). School-age outcomes in children with birth weights under 750 g. *New England Journal of Medicine, 12*(331), 753–759.

Haith, M.M. (1980). *Rules that Babies Look By.* Hillsdale, NJ: Lawrence Erlbaum Associates.

Hanson, M.J. (1984). *Atypical infant development.* Austin, TX: Pro-Ed.

Ichord, R. (1986). *Home care of the high-risk infant: A holistic guide to using technology.* Rockville, MD: Aspen Publishers.

Kopp, C.B. (1994). *Baby steps: The "whys" of your child's behavior in the first two years.* New York, NY: W.H. Freeman & Co.

Meisels, S.J., & Provence, S. (1989). *Screening and assessment: Guidelines for identifying young disabled and developmentally-vulnerable children and their families.* Arlington, VA: NEC*TAS & Zero to Three.

Meisels, S.J., & Shonkoff, J.P. (1992). *Handbook of early childhood intervention.* Cambridge, MA: Cambridge University Press.

Smolack, L. (1986). *Infancy.* New York, NY: Prentice Hall.

Volpe, J. (1989). Intraventricular hemorrhage and brain injury in the premature infant: Diagnosis, prognosis and prevention. *Clinics in Perinatology, 16*(2), 387–411.

ADDITIONAL RESOURCES

Als, H. (1994). Individualized developmental care for the very low birth weight preterm infant. *JAMA, 272*(11), 853–858.

Brazelton, T.B. (1984). *Neonatal behavioral assessment scale* (2nd ed.). Philadelphia, PA: J.B. Lippincott.

Gibbs, E.D., & Teti, D.M. (1990). *Interdisciplinary assessment of infants: A guide for early intervention professionals.* Baltimore, MD: Paul H. Brookes Publishing.

Glascoe, F.P. (1991). Developmental screening: Rationale, methods and applications. *Infants and Young Children, 4*(1), 1–10.

Stroufe, L.A., Cooper, R.G., & Marshall, M. (1988). *Child development: Its nature and course.* New York, NY: Alfred A. Knopf.

Widerstrom, A.H., Mowder, B.A., & Sandall, S.R. (1991). *At-risk and handicapped newborns and infants: Development, assessment and intervention.* Englewood Cliffs, NJ: Prentice Hall.

Chapter 20

Developmental Assessment and Intervention in the Home

Elizabeth Ahmann, ScD, RN, and
Kathleen Lipsi Klockenbrink, MA, EdS

Early intervention programs that address both biological and environmental challenges for the prematurely born infant have been shown to have positive effects on infant developmental outcomes (Als et al., 1994; Barrera, Rosenbaum, & Cunningham, 1986; Infant Health and Development Program, 1990; Shonkoff & Hauser-Cram, 1987). Positive outcomes are more likely when intervention is begun early (Ramey & Campbell, 1987; Shonkoff & Hauser-Cram, 1987), used for prevention rather than remediation (Resnick, Armstrong, & Carter, 1988), and when parental involvement is high (Shonkoff & Hauser-Cram, 1987).

The role of the home care nurse in developmental assessment and intervention will vary based on several factors, including the following: the complexity of the child's medical and developmental problems, the constellation of the home care "team," community resources that can provide early intervention services, and the role played by personnel at the tertiary or chronic care facility that discharges the child. This chapter provides an overview of issues in developmental assessment and intervention for the high-risk infant who is technology-dependent.

FACTORS CONTRIBUTING TO DEVELOPMENTAL PROBLEMS

Preterm infants with multiple medical problems who require the assistance of medical technology are at risk of poor developmental outcomes for a variety of reasons, both medical and environmental:

- a medical history that may include neurological assaults such as intraventricular hemorrhage and periods of oxygen deprivation
- a history of sensory-motor deprivation resulting from long hospital stays coupled with restrictions related to medical fragility and technology dependence
- nutritional inadequacies related to chronic medical conditions
- effects of chronic illness on energy levels and on tolerance for various positions and activities
- continued limitations of activities related to dependence on cumbersome and restrictive medical equipment
- in some cases, going home to a deprived environment.

As discussed in Chapter 19, premature birth places an infant at increased risk for a broad range of developmental and behavioral problems. These include risks in the areas of motor development; cognitive development; visual-motor integration; language development; later learning; and behavioral adjustment, including attentional problems.

The interplay of various medical problems and early development cannot be overemphasized. For example, the premature infant has high calorie needs for catch-up growth.

Source: Excerpts reprinted from *Pediatric Nursing,* Vol. 18, No. 3, pp. 299–305, with permission of Jannetti Publications, Inc., Pitman, New Jersey, © 1992.

The presence of bronchopulmonary dysplasia (BPD) and related cardiac effects (CHF) leads to an energy-demanding work of breathing. As a result, for the infant whose oral intake is poor, or the infant with significant reflux vomiting, adequate caloric intake for supporting body functioning may be difficult to maintain, leaving little energy for developmental activities. At the same time, the infant with BPD or with gastroesophageal reflux may be intolerant of certain positions or activities that might benefit developmental progress. The infant with BPD and CHF may tire easily and tolerate only very short periods of even passive developmental stimulation. Furthermore, the presence of cumbersome tubing and equipment can challenge normal parental-infant interactions that promote the infant's own movement and development in general.

Environmental factors have important effects on development. For one, the restrictions medical equipment places on the infant's interactions with the world, both in the acute hospital and chronic home-based phases, can be profound (Anderson & Auster-Liebhaber, 1984). Secondly, parental involvement has an impact. Several studies have shown that parents who receive no guidance in what to expect for the preterm infant's development or how to observe and interact with their infant have perceptions of and attitudes toward the infant that are different from and more negative than parents receiving guidance (Cusson & Lee, 1993). Studies using modeled interventions have been most effective in improving infant outcomes. Both Resnick and colleagues (1988) and the Infant Health and Development Program (1990) found that when providers model for parent-appropriate techniques for intervening with the infant, improved cognitive outcomes for preterm infants can result.

FAMILY PARTICIPATION IN ASSESSMENT

Family members know the infant or young child most intimately. Family members have a unique perspective on the child's developmental status and needs, and the family has the ultimate responsibility for responding to those needs. For these reasons, families should be invited to participate collaboratively in the developmental assessment and planning process. They should be encouraged to share observations, concerns, and questions about the child. Furthermore, the family should be encouraged to participate in assessing its own resources, limitations, and needs in regard to promoting the child's development. Finally, all information gathered as part of the professional assessment efforts should be shared with the family in terms they can understand. (General issues of parent–professional collaboration are addressed in Chapter 4.)

While numerous formal tools for family assessment are available, few are designed for the purpose of gathering information that will be pertinent in the process of assessing and planning how to promote a child's development. Fur-

ther, few ask families directly for their perceptions and concerns. Exploring the main concern or worry the parents have about the child's development can be particularly useful in both opening a discussion and directing the assessment. Examples of other information families can be asked to provide as part of the assessment process are included in Exhibit 20–1.

A part of the assessment process should include eliciting parental information needs. Potential areas of information needs in relation to growth and development include the potential effect of the child's condition on physical and emotional growth and development; how to provide for the child's emotional needs; discipline and appropriate behavior management strategies; how to plan for the child's future; what services the child may need; and where services can be accessed (Rawlins, Rawlins, & Horner, 1990).

Additionally important in the assessment process is to explore parental hopes and goals for the child (Ahmann & Bond, 1992). Questions such as the following can help determine intervention priorities:

- What are your goals for your child?
- Where do you hope to see your child developmentally a year from now?

Exhibit 20–1 Information Families Can Be Asked To Provide as Part of the Assessment

Observations regarding child's development
  overall development
  specific strengths
  problem areas (explicit observations)
    motor: gross and fine
    cognitive
    feeding/nutrition
    speech/communication
    social/emotional

Observations regarding developmental impact of child's condition
  environmental limitations
  tolerance for activity
  recovery postactivity

Suggestions for intervention plan
  specific activity ideas
  priorities
  desired outcomes
  extent of desire to participate in interventions
  scheduling suggestions
  equipment needs

Other family concerns
  information needs
  long-term concerns
  concerns regarding sibling effects

Preferred methods of information sharing

Source: Copyright © 1990, Elizabeth Ahmann.

Parental goals should direct the assessment process and play a central role in intervention planning.

DEVELOPMENTAL ASSESSMENT

Under ideal circumstances, developmental assessment is a multidisciplinary process. Nurses are often the initial point of contact and frequently serve as the primary case managers for technology-dependent preterm infants. Thus, in the early stages of identification, assessment, and coordination of care, the nurse's role is central. While specialized skills may be called for in many aspects of the assessment, the nurse who possesses a working knowledge of development in the infant and young child and understands the entire assessment process will be a more effective participant. Exhibit 20–2 lists essential aspects of the developmental assessment process.

Relevance of Medical Diagnosis and Health Status

Certain medical conditions will affect how a child should be handled; dictate the signs of stress that should be observed for during handling; and provide insight as to potential developmental conditions that might be expected. Areas of particular concern for the premature infant include respiratory, neurological, and nutritional/feeding status.

Respiratory Status

Information about the child's respiratory status is essential. This information is obtained from both the child's medical record and direct observation.

Exhibit 20–2 Essential Aspects of Developmental Assessment of the Preterm Infant

1. Assessment of family concerns, resources, and priorities
2. Consideration of the child's medical diagnosis, past and current health status, and nutritional status
3. Determination of the child's adjusted age
4. Consideration of
   a. tolerance for position and activity
   b. endurance
5. Assessment of the child's developmental level, both quantitative and qualitative; realms of development to assess include:
   a. cognitive
   b. fine motor
   c. gross motor
   d. communication
   e. adaptive
   f. psychosocial
6. Translation of the developmental assessment data into developmental plans and intervention strategies

Source: Adapted from *Pediatric Nursing,* Vol. 18, No. 3, p. 300, with permission of Jannetti Publications, Inc., Pitman, New Jersey, © 1992.

First, the current diagnosis can provide clues about possible effects of developmental intervention on the child. For example, the child with severe BPD will most likely be less tolerant of physical stimulation and motorically challenging positions than the child with mild BPD or no respiratory impairment. Second, the type of respiratory technology required (e.g., ventilation, oxygen, tracheostomy, suctioning) will indicate environmental limitations that may have an effect on the child's development through restrictions in positioning and mobility. Knowledge of the required technology will also indicate safety precautions that must be adhered to in the treatment process (Ahmann & Lipsi, 1991). Third, observation of the child's resting respiratory and heart rates and respiratory signs and symptoms at rest (nasal flaring, intercostal and/or suprasternal retractions, duskiness) will guide the intensity and duration of intervention planned. Finally, familiarity with the child's medication schedule is important so that both assessment and intervention sessions can be planned for times that the child's respiratory status will be most stable.

Neurological Status

A review of the child's neurological status should also be conducted before any direct handling of the child is attempted. Any neurological disorder or history of neurological complications may be associated with a developmental risk. Conditions of particular concern in infants born prematurely include seizure disorders, hydrocephalus with or without a shunt, and intraventricular hemorrhage (Davis, Tooley, & Hunt, 1987; Revell & Liptak, 1991).

Prior to handling the child with a seizure disorder, it is important to know the type(s) of seizures the child has had. These and any other seizure activity should be observed for during assessment and treatment sessions. (A guide for distinguishing seizure activity from jitteriness is included in Chapter 17.) As fatigue can sometimes precipitate seizures, care should be taken in regard to the intensity and duration of intervention sessions. In addition, intervention sessions should be postponed if the child is ill, has a fever, is otherwise stressed, or if medication dose(s) have recently been missed. Finally, safety precautions for children with seizures should be adhered to during all assessment and treatment sessions. (See Chapter 17.)

Intraventricular hemorrhage is a potential cause of hydrocephalus in early preterm infants (Mantovani & Powers, 1991). Hydrocephalus has a highly variable developmental impact, probably related to the degree of underlying brain injury (Ichord, 1986). Either medication or surgical placement of a shunt can be used to treat hydrocephalus. While it is difficult to damage a shunt, and a shunt will not become dislodged during normal daily activities, the prolonged use of the head-down position should be avoided as part of any intervention plan. (See Chapter 18.)

Nutrition and Feeding Status

Any developmental intervention will require energy expenditure by the infant or young child. At the same time, the infant or young child with respiratory compromise or other chronic illness may be at risk for inadequate caloric intake and poor nutritional status. (See Chapter 9.) For children who are at risk both nutritionally and developmentally, inefficient or excessive expenditure of energy during intervention sessions can compromise weight gain. Further, the inability to gain or maintain weight can signal an energy deficit that will adversely affect the child's ability to tolerate increased developmental stimulation. Prior to planning an intervention program, a nutrition and feeding assessment should be conducted. Data relevant to the intervention plan includes the following:

- child's growth pattern and current growth parameters (weight, length, weight for length, and head circumference)
- a feeding history (including the use of total parenteral nutrition, nasogastric, or gastrostomy tube feedings, and the age of introduction of oral feedings)
- any feeding problems, including behavioral concerns and any early oral-motor concerns.

Common feeding problems in premature and technology-dependent infants are reviewed in Chapter 9.

Other Medical Considerations

A wide variety of other medical conditions can affect the developmental assessment and intervention process for the infant and young child. For this reason, a complete medical history is an invaluable first step in the developmental assessment. Some particular conditions to note are the following:

- visual impairment or risk factors such as retinopathy of prematurity (ROP)
- auditory impairment or related risk factors
- presence of a tracheostomy, which may affect language development
- orthopedic impairment and any necessary adaptive equipment
- reflux vomiting.

(Chapters 21 through 23 address several of these related developmental concerns.)

Determination of Adjusted Age Level

The prematurely born infant who has suffered no serious brain injury will generally follow the same sequence of development as a term infant (Ichord, 1986). However, the degree of prematurity and complications secondary to prematurity can affect the rate of development. For this reason, developmental expectations for the preterm infant (born prior to 37 weeks gestation) are based on an adjusted age level as distinguished from the chronological age. The adjusted age level is calculated as follows:

> 40 weeks (term) minus the gestational age at birth (in weeks) yields the number of weeks of prematurity attributed to the infant. The number of weeks of prematurity is then subtracted from the infant's chronological age (weeks since birth) to determine the adjusted age level.

For example, an 11-month-old infant (44 weeks) born at 28 weeks gestation would have an adjusted age level of 32 weeks, or 8 months. The age level of the prematurely born infant or toddler is typically adjusted until 2 years of age. At this point, only very subtle developmental differences may exist between nonpremature infants and otherwise healthy premature infants. However, continued adjustment may be appropriate even beyond 2 years of age for the chronically ill preterm infant.

Consideration of Tolerance and Endurance

Consideration of both tolerance (for position and activity) and of endurance is necessary for developing an intervention plan that will not overly tax the medically fragile child, leading to adverse medical and developmental consequences. For this reason, close observation of the child's ability to tolerate different positions and activities is an important aspect of the assessment process. Observation of tolerance and endurance can occur in tandem with the assessment of the child's developmental level.

The factors that should be observed for an assessment of tolerance and endurance include the following (Als, 1982):

- autonomic responses, including respiratory status, color changes, and visceral signs
- motor responses, including posturing, tone, and movement
- state and organization responses, such as the ability to transition smoothly from one state to another
- attention-interaction responses, including the child's ability to come to an alert state and respond appropriately to presented stimuli.

These responses, or signs of stress, vary from child to child and should be interpreted individually. The presence of these signs at any time during the assessment or intervention process suggests that the developmental activity or its duration are stressful for the child. If the child appears stressed, an assessment can be completed over several sessions. As a related matter, both assessment and interventions should be planned for times that the child will be most rested and most stable medically. The time required for the child to return to baseline vital signs and comfort level after activity also gives clues about tolerance. Information on recovery after activity can be obtained both from observation and from parental report.

Assessment of Developmental Level

Assessment of the developmental level of the preterm infant involves both a quantitative and qualitative component.

Quantitative Analysis

The developmental level of an infant or young child is assessed by comparing the individual's skills to the normal sequence of skill development. The nurse should first closely observe the child's skills and abilities in play and daily activities. A complete observation will include noting skills in the following realms of development: cognition, fine motor, gross motor, communication, adaptive, and psychosocial.

As a second step in the assessment of developmental level, the nurse should compare the skills and abilities noted in the observation of the child to the normal sequence of development. The nurse who is well versed in developmental theory may find it easy to make this comparison. For nurses with less expertise, charts of developmental sequences can be carried as a reference. The purpose of comparing the child's skills to the sequence of normal development is twofold. First, the nurse can use this comparison to determine the child's "age-equivalent," or the age level at which the child is functioning. This will allow for developmental intervention plans that build on the child's existing skills in a sequential fashion. Of course, when determining the developmental age-equivalent for prematurely born infants and young children, the adjusted age level should be taken into account. That is, skill acquisition should be compared to what is typically expected for the adjusted age of the premature infant or young child.

A second reason for comparing observed skills to a set of norms is to assist the nurse in noting whether certain realms of development are delayed in comparison to others. For example, for a young child with a tracheostomy, the acquisition of expressive language skills may lag behind acquisition of skills in other developmental realms. When this is observed, further assessment as well as intervention can then be targeted to address the child's specific developmental needs.

Various assessment tools are available to assist the nurse in organizing and referencing developmental observations. One of the most efficient and commonly used is the Denver II (Frankenburg & Dodds, 1990). The Denver II is a screening tool that is easy to both administer and interpret. Fur-

thermore, its manual provides information that both assists in identification of children who would benefit from a more extensive evaluation and indicates which discipline(s) should be involved. The *Washington Guide to Promoting Development in the Young Child* (Powell, 1981), while not a screening tool, provides a framework for assessment and includes a listing of suggested activities to promote development. Castiglia and Petrini (1985) review other developmental assessment tools.

When assessment tools are used, several cautions apply (Ahmann & Lierman, 1992; Castiglia & Petrini, 1985):

- The chosen tool should be applicable to the specific assessment need.
- The nurse must be fully trained in the use of the tool to ensure proper use and meaningful interpretation of the findings.
- Screening tools cannot be considered diagnostic.

Qualitative Analysis

For the child who is technology-dependent, a qualitative analysis of developmental performance is essential. A qualitative analysis assesses the specific skills demonstrated by the child to determine *how* the child approaches and completes the presented task (Gorga, Stern, & Ross, 1985; Landry, Fletcher, Zarling, Chapieski, & Francis, 1984; Williamson, Wilson, Lifschitz, & Thurber, 1990). This analysis requires observing the child for the following (examples are provided in parentheses):

- attention to tasks (is it fleeting or extended?)
- approach to activities (do multiple items on a tabletop overwhelm the child?)
- problem-solving efforts (is trial and error used to complete a challenging task?)
- ability to adapt to new circumstances or challenging activities (does the child become easily frustrated?)
- responsiveness to activities that encourage expansion of existing skills

A qualitative analysis assists in distinguishing true deficits from delayed skill acquisition resulting from environmental factors, such as low energy and limitations posed by positioning or medical equipment. A qualitative analysis can also assist in appropriate developmental planning for children with complex conditions and care requirements.

Referrals

Referrals can be made to other professionals that may have valuable input in a multidisciplinary assessment of the developmental status of the technology-dependent infant and young child. These include specialty physicians (e.g., pulmonary neurology and physical medicine); physical therapists; occupational therapists; speech pathologists; audiologists; early interventionists; nutritionists; and, in some cases, child psychologists. (See Chapter 19 for referral criteria.)

FROM ASSESSMENT TO INTERVENTION: THE ROLE OF THE NURSE

The purpose of intervention is to promote normal development in the technology-dependent infant and young child. Toward this end, several factors are important in developing intervention plans. First, family members should be involved in the development and implementation of intervention plans. Second, specific therapeutic activities may be recommended to address deficits or delays noted by the parent, nurse, and/or other assessing professionals. These activities may be recommended by any of a variety of specialists. Third, while specific delays or deficits must certainly be addressed in planning intervention strategies, issues related to normal developmental needs should also be addressed in planning. (See Special Issue, "Normalization: A Guide For Parents.") Fourth, intervention plans should address ways to minimize potential adverse consequences of the required medical technology on the child's development. As a final point, advocacy and program development may be necessary to ensure that the developmental needs of technology-dependent children, both as individuals and as a group, can be adequately addressed.

Involving the Family

The importance of involving the family in early intervention efforts has been repeatedly demonstrated (Huber, Holditch-Davis, & Brandon, 1993; Infant Health and Development Program, 1990; Resnick et al., 1988; Shonkoff & Hauser-Cram, 1987). This involvement can occur in several ways.

First, and perhaps most critical, is for professionals to explain a child's developmental needs to parents in ways that have meaning in the parents' own cultural and socioeconomic framework (Huber et al., 1993). A sensitive, respectful parent–professional relationship can be the first step in helping parents hear and understand the benefits of early intervention for their child (Zeanah & McDonough, 1989). Also, many parents desperately want information about normal development in relation to their own child's medical problems and want to hear about what their child's strengths are and what is normal as well as what is delayed or abnormal (Diehl, Moffitt, & Wade, 1991).

Family goals and priorities for the intervention plan should receive the highest priority. They should be respected, even if they differ from some of the professionally designated goals (Ahmann & Bond, 1992). (Chapter 4 discusses the issue of parent–professional collaboration in detail.)

As part of the developmental intervention plan for the infant, professionals should model and teach intervention practices to parents, from neck flexion during bottle feeding and trunk rotation during diapering to gazing at and talking to the infant. It is also important to assist parents in identifying and responding to infant stress cues. These efforts can help parents learn effective techniques for interacting with their child. Intervention practices that are tied to normal daily activities, such as feeding and diapering, may be easiest for parents to incorporate into a demanding schedule of care.

Addressing Deficits and Delays

The nurse may have several roles in relation to addressing deficits or delays in development. For children who are medically fragile or technology dependent, nurses are often the most appropriate case managers. The nurse as case manager will arrange for multidisciplinary team meetings, to include family members if they desire, as the developmental assessment is translated into an intervention plan. The nurse can facilitate discussion, assist parents in participating in the planning process, and ensure that all activities and procedures are explained to family members. The nurse can help family members advocate for the child by ensuring that the plans for developmental stimulation are balanced appropriately with the child's need to achieve medical stability (Gorski, 1991). In this regard, the timing, intensity, and duration of treatment sessions are very important considerations in planning. The nurse can also assist family members by encouraging intervention activities that can be incorporated into daily routines with relative ease. Finally, as a member of a transdisciplinary team, the nurse may be trained in specific intervention techniques to apply and model when working with the child (Ahmann & Lierman, 1992). In fact, nurses are perhaps best situated to carry out initial intervention strategies in the transdisciplinary model, to ensure that the professional most experienced in monitoring the infant's medical condition can observe the effects of developmental activities early on. Ahmann and Lierman (1992) provide an example of this process.

Monitoring Tolerance for Activities

The child who is medically fragile may easily become overtaxed during activities, and the nurse should help others working with the child to recognize signs of stress. Prior to developmental intervention activities, the child's physiologic status should be observed. Attention should be given to respiratory rate and pattern, nasal flaring and retractions, skin color, and resting muscle tone and state (Ahmann & Lipsi, 1991). Assessing and interpreting autonomic, motoric, state, and attention-interaction responses (see Exhibit 20–3)

Exhibit 20–3 Stress Signals

Stress signals of an infant or young child will be individual and may include the following:
- chest retractions (intercostal and suprasternal)
- nasal flaring
- marked increase in respiratory rate
- difficulty returning to resting respiratory rate
- increased heart rate
- increased duskiness or mottling of skin color
- clammy appearance
- flailing of limbs
- change in muscle tone
- tremors
- hiccoughs
- defecation
- excessive crying
- persistent gaze aversion

Source: Reprinted with permission from Ahmann, E., and Lipsi, K.A. Early Intervention for Technology-Dependent Infants and Young Children. *Infants and Young Children*, Vol. 3, No. 4, pp. 67–77, Aspen Publishers, Inc. © 1991.

during treatment is important, as these are the ways an infant or young child will communicate stress (Als, 1982). Some stress may be acceptable during treatment if recovery to the pretreatment baseline is rapid, but the child should not be overtaxed. Parental feedback about the child's recovery period after intervention sessions will be helpful in gauging the effects of the activities (Ahmann & Lipsi, 1991).

Addressing Common Developmental Needs

The nurse also has an important role to play in ensuring that the developmental needs common to all infants and young children are given attention in planning. This concept is sometimes called *normalization*. (See also Special Issue, "Normalization: A Guide for Parents.") For example, among infants, the development of trust can be facilitated in several ways. Supporting parents in meeting the infant's needs and establishing regular routines is key. Limiting the number of professional caregivers interacting with the infant on a regular basis is also helpful: an important consideration for the nurse as case manager. Utilizing a transdisciplinary approach to treatment can be a way to limit the number of professional caregivers. As another example, among toddlers, attention should be paid to promoting the development of independence by facilitating mobility, encouraging competence in daily activities, and allowing participation in appropriate aspects of medical procedures (for example, holding the saline vial during suctioning). Table 20–1 provides examples of how common developmental needs can be addressed for the child dependent on medical technology.

Reducing Adverse Consequences of Technology

Additionally, the nurse should ensure that the intervention plan includes steps to reduce potential adverse consequences of technology dependence. Some examples of activities in this regard include the following:

- early use of an appropriate pacifier to provide oral-motor stimulation when oral feedings cannot be tolerated in a ventilated or tube-fed infant (see Chapter 9)
- the use of infant seats and blankets or sheets on the floor to provide positioning options for the ventilator-dependent infant (Ahmann & Lipsi, 1991; Anderson & Auster-Liebhaber, 1984)
- the use of portable apnea monitors, wheelchairs modified to carry a ventilator (Steele, 1986), and other similar equipment adaptations to allow the child to experience a variety of environments
- lengthy oxygen tubing or backpacking of nutrition solution to allow toddlers greater mobility (Smith, Danek, & Acree, 1990; Voyles, 1981).

Additional suggestions as well as case examples are provided elsewhere in the literature (e.g., Ahmann & Lipsi, 1991; D'Apolito, 1991; Liakopoulou, Patterson, Samaraweere, & Finnegan, 1983; Nugent, 1989; Vessey, Farley, & Risom, 1991). Of course, any activities should be attempted only if medically safe for the child. The child's tolerance for positions, activities and stimulation should be monitored carefully when any interventions are initiated.

EVALUATION

The nurse as case manager will want to ensure that the developmental intervention program for each infant or child is evaluated and updated on a regular basis. Evaluation meetings should include the family and members of the transdisciplinary team: nurse(s), physical and/or occupational therapist(s), and others. Team meetings are especially important to encourage cross-discipline sharing of both information and strategies that can best promote the child's health and development. Considerations for evaluation of the intervention program are listed in Exhibit 20–4.

Related to evaluation, a final important role of the nurse in promoting normal development of technology-dependent infants and young children is advocacy and program development. Nurses should first become aware of programs in their community that can provide developmentally related services to the high-risk preterm infant. Nurses can also be instrumental in raising awareness of the developmental needs of technology-dependent children in institutional and community settings. Part H of Public Law 99-457, The Education of the Handicapped Amendments of 1986 (since renamed the Individuals with Disabilities Education Act [IDEA]), provides for early intervention services for chil-

Table 20–1 An Overview of Developmental Issues in Pediatric High-Technology Home Care

Developmental stage[a]	Developmental issues	Interventions
Infant (0–1 years)	Sensory experience	• Encourage tactile and verbal interactions by caregivers. • Provide visual and auditory stimulation as tolerated.
	Motor experience	• Vary positioning to encourage freedom of movement.
	Development of trust	• Support parents in efforts to consistently meet infant's needs. • Encourage close relationship with one caregiver.
	Need to suck	• Encourage nonnutritive sucking if necessary and tolerated.
Toddler (1–3 years)	Freedom of mobility	• Arrange equipment to facilitate mobility (e.g., long oxygen tubing, backpacking of nutrition solution). • When mobility must be restricted, provide suitable alternate activities (e.g., reading a story, playing with blocks).
	Need to explore	• Provide safe environment (e.g., cover electric outlet, secure IV poles and pumps, cover knobs and dials on equipment).
	Oppositional behavior	• Allow as much control as possible (e.g., child can hold saline during suctioning). • Do not offer choice when there is none.
	Development of language	• Provide simple explanations. • Use repetition. • Assist tracheotomized or ventilator-dependent child with alternate expressive modality.
Preschool (4–6 years)	Vivid fantasy life	• Use dolls and stuffed animals to elicit child's understanding and to explain conditions and procedures. • Allow to play nurse or doctor on dolls using realistic but safe supplies. • Accept invisible playmates.
	Fears of contagion, intrusive procedures, castration	• Reassure with simple, honest explanations.
	Development of guilt and conscience	• Avoid bribing and threatening. • Praise as appropriate. • Provide acceptable outlet for anger and frustration (e.g., hitting a pillow, knocking down blocks). • Assure child that treatments are not a punishment.
	Mastery of new skills	• Encourage child to assist with treatments in simple ways (e.g., arranging supplies, opening packages). • Continue to facilitate mobility and exploration of environment (e.g., put ventilator on wheelchair so that child can go outside).
Schoolage (7–11 years)	Self-esteem concerns	• Provide opportunities for child to master tasks (e.g., learn to suction own trach tube, remove tape from IV site). • Encourage child to help with family chores.
	Understanding of rules	• Teach rules of safety relevant to equipment. • Train child in emergency procedures (e.g., clamping catheter).
	Need to succeed and enjoyment of competition	• Encourage use of board games, computer games, and puzzles when mobility must be restricted.
	Peer group becomes important	• Assist in reintegration into peer group (e.g., inservice teachers and students before return to school). • Assist in identifying supportive friends. • Discuss people's reactions with child. • Support child when teased and rejected. • When outside of home, ensure that child carries emergency supplies and identification, including telephone numbers of parents and pediatricians.
Adolescents (12–18 years)	Rationalization and intellectualization	• Approach discussions on an adult level. • Provide honest information as desired about condition, treatments, and prognosis.
	Vacillation between independence and dependence	• Allow adolescent to decide if parents should be present during appointments. • Involve adolescent in decision making regarding various aspects of care.

Table 20–1 continued

Developmental stage[a]	Developmental issues	Interventions
	Egocentrism and belief in own unlimited powers; rebellion	• Allow adolescent to participate in own care and provide necessary training. • Monitor self-care from afar. • Monitor self-care to ensure adolescent receives necessary treatments. • Explain need for therapies and equipment. • Accept rebellion in other realms.
	Peer acceptance important	• See suggestions for school age child. • Help adolescent focus on similarities with peers. • Help conceal differences when possible (e.g., hide tubing under clothing). • Introduce adolescent to others who are technology-dependent. • Become an ally to adolescent.
	Concern with body image, changes, and sexuality	• See suggestions regarding peer group acceptance. • Help adolescent focus on strengths and good qualities. • Obtain information about possible sexual limitations (e.g., in spinal cord injury). • Address questions honestly. • Provide support for developing identity.

[a]Children may have characteristics of more than one stage simultaneously, and ages are approximate.

Source: Copyright © 1990 Elizabeth Ahmann.

dren from birth to 3 years with disabilities. (See Special Issue, "Early Intervention Services for the High-risk Infant.") Nurses can help train early interventionists in working with children who are medically fragile and technology dependent.

CONCLUSION

Nurses have a key role to play in ensuring a complete and family-centered developmental assessment of the technology-dependent infant and young child. This should include a quantitative and qualitative assessment and may incorporate evaluations by other professionals as needed. As the assessment is translated into intervention plans, the nurse's role remains important and can include case management, parent education, intervention as part of a transdisciplinary team, advocacy for special needs of both the infant or child and the family, and even program development. In all phases of developmental assessment and planning, the nurse must remain attentive to balancing the child's needs for appropriate developmental stimulation and for medical stability. The nurse must also recognize and support the family's central role in the assessment and planning process.

Infants and young children who are medically fragile and technology-dependent present with multiple and complex needs. In the midst of addressing their complex medical and nursing needs, their developmental needs can easily be overlooked. Nurses can play an important role in ensuring that this does not happen.

Exhibit 20–4 Aspects of Evaluation of the Treatment Program

- statement of goals for the child and family
- statement of measurable short- and long-term objectives
- documentation of actual treatment strategies
- documentation of actual progress on goals and objectives
- identification of factors interfering with treatment
- identification of differences in goals of different parties
- identification of possible conflicts in aspects of treatment
- assessment of communication between providers and family
- revision of goals, objectives, treatment strategies, and communication plans
- documentation of revisions in treatment program

Source: Reprinted from Ahmann, E. and Lipsi, K.A. Early Intervention for Technology-Dependent Infants and Young Children, *Infants and Young Children,* Vol. 3, No. 4, pp. 67–77, Aspen Publishers, Inc., © 1991.

REFERENCES

Ahmann, E., & Bond, N.J. (1992). Promoting normal development in school-age children who are technology-dependent: A family-centered model. *Pediatric Nursing, 18*(4), 399–405.

Ahmann, E., & Lierman, C. (1992). Promoting normal development in technology dependent children: An introduction to the issues. *Pediatric Nursing, 18*(2), 143–148.

Ahmann, E., & Lipsi, K.A. (1991). Early intervention for technology-dependent infants and young children. *Infants and Young Children, 3*(4), 67–77.

Als, H. (1982). Towards a synactive theory of development: Promise for the assessment and support of infant individuality. *Infant Mental Health Journal, 3,* 229–243.

Als, H., Lawhorn, G., Duffy, F.H., McAnulty, G.B., Gibes-Grosman, R., & Blickman, J.G. (1994). Individualized developmental care for the very low-birth-weight preterm infant. *JAMA, 272*(11), 853–857.

Anderson, J., & Auster-Liebhaber, J. (1984). Developmental therapy in the neonatal intensive care unit. *Physical and Occupational Therapy in Pediatrics, 4,* 89–106.

Barrera, M.E., Rosenbaum, P.L., & Cunningham, C.E. (1986). Early home intervention with low birthweight infants and their parents. *Child Development, 57,* 20–33.

Castiglia, P., & Petrini, M.A. (1985). Selecting a developmental screening tool. *Pediatric Nursing, 11*(1), 8–17.

Cusson, R.M., & Lee, A.L. (1993). Parental interventions and the development of the preterm infant. *Journal of Obstetric, Gynecologic, and Neonatal Nursing, 23*(1), 60–68.

D'Apolito, K. (1991). What is an organized infant? *Neonatal Network, 10*(1), 23–28.

Davis, S.L., Tooley, W.H., & Hunt, J.V. (1987). Developmental outcome following posthemorrhagic hydrocephalus in preterm infants: Comparison of twins discordant for hydrocephalus. *American Journal of Diseases of Children, 141,* 1,170–1,174.

Diehl, S.F., Moffitt, K.A., & Wade, S.M. (1991). Focus group interview with parents of children with medically complex needs: An intimate look at their perceptions and feelings. *Children's Health Care, 20,* 170–178.

Frankenberg, W.K., & Dodds, J.B. (1990). *Denver II.* Denver, CO: Denver Developmental Materials Inc.

Gorga, D., Stern, F. M., & Ross, G. (1985). Trends in neuromotor behavior of preterm and fullterm infants in the first year of life: A preliminary report. *Developmental Medicine and Child Neurology, 27,* 756–766.

Gorski, P. (1991). Promoting infant development during neonatal hospitalization: Critiquing the state of the science. *Children's Health Care, 20*(4), 250–257.

Huber, C., Holditch-Davis, D., & Brandon, D. (1993). High-risk preterm infants at 3 years of age: Parental response to the presence of developmental problems. *Children's Health Care, 22*(2), 107–124.

Ichord, R. (1986). Developmental issues in care of the high risk infant. In E. Ahmann (Ed.), *Home care for the high risk infant: A holistic guide to using technology.* Rockville, MD: Aspen Publishers.

Infant Health and Development Program. (1990). Enhancing outcomes of low-birth-weight, premature infants: A multisite, randomized trial. *JAMA, 263,* 3,035–3,042.

Landry, S.H., Fletcher, J.M., Zarling, C.L., Chapieski, L., & Francis, D.J. (1984). Differential outcomes associated with early medical complications in premature infants. *Journal of Pediatric Psychology, 9*(3), 385–401.

Liakopoulou, M., Patterson, A., Samaraweere, S., & Finnegan, L. (1983). Developmental interventions in infancy during lengthy hospitalizations. *Developmental and Behavioral Pediatrics, 4*(3), 213–217.

Mantovani, J.F., & Powers, J. (1991). Brain injury in premature infants: Patterns on cranial ultrasound, their relationship to outcome, and the role of developmental intervention in the NICU. *Infants and Young Children, 4*(2), 20–32.

Nugent, K.E. (1989). Routine care: Promoting development in hospitalized infants. *MCN: The American Journal of Maternal/Child Nursing, 14,* 318–321.

Powell, M.L. (1981). Use of the Washington guide to promoting development in the young child. In M.L. Powell (Ed.), *Assessment and management of developmental changes and problems in children.* St. Louis, MO: Mosby.

Ramey, C.T., & Campbell, F.A. (1987). The Carolina abecedarian project. In J.J. Gallagher & C.T. Ramey (Eds.), *The malleability of children.* Baltimore, MD: Paul H. Brookes Publishing.

Rawlins, P.S., Rawlins, T.D., & Horner, M. (1990). Development of the family needs assessment tool. *Western Journal of Nursing Research, 12*(2), 201–214.

Resnick, M.B., Armstrong, S., & Carter, R.L. (1988). Developmental intervention program for high-risk premature infants: Effects on development and parent-child interaction. *Journal of Developmental and Behavioral Pediatrics, 9,* 73–78.

Revell, G.M., & Liptak, G.S. (1991). Understanding the child with special health care needs: A developmental perspective. *Journal of Pediatric Nursing, 6*(4), 258–268.

Shonkoff, J.P., & Hauser-Cram, P. (1987). Early intervention for disabled infants and their families: A qualitative analysis. *Pediatrics, 80,* 650–658.

Smith, D., Danek, G., & Acree, B. (1990). *Toddler backpacking of nutrition support solutions to facilitate normal development.* Poster presentation at the 25th Annual Conference of the Association for the Care of Children's Health, Washington, DC.

Steele, N.F. (1986). Wheelchair modifications for a ventilator. *Journal of Pediatric Nursing, 1,* 206–207.

Vessey, J.A., Farley, J.A., & Risom, L.R. (1991). Iatrogenic developmental effects of pediatric intensive care. *Pediatric Nursing, 17,* 229–232.

Voyles, J.B. (1981). Bronchopulmonary dysplasia. *American Journal of Nursing, 81,* 510–514.

Williamson, W.D., Wilson, G.S., Lifschitz, M.H., & Thurber, S.A. (1990). *Pediatrics* (Suppl.), 405–410.

Zeanah, C.H., & McDonough, S. (1989). Clinical approaches to families in early intervention. *Seminars in Perinatology, 13,* 513–522.

ADDITIONAL RESOURCES

Brandt, P.A., & Magyary, D.L. (1989). Preparation of clinical nurse specialists for family-centered early intervention. *Infants and Young Children, 1*(3), 51–62.

Bredekamp, S. *Developmentally appropriate practice in early childhood programs serving children from birth through age 8.* Washington, DC: National Association for the Education of Young Children.

Caputo, D. (1979). The development of prematurely born children through middle childhood. In T. Field (Ed.), *Infants born at risk.* New York, NY: SP Medical Books.

Davis, P.B., & May, J.E. (1991). Involving fathers in early intervention and family support programs: Issues and strategies. *Children's Health Care, 20*(2), 87–91.

Gottfried, A. (1986). *Playful: A guide to counseling parents on healthy infant development.* Evansville, IN: Mead Johnson & Co.

Hall, S.S., & Weatherly, K.S. (1989). Using sign language with tracheotomized infants and children. *Pediatric Nursing, 15,* 362–367.

Hanft, B. (1988). The changing environment of early intervention services: Implications for practice. *American Journal of Occupational Therapy, 42,* 724–731.

Hansen, S., Holaday, B., & Miles, B.S. (1990). *Journal of Pediatric Nursing, 5*(4), 246–251.

Hussey, B. (1988). *Understanding my signals: Help for parents of premature infants.* Palo Alto, CA: Vort Corp.

Kelly, J.F., & Barnard, K.E. (1988). Early intervention. In H.M. Wallace, G. Ryan, & A.C. Oglesby (Eds.), *Maternal and child health practices* (3rd ed.). Oakland, CA: Third Party Publishing.

Lerner, H., & Ross, L. (1991). Community health nurses and high risk infants: The current role of Public Law 99-457. *Infants and Young Children, 4*(1), 46–53.

Lipsi, K., Clements-Shafer, K., & Rushton, C.H. (1991). Developmental rounds: An intervention strategy for hospitalized infants. *Pediatric Nursing, 17*(5), 433–438+.

Long, T., Katz, K., & Pokorni, J. (1989). Developmental intervention with the chronically ill infant. *Infants and Young Children, 1*(4), 78–88.

MacPhee, M., & Mott, C. (1991). Teaching nurses about neuromotor development: An evaluative study. *Pediatric Nursing, 17*(5), 438–444.

National Information Center for Children and Youth with Disabilities. (1991). The education of children and youth with special needs: What do the laws say? *NICHCY News Digest, I*(1). Washington, DC.

Saylor, C.F., Elksnin, N., Farah, B.A., & Pope, J.A. (1990). Depends on who you ask: What maximizes participation of families in early intervention programs. *Journal of Pediatric Psychology, 15,* 557–569.

Sherman, L.P., & Rosen, C.D. (1990). Development of a preschool program for tracheostomy dependent children. *Pediatric Nursing, 16,* 357–361.

Chapter 21

Hearing Loss in the High-risk Infant

Revised by B. Patrick Cox, PhD, CCC-A

Hearing is integrally related to an infant's communication, speech and language, intellectual, and psychosocial development. This is especially true for infants raised in the majority aural-oral culture. Optimal development in all areas of infant development is dependent on early detection of hearing loss with concomitant appropriate intervention. Failure to identify an infant's hearing loss may lead to delayed expressive and receptive language, speech problems, psychosocial problems, and diminished academic achievement. Nurses in all settings play an important role in early detection of hearing loss and in helping parents with appropriate referrals for intervention.

This chapter has the following purposes:

- to introduce important terminology related to hearing loss
- to explore the current state of identifying infants with hearing loss (including electrophysiologic procedures and "high-risk" indicators)
- to discuss the complete audiologic evaluation
- to describe intervention techniques, with specific reference to related federal legislation.

Particular focus is given to the nurse's role in early identification and intervention with infants having hearing loss.

IMPORTANT AUDIOLOGIC TERMINOLOGY

The terms *deaf, hard of hearing,* and *hearing impaired* are sometimes used interchangeably. The terms may have both audiologic and cultural meanings. Although the nurse and other health care team members must remain sensitive to the ambiguity of these words and to the issue of labeling, especially on an individual level, the following definitions are provided for use here:

- *Deaf* refers to individuals whose hearing loss is sufficient to preclude their making meaningful use of everyday oral-auditory communication even with amplification and/or those who choose to be members of the Deaf culture regardless of the degree of hearing loss.

- *Hard of hearing* refers to individuals with mild to profound hearing loss who, with or without a hearing aid, are successful at using everyday oral-auditory communication and who choose not to be members of the Deaf culture.

- *Hearing impaired* is often used as an inclusive term for all persons with hearing loss. The word "impaired" is considered by some people to be offensive and pejorative. Use of this term in this text will be limited to quotations of other authors cited.

Types of Hearing Loss

Another important area of terminology relates to the type of hearing loss present. There are three types of hearing loss: (1) conductive, (2) sensorineural, and (3) mixed.

Conductive

Conductive hearing loss involves the outer (external) ear or the middle ear (the spaces beyond the tympanic membrane with the three tiny bones or ossicles), or both. It is characterized by a decrease in perceived loudness of sound that ranges in degree from mild to moderately severe. Causes of conductive hearing loss include wax accumulation, perforated tympanic membrane, middle ear infection (otitis media), otosclerosis, and more serious congenital conditions in which there is partial or total absence of one or more of the structures of the outer and/or middle ear. A number of syndromes (such as Treacher-Collins, Pierre Robin, and Apert syndromes) are also associated with conductive hearing loss (Northern & Downs, 1991).

Conductive disorders that cannot be remedied by medical or surgical intervention require vigorous nonmedical intervention, such as hearing aid amplification and aural habilitation (including auditory training and parent teaching and counseling). Infants with conductive hearing loss must be monitored frequently. Hearing loss may delay speech and language development and markedly affect the infant's ability to learn.

Sensorineural

Sensorineural hearing loss involves the inner ear (the delicate structures of the cochlea and the auditory nerve fibers leading to the brain). Sensorineural hearing loss occurs when the inner ear structures fail to develop, develop only partially, or are damaged after normal development. Sensorineural hearing loss often includes both a decrease in sound loudness (as is true for people with conductive hearing loss) and a diminution in the ability to understand speech. As a result, it cannot be assumed that two persons with the same pure-tone audiogram understand speech equally well. One might understand 100% of words spoken during the audiologic test, and another might understand 0% of words without visual cues. For this reason, the presence of a hearing aid should not lead the nurse to believe that the person understands everything that is said through audition alone.

The majority of infants with sensorineural hearing loss will not benefit from traditional medical or surgical intervention. An exception is the surgical procedure involved in the cochlear implant. While the cochlear implant is performed more often now than 10 years ago, the decision to implant an infant or child is complex. Issues include whether the infant or child would benefit more from traditional amplification, the medical risks involved in implantation, informed consent, and the value the family places on making all possible uses of audition.

Mixed

Mixed hearing loss involves components of sensorineural and conductive hearing loss. An example is an infant born with Waardenburg's syndrome who also has otitis media. Mixed hearing loss results from a problem in the outer or middle ear as well as the inner ear and may occur at all or some of the frequencies important for human communication.

Degree and Configuration of Hearing Loss

In addition to knowledge of an infant's type of hearing loss, the nurse or other health care provider needs to know about the *degree* and *configuration* of hearing loss present. Regardless of its cause or origin, hearing loss varies substantially in degree. The hearing loss may be *unilateral* (one ear affected) or *bilateral*. The *configuration* may be symmetrical, with equal loss over the entire range of hearing, or the loss may be more pronounced in a particular frequency range (e.g., high-frequency hearing loss).

Audiologists average the hearing loss at three frequencies (500 Hz, 1,000 Hz, and 2,000 Hz) on the pure-tone audiogram to derive the *pure-tone average (PTA)*. A person's PTA is then converted into a descriptive term for the degree of hearing loss. Table 21-1 shows the generally accepted terminology relating the PTA to the degree of hearing loss. Using this guide, one would say that a person with PTAs of 60 dB in the left ear and 100 dB in the right ear has a moderately severe loss in the left ear and a profound loss in the right ear.

IDENTIFICATION OF INFANTS WITH HEARING LOSS

The *NIH [National Institutes of Health] Consensus Statement: Early Identification of Hearing Impairment in Infants and Young Children* (National Institutes of Health, 1993b, p. 9) states, "Identification of hearing impairment must be seen as imperative for all infants and as an important adjunct to child health care. Since 20–30 percent of children who subsequently have hearing impairment will develop hearing loss during early childhood, an ever-vigilant pluralistic approach must be taken to hearing screening and identification of young children." Infants born prematurely may be at an

Table 21-1 Relationship between the Pure Tone Average (PTA) on the Audiogram and the Degree of Hearing Loss

PTA (in db)	Classification of hearing loss
−10–15	None
16–25	Slight
26–40	Mild
41–55	Moderate
56–70	Moderately severe
71–90	Severe
91–120+	Profound

increased risk of hearing loss. Risk factors include low birth weight, low Apgar scores, mechanical ventilation, and ototoxic medications, among others (Joint Committee, 1994). Early detection is dependent on cooperation among the infant's family; local, state, or national health care systems; and the health care professionals who have contact with the infant and family. Because the majority of children with acquired hearing impairments are initially identified by parents, nurses should encourage parents or caregivers to share immediately any concerns they may have about the infant's hearing and/or delay of early communication and developmental milestones.

Universal Screening

Universal hearing screening of all infants before 3 months of age is recommended in the 1993 *NIH Consensus Statement* (National Institutes of Health, 1993b) and the 1994 *Joint Committee on Infant Screening Position Statement.* However, identification audiometry policies and procedures vary from state to state, and nearly half the states have no official mandated or nonmandated newborn hearing screening program or policy (Blake & Hall, 1990). A comprehensive program for early detection of hearing loss includes hearing screening (identification audiometry), referral for complete audiologic evaluation of those infants who fail the hearing screening, referral for appropriate intervention services, systematic and periodic follow-up, and public education regarding hearing loss in infants and children.

High-risk Indicators

In locales where universal screening of infants has not been implemented, high-risk indicators associated with sensorineural and/or conductive hearing loss can be used as a first step in screening (Joint Committee, 1994). Exhibit 21–1 provides indicators for use with neonates. Exhibit 21–2 lists indicators for use with infants when certain health conditions develop that require rescreening. Exhibit 21–3 provides indicators for use with infants and toddlers (29 days–3 years) who require monitoring of hearing. This category includes those newborns who may pass initial hearing screening but require periodic monitoring at least every 6 months until age 3 years and at appropriate intervals after that age.

High-risk indicators have disadvantages if used as the sole method of screening. Disadvantages include the following:

- Fifty percent of newborns with congenital hearing losses are not found by the sole use of high-risk indicators and are missed.

- Children born in smaller hospitals may not be routinely identified.

Exhibit 21–1 Recommended Indicators for Neonates (Birth–28 Days)

1. Family history of hereditary childhood sensorineural hearing loss
2. In utero infection (i.e., cytomegalovirus, rubella, syphilis, herpes, and toxoplasmosis)
3. Craniofacial anomalies, including those with morphological abnormalities of the pinna and ear canal
4. Birth weight less than 1,500 grams (3.3 lbs)
5. Hyperbilirubinemia at serum level requiring exchange transfusion
6. Ototoxic medications, including but not limited to the aminoglycosides, used in multiple courses or in combination with loop diuretics
7. Bacterial meningitis
8. Apgar scores of 0–4 at 1 minute or 0–6 at 5 minutes
9. Mechanical ventilation lasting 5 days or longer
10. Stigmata or other findings associated with a syndrome known to include sensorineural and/or conductive hearing loss

Source: American Academy of Pediatrics Joint Committee on Infant Hearing Screening, Position Statement 1994.

Exhibit 21–2 Indicators for Use with Infants and Toddlers (Age 29 Days through 2 Years) when Certain Health Conditions Develop that Require Rescreening

1. Parent/caregiver concern regarding hearing, speech, language, and/or developmental delay
2. Bacterial meningitis and other infections associated with sensorineural hearing loss
3. Head trauma associated with loss of consciousness or skull fracture
4. Stigmata or other findings associated with a syndrome known to include a sensorineural and/or conductive hearing loss
5. Ototoxic medications, including but not limited to chemotherapeutic agents or aminoglycosides, used in multiple courses or in combination with loop diuretics
6. Recurrent or persistent otitis media with effusion for at least three months

Source: American Academy of Pediatrics Joint Committee on Infant Hearing Screening, Position Statement 1994.

- Follow-up is less than optimal in most programs currently in use, resulting in only a small proportion of cases being identified (National Institutes of Health, 1993a).

Optimally, universal screening should utilize electrophysiologic procedures as well as high-risk indicators.

Technological Considerations in Screening

Early efforts to detect newborn hearing loss were focused mainly on the use of parent questionnaires; high-risk crite-

Exhibit 21–3 Indicators for Use for Infants and Toddlers (29 Days–3 Years) Who Require Periodic Monitoring of Hearing

Indicators associated with delayed-onset sensorineural hearing loss include:
1. Family history of hereditary childhood hearing loss
2. In utero infection, such as cytomegalovirus, rubella, syphilis, herpes, or toxoplasmosis
3. Neurofibromatosis Type II and neurodegenerative disorders

Indicators associated with conductive hearing loss include:
1. Recurrent or persistent otitis media with effusion
2. Anatomic deformities and other disorders that affect eustachian tube function
3. Neurodegenerative disorders

Source: American Academy of Pediatrics Joint Committee on Infant Hearing Screening, Position Statement 1994.

ria; formal and informal observation; and portable, hand-held, limited-intensity screening instruments. These procedures relied heavily on behavioral observation of the infant and parent report. As an outgrowth of looking at an infant's physiologic responses to sound, clinicians and researchers sought procedures that would more objectively define the presence of a hearing loss.

A number of electrophysiologic procedures (e.g., procedures that involve measuring some aspect of infant physiology such as heart rate, breathing, brain activity, or change in body movement that is temporally related to a specified test stimulus) were developed. The two procedures used most extensively are auditory brainstem response audiometry (ABR) and otoacoustic emissions (OAE). Although the nurse may not be directly involved in ABR or OAE protocols, a basic understanding of the two procedures will facilitate explaining the procedures to parents.

ABR

The ABR procedure has been recommended for use in newborn hearing screening for 15 years (Schulman-Galambos et al., 1979). ABR is a procedure designed to look at the infant's response to sound using ongoing brain-wave activity similar to an electroencephalogram (EEG). The audiologist is particularly interested in the following: the appearance of soundwaves in the first 10 msec after a sound is presented, the morphology of the wave, the time each wave appears, and its relationship to other waves. The audiologist looks for responses to sound at various intensity levels down to a minimum level of 30 dB HL (hearing level).

OAE

The OAE procedure is newer in its potential use for hearing screening. Despite this, the OAE procedure was selected by the 1993 NIH Consensus Development Conference as

the procedure of choice in newborn hearing screening (National Institutes of Health, 1993a). (ABR was recommended as a follow-up for any infant who failed the OAE.) The OAE procedure is based on our knowledge that some of the sound that reaches the cochlea is "reflected" back from the cochlea into the middle ear. By placing a noninvasive probe tube microphone into the external ear canal, the audiologist can measure patterns of "reflected" sound at intensities as low as 30 dB HL. The OAE procedure is assumed to be sensitive, specific, and cost-effective.

NURSES' ROLE IN EARLY IDENTIFICATION AND REFERRAL

Nurses are in a particularly advantageous position to conduct hearing screenings and identify infants at risk of hearing loss. Until universal hearing screening of all newborns is a reality, the neonatal intensive care nurse is critical in assessing high-risk factors and helping the family obtain an appropriate referral to a certified audiologist. Additionally, the nurse practitioner who takes a developmental history and has the opportunity to observe the infant carefully in the home or office, the nurse in a pediatrics practice who sees infants on a routine basis for well-baby visits, the community health nurse, and the home care nurse—all play pivotal roles in both identification (by obtaining a detailed history and conducting an informal auditory behavioral screening) and in referral.

History

A complete history should address the risk factors enumerated in Exhibits 21–1, 21–2, and 21–3. If the family does not have all of the necessary information, hospital and physicians' records can be obtained and reviewed. History taking should also address any parental or caregiver concerns and include careful questioning regarding their observations. A list of age-appropriate questions to elicit parent/caregiver observations about the infant's hearing and developmental/communication milestones is provided in Appendix 21–A. (For nurses who already use another questionnaire for development and communication, it is suggested that the "Hearing" items for each age category from Appendix 21–A be incorporated into that questionnaire.)

The nurse should be alert to the fact that to many parents/caregivers, infant vocalizations are a sign of normal hearing. In fact, however, infants with the most profound hearing loss often engage in automatic, reflexive babbling. In many cases, it is not until later, when babbling fails to lead to speech, that parents become concerned. Thus, neither the fact that an infant is vocalizing nor the lack of parental concern about hearing loss rule out hearing loss in an at-risk infant.

Informal Screening

After a complete history has been taken, the nurse's assessment continues with an informal auditory behavioral screening of the infant. Casual observation of the infant's apparent responses to sound, however, may be misleading to the parents/caregivers as well as to the nurse. At birth and in the early months of life, infants attend best to sounds that contain multiple frequencies, such as speech, noisemakers, and environmental sounds. On the basis of reactions to these sounds alone, it is impossible to state unequivocally that the infant hears at all the frequencies important for human communication. For example, an infant may have hearing only in the lower frequency range yet may still appear to startle to a hand clap, especially if it is near the ear.

To conduct an informal observation of an infant's response to sounds, the nurse can optimize the observation by attending to the following:

1. Observe the infant in his or her bassinet or while seated on the parent's lap.
2. Observe the infant's behavior prior to presentation of sound. It is best to observe when the infant is reasonably quiet, has just fallen asleep, or is between feedings.
3. Present interesting and familiar sounds (noisemakers, animal sounds, soft whisper, everyday conversational level speech) out of the infant's visual field, about 6 inches from the infant's ear.
4. Change the sounds frequently so that the infant does not adapt to the sound. Be careful not to present sounds in a rhythmical pattern.
5. For infants old enough to be seated on the parent's lap and who are visually alert, use a screening assistant to provide a quiet visual distraction (i.e., toy) to keep the infant facing forward between responses.
6. Make observations in a quiet room that is free of visual distractions.
7. Make repeated observations to estimate the reliability of responses.
8. Make sure that the airflow from a squeeze toy does not reach the infant. Take care not to touch the infant's ear immediately before or during the presentation of a sound.

Auditory Developmental Guidelines

Finally, observation of an infant's responses to sounds will be more meaningful if the nurse uses recognized auditory developmental guidelines. In this way, the nurse can ascertain if the child is responding in an age-appropriate manner. Table 21–2 summarizes the maturation of an infant's orientation behavior. An infant who is developing

Table 21–2 Development of Infant's Orienting Responses to Noisemakers

Age (months)	Responses
0 to 4 months	Eye widening, eye blink (in a very quiet environment), or arousal from sleep as in newborn testing. Startle response to loud speech.
4 to 7 months	By 4 months, a "rudimentary" head turn is seen: a "wobble" of the head even slightly toward the sound.
	This response gradually matures until at 6 months the head turn is definite, toward the side of the sound, but only on a plane level with the eyes. He does not fixate the sound source in the lower level where it comes from.
	By 7 months there is an inclination to find the sound source on the lower level; the child will look first to the side and then down. He may even be mature enough to find the source directly.
7 to 9 months	At the beginning of this period he should soon find the sound source on the lower level directly, but if the sound is presented on a level above his head, he will only look toward the side. At the end of this period he may begin to look toward the side and then up, to fixate the higher sound source.
9 to 13 months	At 9 months, the beginning indirect localization of the higher level will be seen which soon turns to direct localization. We thus see shortly after 1 year of age a direct localization of sounds in any plane.
13 to 24 months	The same type of orientation prevails for the older child as was seen for the 13-month-old. In other words, the full maturation of the auditory behavior of the child occurs at about 13 months and does not change significantly after that.

Source: Excerpted from *Hearing in Children*, 4th ed., by J.L. Northern and M.P. Downs, pp. 253–254, with permission of Williams & Wilkins, © 1991.

normally will orient to sound by a rudimentary head turn at age 4 months. An infant of 8 months should quickly find the sound source at an angle below the ear and begin to find it when presented on a level above the ear.

Specialized Screening Instruments

In today's health care practice, nurses may have specialized screening equipment available to assess hearing. One such instrument is a portable, hand-held hearing screening tool designed to provide a limited number of frequencies (i.e., 500 Hz, 1,000 Hz, 2,000 Hz, and 4,000 Hz) and intensities (i.e., 40 dB HL and 25 dB HL screening levels) important to human hearing. The nurse presents the tone through the portable headphone and observes the infant's responses.

Because the presence of a middle-ear infection can affect the results of hearing screening, a portable, hand-held instrument referred to as a tympanometer can be used to augment the nurse's examination. Screening tympanometers allow the nurse to seal the infant's ear canal quickly with an inflatable probe tip and chart the mobility of the middle ear. The tympanogram will show the presence of abnormal middle-ear conditions, such as otitis media, a poorly functioning eustachian tube, or problems with the tympanic membrane or ossicles. Such problems clearly affect the infant's health and may themselves contribute to delayed development of speech and language.

Referrals

Regardless of the nurse's observation of infant responses, every infant with a high-risk indicator, parent/caregiver concern, or an abnormal tympanogram should be referred to a certified audiologist and board-certified otologist. When referrals are made, the nurse should continue to be the advocate for the infant and to encourage the family to follow through with the recommendations for medical evaluation. If intervention is warranted, the nurse can also facilitate its implementation.

AUDIOLOGIC AND MEDICAL EVALUATION

When an infant is referred by the nurse for suspected hearing loss, the infant should receive a complete audiologic and medical evaluation.

Audiologic Examination

The audiologic evaluation includes a complete history, which amplifies the nurse's history in the areas of particular concern to the pediatric audiologist. The infant is observed by the audiologist to determine overall responsivity to sound and the degree to which developmental milestones are being achieved.

The infant is then given a complete diagnostic hearing evaluation. Unlike screening audiometry conducted by a nurse or audiologist, the complete evaluation is designed to provide information regarding the degree and type of hearing loss. In a sound-controlled environment with more precise methods, the audiologist can obtain exact threshold values for hearing. Procedures include pure tone and speech audio-

metry, special tests such as immittance (designed to provide information regarding middle-ear status and the presence or absence of the acoustic reflex), and the ABR or OAE.

The pediatric audiologist must choose a particular methodology in order to obtain this information. In addition to the ABR and OAE (which rely on the objective measurement of changes in EEG activity or the sound energy reflected back from the cochlea, respectively), the audiologist selects one of several behavioral methodologies. (See Exhibit 21–4.) The selection is dependent on a number of factors, including chronological and developmental age, motor abilities, and general attention level of the infant.

Following the completion of these formal and informal tests, the audiologist reviews the results of the evaluation with the parents and other family members. It is desirable to have the parents present during the evaluation. Their observations and feelings about how the infant responds are critical to the audiologist, providing information about how typical that day's results are in their minds. It also allows the pediatric audiologist to learn more about the individual family members and how they interact. In addition, this time together provides a solid basis for future counseling.

Medical Evaluation

Any infant found to have a hearing loss must be referred for a complete medical evaluation. This includes a review of

Exhibit 21–4 Behavioral Audiology Methods for the Infant and Young Child

---

Behavior Observation Audiometry (BOA)
BOA is similar to the informal screening described earlier, but uses more carefully specified signals in a sound-treated room and is conducted by an audiologist or team of audiologists. Method is used from birth until the child is able to perform one of the methods listed below.

Animated Visually Reinforced Audiometry (AVRA)
Child is rewarded with a lighted, animated toy when he or she responds to sound. Method has been demonstrated to be reliable as young as 4 months of age; it is often used for older children when hearing loss or a developmental disability precludes using conditioned play audiometry.

Conditioned Play Audiometry (CPA)
Child is taught to perform a motor act (e.g., to put a peg in a pegboard) when sound is heard. This method is used successfully with children as young as 18 months of age.

Tangible Reinforced Operant Conditioned Audiometry (TROCA)
Child is taught to push a button when he or she hears the sound and is rewarded with an edible or nonedible reinforcer. This method is particularly helpful with children above 2 years of age and children with low verbal skills or developmental delay.

the audiologic, developmental, and medical histories, as well as a thorough physical examination of the ears, head, and neck to identify any observable abnormalities. Also, the otologist, or otolaryngologist, must evaluate the infant's susceptibility for otitis media. Otitis media is a health problem in its own right, and, of equal importance, chronic otitis media has serious effects on speech and language development. Otitis media combined with permanent hearing loss places the infant in double jeopardy.

The otologist may also order laboratory tests that help to detect the cause of the hearing loss and that determine both its progression and the prognosis. The otologist also certifies that the infant with a hearing loss has no physical problems that preclude the use of a hearing aid if this is indicated.

Other Specialists

The otologist, nurse, and audiologist must also make referrals to other medical and nonmedical specialists. Current practice dictates that all infants identified as having a permanent hearing loss be referred to a clinical geneticist (or genetic team) with particular expertise in the genetic factors associated with hearing loss. Referral provides the family with valuable information about the infant possibly having a syndrome associated with progressive hearing loss or other developmental issues. Also, the geneticist will explore the possibility of a familial genetic component. (See Chapter 24 for an indepth discussion of genetic issues.) Families vary in their decision making as to whether the birth of one child with hearing loss precludes having additional children. However, hearing health care practitioners have an ethical and legal obligation to provide information to families about the possibility of hearing loss in subsequent children. Occupational and physical therapy and speech-language pathology are other possible referrals.

INTERVENTION

The intervention plan developed for an infant with hearing loss must be individualized to his or her needs and those of the family. Such intervention is facilitated by important federal legislation enacted since the mid-1970s.

Federal Legislation

In 1975, Public Law (P.L.) 94-142 (known as the Education for All Handicapped Children Act) introduced landmark equal education rights for all handicapped children. In 1985, P.L. 99-457 (known as the Education of the Handicapped Act Amendments) was enacted. This law reauthorized the earlier Education of the Handicapped Act. More specifically, the law recognized the importance of infant and preschool education and the unique role of families in developmental care of children with disabilities. (See also Special Issue, "Early Intervention Services for the High-risk Infant.")

According to Sass-Lehrer and Bodner-Johnson (1989), the enactment of 99-457 ". . . provides a challenge to the field of education of the deaf and to early childhood educators to re-examine basic assumptions about the range of services, the professionals providing those services, and the role of families who have children with hearing (loss)" (p. 74). Audiology is one of the services addressed in P.L. 99-457. The provision of intervention services by the audiologist, nurse, and other members of the team allows the opportunity for rich interaction between the practitioners. This results in the delivery of the best available hearing intervention services.

Collaboration

An example of the need for collaboration relates to the selection and use of hearing aids by the infant with hearing loss. Hearing aids are often difficult to keep on an infant and need constant monitoring to ensure that they are fully functioning. Parents are sometimes reluctant to put hearing aids on an infant as this is visible evidence of hearing loss.

The audiologist may share applied hearing aid use tips with the family and the nurse. If the nurse is the case manager, it is likely that he or she will have more frequent contact with the infant/family than the audiologist and can thereby monitor hearing aid functioning and use. Nurses also can provide support to the parents in relation to their feelings about hearing aid use. By keeping in close contact with the audiologist, the nurse can alert the audiologist to any problems that may develop with the hearing aids or changes in the responsivity of the infant.

The audiologist and nurse also may collaborate on the infant's ongoing otologic status. As noted before, it is crucial that the infant with hearing loss have frequent middle-ear checks. This is especially true if the infant has had a history of otitis media in the first year of life. If the community health or home care nurse has screening tympanometry, she or he can provide screening checks at home as often as necessary. Also, the nurse can be extremely helpful in noting the need for new hearing aid earmolds (the custom-made device that couples the hearing aid to the infant's external ear canal). As the infant's ear canal size changes dramatically during the first 2 years of life, new earmolds are often needed every 6 to 8 weeks. The nurse can note acoustic feedback from the hearing aid and make certain that the audiologist sees the infant immediately for a new earmold.

Home Programs

Home stimulation or early intervention programs also are an important component of care for the infant with hearing loss. Such programs are often directed by trained educators of the deaf/hard of hearing, pediatric audiologists, or speech-language pathologists. The programs are reinforced by stimulation programs conducted by nurses or child development specialists.

Home-based parent–infant programs teach parents how to optimize communication with the infant. Parent education and counseling are needed for topics like getting the infant's attention, making good use of visual cues, providing continuing use of the hearing aid, and understanding the nature of communication when one person in the family has a hearing loss.

Parents may need support in relation to both speech and language development and the effect of hearing loss on speech and language. They need to be encouraged to continue to communicate with the infant regardless of the degree of hearing loss. It is important for parents, even those with other children, to understand the nature of language, specifically, that receptive input of language occurs in all infants many months before expressive language is intelligible.

Intervention Goals

The specific goals of intervention will vary from infant to infant and depend on many factors including but not restricted to the following: the degree of hearing loss, the family's goals for the infant, the team's recommendations, the availability of parent–infant and preschool programs, the health of the infant, and the presence of other developmental challenges. In all of the goals set by the multidisciplinary team, the nurse plays a vital role in many ways, including team facilitator, home-visit coordinator, direct service provider, health care advocate, and family advocate.

REFERENCES

Blake, P.E., & Hall, J.W. (1990). The status of statewide policies for neonatal hearing screening. *Journal of the American Audiologic Association, 1,*(2) 67–74.

Joint Committee on Infant Hearing. (1994). Joint Committee on Infant Hearing 1994 Position Statement. *Audiology Today, 6*(6), 6–9.

National Institutes of Health. (1993a). *NIH consensus development conference: Early identification of hearing impairment in infants and young children (program and abstracts),* Bethesda, MD: Author.

National Institutes of Health. (1993b). *NIH Consensus Statement: Early identification of hearing impairment in infants and young children* (11 [1]). Bethesda, MD: Author.

Northern, J., & Downs, M. (1991). *Hearing in children.* Baltimore, MD: Williams & Wilkins.

Sass-Lehrer, M., & Bodner-Johnson, B. (1989). Public law 99-457: A new challenge to early intervention. *American Annals of the Deaf, 134*(2) 71–77.

Schulman-Galambos, C., and Galambos, R. (1979). Brainstem evoked response audiometry in newborn hearing screening. *Archives of Otolaryngology, 105,* 86–90.

ADDITIONAL RESOURCES

American Speech-Language-Hearing Association. (1991). Guidelines for the audiologic assessment of children from birth through 36 months of age. *Asha, 33*(Suppl. 5), 37–43.

Bess, F., & Hall, J. III (Eds.). (1992). *Screening children for auditory function.* Nashville, TN: Bill Wilkerson Center Press.

(1989). Early intervention program for infants and toddlers with handicaps: Final regulations. *Federal Register, 54,* 26,306–26,348.

Kramer, S., & Williams, D. (1993). The hearing-impaired infant and toddler: Identification, assessment and intervention. *Infants and Young Children, 6,* 35–49.

Ling, D. (1989). *Foundations of spoken language for hearing-impaired children.* Washington, DC: Alexander Graham Bell Association for the Deaf.

Martin, F. (1994). *Introduction to audiology.* Englewood Cliffs, NJ: Prentice-Hall.

Mauk, G.W., White, K.R., Mortensen, L.B., & Behrens, T.R. (1991). The effectiveness of screening programs based on high-risk characteristics in early identification of hearing impairment. *Ear and Hearing, 12,* 312–319.

Simmon-Martin, A., & Rossi, K. (1990). *Parents and teachers: Partners in language development.* Washington, DC: Alexander Graham Bell Association for the Deaf.

Turner, R. (1990). Analysis of recommended guidelines for infant hearing screening. *Asha, 32,* 57–61.

Turner, R. (1992). Comparison of four hearing screening protocols. *Journal of the American Academy of Audiology, 3,* 200–207.

Watkins, S., & Clark, T. (1993). *The SKI-HI model: A resource manual for family centered, home-based programming for infants, toddlers, and preschool-aged children with hearing impairment.* Logan, UT: HOPE, Inc.

Questions To Ask Parents about the Infant's Hearing

2 MONTHS		
Hearing		
1. Have you had any worry about your child's hearing?	Yes	No
2. When he's sleeping in a quiet room, does he move and begin to wake up when there's a loud sound?	Yes	No
Developmental and Communication		
3 Does he lift up his head when he's lying on his stomach?	Yes	No
4. Does he smile at you when you smile at him?	Yes	No
5. Does he move both hands together in the same way?	Yes	No
6. Does he look at your face without your making gestures to him?	Yes	No
4 MONTHS		
Hearing		
1. Have you had any worry about your child's hearing?	Yes	No
2. When he's sleeping in a quiet room, does he move and begin to wake up when there's a loud sound?	Yes	No
3. Does he try to turn his head toward an interesting sound or when his name is called?	Yes	No
Developmental and Communication		
4. Does he lift his head up to 90° and look straight ahead?	Yes	No
5. Does he touch his hands together and play with them?	Yes	No
6. Does he laugh and giggle without being tickled or touched?	Yes	No
7. Does he coo to himself and make noises when he's alone?	Yes	No
6 MONTHS		
Hearing		
1. Have you had any worry about your child's hearing?	Yes	No
2. When he's sleeping in a quiet room, does he move and begin to wake up when there's a loud sound?	Yes	No
3. Does he turn his head toward an interesting sound or when his name is called?	Yes	No
Developmental and Communication		
4. Does he lift up his head and chest with his arms?	Yes	No
5. Does he keep his head steady when sitting?	Yes	No
6. Does he roll over in his crib?	Yes	No

7. Does he reach for objects within his reach and hold them?	Yes	No
8. Does he see small objects like peas or raisins?	Yes	No

8 MONTHS

Hearing

1. Have you had any worry about your child's hearing?	Yes	No
2. When he's sleeping in a quiet room, does he move and begin to wake up when there's a loud sound?	Yes	No
3. Does he turn his head directly toward an interesting sound or when his name is called?	Yes	No
4. Does he enjoy ringing a bell or shaking a rattle?	Yes	No

Developmental and Communication

5. Does he support most of his weight on his legs?	Yes	No
6. Can he sit alone unaided for 5 minutes?	Yes	No
7. Can he sit and look for objects that have fallen out of sight?	Yes	No
8. Can he pick up two objects, one in each hand?	Yes	No
9. Can he transfer an object from one hand to the other?	Yes	No
10. Can he feed himself a cracker?	Yes	No
11. Does he make a number of different sounds and change their pitch?	Yes	No
12. Does he clap his hands in imitation and make noises at the same time?	Yes	No

10 MONTHS

Hearing

1. Have you had any worry about your child's hearing?	Yes	No
2. When he's sleeping in a quiet room, does he move and begin to wake up when there's a loud sound?	Yes	No
3. Does he turn his head directly toward an interesting sound or when his name is called?	Yes	No
4. Does he try to imitate you if you make his own sounds?	Yes	No

Developmental and Communication

5. Does he play peekaboo with you?	Yes	No
6. Can he stand for at least 5 seconds, holding onto a crib or chair?	Yes	No
7. Does he try to hold a toy when it's pulled away?	Yes	No
8. Is he shy or afraid of strangers?	Yes	No
9. Can he pull himself to standing position alone?	Yes	No

12 MONTHS

Hearing

1. Have you had any worry about your child's hearing?	Yes	No
2. When he's sleeping in a quiet room, does he move and begin to wake up when there's a loud sound?	Yes	No
3. Does he turn his head directly toward an interesting sound or when his name is called?	Yes	No
4. Is he beginning to repeat some of the sounds that you make?	Yes	No

Developmental and Communication

5. Can he pick up a raisin or a pea?	Yes	No
6. Can he get to a sitting position without help?	Yes	No
7. Does he wave bye-bye or pat-a-cake when you tell him to?	Yes	No
8. Can he say "mamma" or "dadda?"	Yes	No

Source: Reprinted from *Hearing in Children,* 4th ed., by J.L. Northern and M.P. Downs, pp. 256–257, with permission of Williams & Wilkins Company, © 1991.

Chapter 22

Speech and Language Development in the Chronically Ill Preterm Infant

Revised by Deirdre F. Jackson, MSN, CCRN, CPN

The ability to communicate is important in the young child's establishment of social relationships, development of self-image, and formation of skills essential to future academic success. Therefore, careful screening and timely intervention are important in the prevention of long-term communication impairment in the high-risk infant.

This chapter introduces the community health or home care nurse to the following pertinent issues:

- the communication process and its development
- factors contributing to speech and language problems in the high-risk infant
- identification of specific problems and guidelines for referral to a speech-language pathologist or otolaryngologist
- special issues for tracheotomized and ventilator-dependent children
- recommendations for language stimulation
- alternative and augmentative communication systems.

COMMUNICATION DEVELOPMENT

Communication development is dependent on multiple factors. For example, normal anatomy and function of structures in the mouth and nasal cavity are needed for articulation and resonance. Adequate function of the respiratory system is required to provide breath support for speech. Normal hearing is necessary to synthesize auditory input. Certain cognitive skills (e.g., object permanence, understanding of cause and effect relationships, imitation, intention, anticipation, and representation), are essential precursors to the development of verbal or gestural communication. These concepts are generally acquired during the first year of life (Ryan, 1988). Communication development is also a social phenomenon.

Communication development begins immediately after birth and continues as the child synthesizes information received through environmental interactions. Each child develops speech and language skills at his or her own individual pace. Nonetheless, each child is expected to achieve certain communication milestones by specific ages. (See Table 22–1.)

Communication development can be analyzed in terms of two systems: (1) reception and (2) expression. A child may develop normal receptive skills but demonstrate a specific expressive speech disorder. Conversely, a child with an auditory deficit may have normal speech potential that cannot develop until receptive skills begin to emerge.

Reception

Reception involves the ability to comprehend the language and symbols of one's environment. Receptive functioning develops as a child begins to respond to auditory stimuli in the environment. (See Chapter 21, Hearing Loss in the High-risk Infant.) During the first few months of life,

Table 22–1 Selected Language Milestones, 0 to 24 Months

Months[a]	Language skills[b]
0–3	Cries become differentiated
	Turns to sound
	Coos, chuckles
4–6	Babbles, squeals
	Laughs aloud
	Recognizes familiar voice
	One-syllable imitative utterances
7–9	Imitates speech sounds
	Responds to inflection in caregiver's command
10–12	First word (e.g., dada, mama)
	Uses jargon
	Recognizes some objects by name
	Imitates some animal sounds
13–15	Vocabulary of 3–5 words
	Responds to simple commands
18–24	Rapid increase in vocabulary from 10–300 words
	Forms 2–3-word phrases
	Uses "I," "me," and "you"
	Articulation lags behind vocabulary

[a] Age corrected for prematurity.
[b] There is a range of *normal* in development.

Source: Adapted with permission of Mosby-Year Book from Marino, B.L., Rogers, J.E., and Aruda, M.M., Assessing Development, in *Comprehensive Child and Family Nursing Skills*, D.P. Smith, ed., © 1991, pp 131–136, and from Essentials of Pediatric Nursing, 3rd ed., by L.F. Whaley and D.L. Wong, © 1989.

an infant refines this ability to respond to relevant auditory stimuli and learns to block out what is not needed. With continued maturation of auditory skills, a child begins to symbolize, and the ability to comprehend language develops. By 12 to 15 months of age, toddlers recognize familiar environmental elements and respond to simple directions.

Expression

Expression involves any form of communicating needs or ideas, whether verbally or nonverbally. The infant's first cry begins expressive communication with the environment. Parents learn to differentiate the reasons for their infant's cries—hunger, discomfort, or boredom (Whaley & Wong, 1991). Cooing is followed by the emergence of babbling at 4 months of age. Babbling can persist until the child is 12 months of age, then it gradually becomes interspersed with meaningful words. The next stage of prespeech communication is labeled *jargon*. Jargon can be defined as meaningless, unintelligible sound sequences. This early form of purposeful communication has been described by parents as sounding like a foreign language. It occurs simultaneously with the development of meaningful words and can continue

throughout the child's 2nd year of life. By 18 months of age, echolalia is seen. *Echolalia* is the imitative production of words, phrases, or sentences. It can be present with or without comprehension of the utterances. By the age of 3 years, echolalia decreases, and the young child's communication consists of simple sentences. The 3-year-old child is generally intelligible to the family and usually is understood by peers.

By the 3rd year of life, it is important to differentiate between speech and language. Speech involves the oral-motor coordination of the jaw, tongue, lips, and palate, with respiration and phonation. A child's speech development is analyzed in terms of the ability to be understood and the specific ability to produce phonologic sequences (consonant and vowel combinations). Language involves word order and the ability to combine meaningful words into comprehensible sentences. A child's language development is judged in terms of vocabulary, syntax (grammatical structures), word order, and sentence length. Language development is also described in terms of pragmatic skills or the appropriateness of language use.

REASONS FOR SPEECH AND LANGUAGE DELAY

Any child who has had a difficult neonatal course may be at risk for speech or language difficulties. Medical problems such as neurologic insults or respiratory disorders predispose high-risk infants to inactivity. They may also have feeding disorders or oral defensiveness. (See Chapter 9, Nutrition and Feeding of the Chronically Ill Infant.) Additionally, severely ill infants are often not positioned prone. These circumstances predispose the infant to poor development of muscles used in respiration and speech.

Many high-risk infants are hospitalized repeatedly or for an extended time. Hospitalized infants usually have inconsistent caregivers and limited opportunity for appropriate exploration of their environments. Many intensive care units have high ambient noise levels and excessive visual stimulation that create an artificial and unfavorable developmental milieu. Difficulties in learning to attend to relevant auditory and visual stimuli may develop if the young child cannot learn to differentiate important from unimportant stimuli. Some infants respond by overreacting to the excessive environmental stimulation, whereas others become unresponsive and listless.

The high-risk infant may also be at risk for becoming a passive communicator (Simon, Fowler, & Handler, 1983). Chronically ill infants often require extensive attention from medical and nursing personnel or parents. They may express themselves only when asked questions. Communicative passivity arises not only because of the young child's inability to communicate but also because of inexperience and the absence of an environmental need for expression.

COMMUNICATION PROBLEMS IN CHILDREN WITH A TRACHEOSTOMY

The presence of a tracheostomy tube can create *aphonia,* or the inability to produce voice. Since the tracheostomy tube is placed above the vocal cords, a leak of air around the cannula and through the vocal cords is necessary to obtain vocalization. If there is no space around the tracheostomy tube because of a tight-fitting cannula, or if the upper airway is narrowed as a result of subglottic stenosis or congenital anomaly, air will not pass through the vocal cords, and aphonia occurs (Fowler, Simon, & Handler, 1985). Voice can sometimes be obtained if some air can leak around the cannula, the child's respiratory muscles are strong, the upper airway is patent, and there is good vocal cord movement.

Communicative passivity is even more of a problem for children with tracheostomies because audible crying and other vocalizations are not produced. When a child cannot respond vocally, parents talk to them less frequently and do not leave time for the child to respond. It may also be harder to sustain conversation. Parents may become frustrated because they cannot accurately interpret the child's needs. The child may experience frustration and isolation. This lack of reciprocal exchange alters the quality of parent–child interactions and creates an environment that is less supportive of language development (Aradine, 1983; Jackson & Albamonte, 1994).

As the size of the tracheostomy tube is changed to accommodate normal growth, the ability to vocalize also changes. The child must adjust to these alterations. The child who has a tracheostomy and is also ventilator dependent faces additional problems. Vocalizations aided by the ventilator are produced on inhalation; those produced independent of the ventilator require exhalation. Breaths provided by the ventilator must be coordinated with self-initiated breaths. It may become difficult for the infant or young child who is being weaned from the ventilator, or who requires only intermittent ventilation, to adapt to continually changing vocalization mechanisms. These confusing vocal experiences can contribute to delayed vocalization in a young tracheotomized or ventilator-dependent child long after the ability to produce voice has developed.

Specific communication problems commonly seen in children with tracheostomies include hoarseness and weakened breath support. Hoarseness decreases vocal intensity or the loudness of the child's voice. Weakened breath support affects not only intensity levels but also the initiation of vocalizations, duration of phonation, and verbal intelligibility. Vocalizations may be limited to 2 to 3 sec and 2 to 3 syllables. Sound production may be delayed or disordered, and voices often sound breathy. Weakened breath support is even more of a problem for children with underlying respiratory or neuromuscular disorders (Jackson & Albamonte, 1994). Pitch can also vary, but inappropriate pitch is not as significant a problem as hoarseness or weakened breath support.

These problems with vocal quality may be temporary or permanent, depending on the child's underlying condition and on the frequency and length of intubation or cannulation.

IDENTIFICATION OF SPEECH AND LANGUAGE PROBLEMS

The family should have an active role in assessment of speech and language problems. Their perception of the significance of the problem can influence the selection of specific interventions. If delays are identified, the community health nurse can assist the family by explaining the roles of specialists, such as audiologists, speech-language pathologists, or otolaryngologists. The nurse can also help the family in coordinating necessary evaluations and services.

Response to Environment

The high-risk infant's ability to respond to the environment, both through auditory responsiveness and through prespeech communication, must be monitored throughout early childhood. Any infant who does not appear to respond consistently to noises or to the human voice should be referred for further diagnostic assessment by an audiologist. This assessment should be coordinated with otolaryngologic consultation. (See Chapter 21, Hearing Loss in the High-risk Infant.)

Expressive Disorders

Expressive speech and language disorders are more difficult to identify at an early age because of the variability of developmental patterns among children. Most children use a few meaningful words and symbolize or comprehend language by 12 to 15 months of age. Most have a vocabulary of more than 10 words by 18 months of age. Other children, however, do not begin talking until 15 to 18 months of age or later. These late talkers may demonstrate normal speech and language development at a more rapid pace once speech begins to emerge. Certainly by 18 months of age, all children should be able to follow simple directions without gestural and situational cues. They should also recognize family members and favorite toys. If specific hearing problems are not obvious, but the child does not appear to have reached age-appropriate language milestones, a full diagnostic developmental assessment should be considered to determine why the child's development of comprehension and cognitive functioning is delayed. If communication delay is expected, referral to a speech-language pathologist should be initiated to aid in identifying possible contributing factors and to select the appropriate interventions for speech and language therapy.

Resonance Problems

Resonance problems (hyponasality, hypernasality) do not occur more frequently in the tracheotomized population than in the normal population. Consequently, any child with questionable resonance problems should be referred to an otolaryngologist for further assessment of palatal functioning and upper airway status. Exhibit 22–1 offers further criteria for identifying potential speech and language disorders.

Child with a Tracheostomy

Children with tracheostomies usually require formal intervention from a speech-language pathologist because of their complex speech and language problems. These children must be taught to use a functional communication system appropriate for both inconsistent verbal attempts and changing respiratory needs. Goals of formal speech and language intervention programs include increasing receptive language skills, stimulating and maintaining voice production, stimulating oral movements and encouraging oral play, and teaching functional expressive language systems (Kaslon & Stein, 1985). Formal programs should be developed by speech-language pathologists trained to work with these children.

LANGUAGE STIMULATION SUGGESTIONS

Speech and language development is a continual process that occurs during all social interactions. To maximize the need for communication, parents and nurses should use appropriate techniques of speech and language stimulation. To decrease communicative passivity and related frustration, any attempt at communication should be accepted. The

Exhibit 22–1 Criteria for Identifying Potential for Speech and Language Disorders

---

1. Does the child seem to comprehend more than suggested by the ability to speak? Is there a gap between expressive and receptive skills?
2. Does the child appear to respond by demonstrating awareness of sound?
3. Does the child seem to be frustrated by an inability to communicate his or her needs?
4. Does the family or caregiver appear to be frustrated by the child's limited capacity for self-expression?
5. Is the child difficult to understand although able to speak?
6. Do the child's communication skills seem disproportionate to (or below) developmental levels?
7. Are there feeding problems?

Exhibit 22–2 Interventions To Stimulate Language Development

---

1. Talk to the child often.
2. Talk to the child normally and use simple sentences.
3. Listen to what the child says.
4. Leave time for the child's response during conversations.
5. Encourage the child to use his voice to indicate wants and needs.
6. Tell the child what you are doing during all direct care. Name body parts during bathing and dressing.
7. Point out and name new and familiar objects and people in the child's environment.
8. Read age-appropriate books.
9. Watch age-appropriate, child-oriented television programs with the child (e.g., Mr. Rogers' Neighborhood, Sesame Street; Rice & Haight, 1986)
10. Play social games such as peek-a-boo and pat-a-cake.
11. Encourage reciprocal vocal play. Play games that include sound imitations (e.g., animal sounds, car sounds, sound-making toys).
12. Sing with and to the child. Listen to child-oriented audiotapes.
13. Include the child in normal family social activities like mealtimes.

Source: Adapted from *Pediatric Nursing,* Vol. 20, No. 2, p. 152, with permission of Jannetti Publications, Inc., Pitman, New Jersey, © 1994.

---

child should be encouraged to initiate communication, and all vocal attempts should be imitated by an adult to encourage their recurrence. Verbalization of a young child's activities and the activities of others in the immediate environment helps the child to learn appropriate words and to expand language concepts. In this regard, language stimulation activities should be coordinated with daily care (i.e., eating, bathing, and dressing) and play. The repetition involved in these activities enables more effective language learning. Even the chronically ill child who is unable to vocalize requires continuous language stimulation both for the development of receptive skills and as preparation for later verbal development. Refer to Exhibit 22–2 for specific language stimulation suggestions.

Normal language stimulation should merely provide an accepting environment for facilitating any communicative attempts. It is important, however, to stress that no child should be forced to communicate. If forcing persists, verbal withdrawal may occur. The community health nurse can promote family-centered care by providing parents with information to assist them in selection of developmentally appropriate language stimulation tools. Parents should be involved in the development of the plan for language stimulation interventions. They can participate by selecting books, toys, and audiotapes. They can also decide the amount and type of television programming that is watched by the child.

ALTERNATIVE AND AUGMENTATIVE COMMUNICATION SYSTEMS

Nonvocal, gestural systems are often developed by the child in an attempt to have needs met. In infants, common nonverbal communication attempts include smiling, reaching, pointing, changing facial expressions, and showing excitement with arm and leg movements in recognition of familiar people or favorite toys. Some infants with tracheostomies may learn to communicate with tongue clicks or lip smacking. Others learn to lower their chins and coordinate exhalation with covering the stoma site to create sounds. This, however, may strain the child's vocal cords (Jackson & Albamonte, 1994).

Parents and the nurse can learn to interpret gestures frequently used by the child. As the child matures, however, these primitive methods may not be sufficient for effective communication. Once the child shows a need for more complex communication and appears to demonstrate a comprehension of the environment, a more formal mode of communication, even if temporary, may be required. Alternative or augmentative communication systems may be helpful for the child who is aphonic, inconsistent in vocal attempts, or ineffective in spoken communication. These systems may also decrease frustration both the child and family experience as a result of inability to understand the child's wants and needs.

Close contact with a speech-language pathologist is essential whenever an alternative or augmentative communication system is used. Parents should collaborate with these professionals and be involved in the selection of an alternative system of communication. Language stimulation interventions should continue to be used with the alternative system as expressive communication develops.

Five alternative or augmentative communication systems can be considered (Jackson & Albamonte, 1994; Simon et al., 1983):

1. esophageal speech
2. spoken language through artificial voice (electrolaryngeal speech)
3. manual or electronic communication systems
4. sign language
5. tracheostomy speaking valve.

Esophageal Speech

Esophageal speech is one of the least restrictive systems of communication for an older child (Kaslon, Grabo, & Ruben, 1978), but it also is the most difficult to initiate for very young children. In an occasional young child with severe subglottic stenosis, however, it has been seen to emerge spontaneously. Esophageal speech also is difficult for the ventilator-dependent child because of the need to coordinate air injection into the esophagus with the breaths from the ventilator (Simon et al., 1983).

Electrolaryngeal Speech

Artificial voice through an electrolarynx can be used for children with long-term or permanent tracheostomies (Fowler et al., 1985). It is helpful in aiding children with early prespeech imitation, especially those who will be able to produce vocalizations. It is also useful for children who cannot learn esophageal speech because of structural problems or poor motor coordination. In some children, the electrolarynx can augment an alternative form of communication, such as sign language, and can prepare the child for eventual speech production following decannulation. A variety of electrolarynges is available for use with adults. Specific considerations for children, including unit size, loudness level, and the ability to hold and initiate the artificial vocal sound, must be assessed in the choice of an appropriate instrument.

Manual or Electronic Communication Systems

The third alternative mode of communication is a manual or electronic communication system that synthesizes speech, thus improving the child's ability to be understood (Fowler et al., 1985). Use of these systems is appropriate only for children who are physically disabled or for those who are unable to produce intelligible or consistent verbalizations. Such systems are expensive and cumbersome and require complex programming in conjunction with the assistance of a specially trained speech-language pathologist.

Sign Language

Sign language uses the young child's natural self-generating gestures and expands them into more standard signs. Sign language can be an enjoyable system for siblings and young peers as well as for the child with a tracheostomy. It must be emphasized to parents and other professionals that sign language does not inhibit verbal communication. Rather, it aids verbal communication when vocalizations begin to occur. Once the child begins to develop spoken communication and can be understood by a listener, sign language rapidly disappears from the communicative repertoire (English & Prutting, 1979; Simon et al., 1983). There are, however, disadvantages to the use of sign language. The child, family, and other caretakers require extensive training. The child's hands cannot be used for other developmentally important activities, like play, while signing. Also, children with significant motor or visuoperceptual problems may have difficulty using sign language (Jackson & Albamonte, 1994).

Tracheostomy Speaking Valve

The Passy-Muir Tracheostomy Speaking Valve is the only speaking valve currently being used with pediatric tracheostomy and ventilator patients (S. Albamonte, personal communication, December 9, 1994). With the Passy-Muir valve in place, air flows through the valve into the tracheostomy tube during inspiration. During exhalation, the valve closes, directing exhaled air through the vocal cords and upper airway. This air stream creates voice (Passy-Muir, Inc., 1994).

Medical stability, adequate airway above the tracheostomy, and adequate cognitive awareness are necessary for successful use of the valve (Passy, 1986). Passy-Muir valves can be used or adapted for use with most types of tracheostomy tubes. A special valve is required for use with ventilators. Valves can be ordered through medical suppliers or directly from Passy-Muir Inc., 4521 Campus Drive, Suite 273, Irvine, CA (Jackson & Albamonte, 1994; Passy-Muir, Inc., 1994).

During initial trials, children should be monitored for adverse changes in the following:

- heart rate; respiratory rate, rhythm, and effort; and oxygen saturation using a cardiorespiratory monitor and pulse oximeter
- effectiveness of cough and ability to clear secretions
- adequacy of air passages in the oral cavity
- subjective expression of comfort.

Peak inspiratory pressure, exhaled volume, presence of high-pressure alarm, and presence of water condensation should also be monitored with mechanically ventilated patients. If any of these adverse changes occur, the trial should be discontinued immediately. Ventilator settings may need to be adjusted, or the tracheostomy tube may need to be resized (Jackson & Albamonte, 1994).

Some children adjust immediately to the use of the Passy-Muir valve. Others require considerable encouragement and distraction during use. Their tolerance of the speaking valve can be improved by gradually increasing the amount of time it is worn. Clinical experience with the valve has shown that young children who use the valve exhibit increased cooing and babbling and have an earlier onset of vocalization than tracheostomized children who do not use the valve. The Passy-Muir valve allows for a more normalized method of communication. Because the valve improves breath support and decreases vocal strain, the child's voice and speech have more normal characteristics. Children can also use their hands for play and other everyday activities (Jackson & Albamonte, 1994).

LONG-TERM OUTCOMES AND POST-DECANNULATION FOLLOW-UP

Overall, premature infants show a higher incidence of receptive and expressive delays than do full-term infants. Long-term outcomes are affected by complex and multifactorial issues. These include short gestation, neurologic status at 8 months, severity of intraventricular hemorrhage, length of hospital stay, presence of chronic lung disease, lower socioeconomic status, and poor maternal education (Casiro et al., 1990; Grunau, Kearney, & Whitfield, 1990; Seidman, Allen, & Wasserman, 1986; Vohr, Garcia-Coll, & Oh, 1988). While language skills generally improve by 3 years of age, problems such as articulation defects, stuttering, dysgrammatism (incomplete or distorted syntactical structure), shorter utterances, poorer vocabularies, less social initiative, and less focused play may continue into the preschool and school-age years (Casiro, Moddemann, Stanwick, & Cheang, 1991; Largo, Molinari, Kundu, Lipp, & Duc, 1990; Seidman et al., 1986; Vohr, Garcia-Coll, & Oh, 1989).

Parents and professionals may be encouraged to know that follow-up assessment in a large population of tracheotomized children revealed that those who were decannulated before the establishment of symbolic communication were able to master communication skills commensurate with their developmental level (Simon et al., 1983). The communication skills of those children who were decannulated after the initiation of comprehension and the use of language were more severely impaired. This more mature population of children exhibited a greater need for speech and language intervention for longer periods of time. Other follow-up has found that voice problems (hoarseness, weakened breath support, and pitch disturbances) and articulation defects are common findings in children who were tracheotomized (Simon & McGowan, 1989; Singer et al., 1989).

The need for speech-language therapy does not cease once the tracheotomized child is decannulated. Speech and language therapy may be even more important after decannulation, since the child must learn to transfer skills learned in alternative modes of communication to the spoken language system.

REFERENCES

Aradine, C.R. (1983). Young children with long-term tracheostomies: Health and development. *Western Journal of Nursing Research, 5*(2), 115–124.

Casiro, O.G., Moddemann, D.M., Stanwick, R.S., & Cheang, M.S. (1991). The natural history and predictive value of early language delays in very low birth weight infants. *Early Human Development, 26,* 45–50.

Casiro, O.G., Moddemann, D.M., Stanwick, R.S., Panikkar-Theissen, V.K., Cowan, H., & Cheang, M.S. (1990). Language development of very low birth weight infants and fullterm controls at 12 months of age. *Early Human Development, 24,* 65–77.

English, S.T., & Prutting, C.A. (1979). Teaching American sign language to a normally hearing infant with tracheostenosis. *Clinical Pediatrics, 14,* 1,141–1,145.

Fowler, S.M., Simon, B.M., & Handler, S.D. (1985). Communication development in children. In E.N. Meyers, S.E. Stool, & I.T. Johnson (Eds.), *Tracheostomy*. New York, NY: Churchill Livingstone.

Grunau, R.V.E., Kearney, S.M., & Whitfield, M.F. (1990). Language development at 3 years in pre-term children of birth weight below 1000 g. *British Journal of Disorders of Communication, 25*, 173–182.

Jackson, D., & Albamonte, S. (1994). Enhancing communication with the Passy-Muir valve. *Pediatric Nursing, 20*, 149–153.

Kaslon, K.W., Grabo, D.E., & Ruben, R. (1978). Voice, speech, and language habilitation in young children without laryngeal function. *Archives of Otolaryngology—Head and Neck Surgery, 104*, 737–739.

Kaslon, K.W., & Stein, R.E. (1985). Chronic pediatric tracheostomy: Assessment and implications for habilitation of voice, speech and language in young children. *International Journal of Pediatric Otorhinolaryngology, 9*, 165–171.

Largo, R.H., Molinari, L., Kundu, S., Lipp, A., & Duc, G. (1990). Intellectual outcome, speech and school performance in high risk preterm children with birth weight appropriate for gestational age. *European Journal of Pediatrics, 149*, 845–850.

Passy, V. (1986). Passy-Muir tracheostomy speaking valve. *Otolaryngology—Head and Neck Surgery, 95*, 247–248.

Passy-Muir, Inc. (1994). *Passy-Muir tracheostomy speaking valve* (Product monograph). Irvine, CA: Author.

Rice, M.L., & Haight, P.L. (1986). "Motherese" of Mr. Rogers: A description of the dialogue of educational television programs. *Journal of Speech and Hearing Disorders, 51*, 282–287.

Ryan, J. (1988). Hearing and speech assessment. In R.A. Ballard (Ed.), *Pediatric care of the ICN graduate*. Philadelphia, PA: W.B. Saunders.

Seidman, S., Allen, R., & Wasserman, G.A. (1986). Productive language of premature and physically handicapped two-year-olds. *Journal of Communication Disorders, 19*, 49–61.

Simon, B.M., Fowler, S.M., & Handler, S.D. (1983). Communication development in young children with long-term tracheostomies: Prelimi-nary report. *International Journal of Pediatric Otorhinolaryngology, 6*, 37–50.

Simon, B.M., & McGowan, J.S. (1989). Tracheostomy in young children: Implications for assessment and treatment of communication and feeding disorders. *Infants and Young Children, 1*, 1–9.

Singer, L.T., Kercsmar, C., Legris, G., Orlowski, J.P., Hill, B.P., & Doershuk, C. (1989). Developmental sequelae of long-term infant tracheostomy. *Developmental Medicine and Child Neurology, 31*, 224–230.

Vohr, B.R., Garcia-Coll, C., & Oh, W. (1988). Language development of low-birthweight infants at two years. *Developmental Medicine and Child Neurology, 30*, 608–615.

Vohr, B.R., Garcia-Coll, C., & Oh, W. (1989). Language and neurodevelopmental outcome of low-birthweight infants at three years. *Developmental Medicine and Child Neurology, 31*, 582–590.

Whaley, L.F., & Wong, D.L. (1991). *Nursing care of infants and children* (4th ed.). St. Louis, MO: Mosby Year Book.

ADDITIONAL RESOURCES

Albamonte, S., & Jerome, A.M. (1993). Pediatrics. In M.F. Mason (Ed.), *Speech pathology for tracheotomized and ventilator dependent patients*. Newport Beach, CA: Voicing.

Bond, N., Phillips, P., & Rollins, J.A. (1994). Family-centered care at home for families with children who are technology dependent. *Pediatric Nursing, 20*(2), 123–130.

Hall, S.S., & Weatherly, K.S. (1989). Using sign language with tracheotomized infants and children. *Pediatric Nursing, 15*, 362–367.

Peterson, H.A. (1973). A case report of speech and language training for a two year old laryngectomized child. *Journal of Speech and Hearing Disorders, 38*, 275.

Simon, B.M., & Handler, S.D. (1981). The speech pathologist and management of children with tracheostomies. *Journal of Otolaryngology, 10*, 440–448.

Chapter 23

Visual Impairment in the Preterm Infant

Revised by Barbara D. Schraeder, PhD, RN, FAAN

Premature and low birth weight (LBW) infants are at risk for visual impairments, including refractive errors, ocular muscle imbalance, and blindness. Vision screening and in some cases careful regular eye examinations by an ophthalmologist should be a routine part of follow-up evaluation of premature infants. Since visual stimulation is an integral component of normal development, visual deficits should be corrected or compensated for early in order to promote optimal development of the infant. Uncorrected eye problems in infants and young children are more likely to lead to irreversible vision loss than are similar problems in the mature vision system of adults (Pediatric Evaluation Preferred Practice Pattern of the American Academy of Opthalmology Quality of Care Committee, 1993). Parents have an important role to play in ensuring vision health for their children. Education and support for parents in detecting visual deficits and scheduling ongoing professional evaluations are essential components of family-centered vision care.

COMMON VISION PROBLEMS

Retinopathy of prematurity is a potential problem for early premature and LBW infants. Ocular muscle imbalance and cortical deficits may also be noted. Many of the terms referred to in the following discussion are defined in Exhibit 23–1.

Retinopathy of Prematurity

Retinopathy of prematurity (ROP) or retrolental fibroplasia (RLF) is a frequent cause of severe vision problems in premature infants. Its prevalence is highest in infants born weighing less than 1,500 g. After a period of decline, it is now believed to be on the rise because of the increasing birth-weight-specific survival of infants weighing between 500 and 1,000 g (Gibson, Sheps, Uh, Schnechter, & McCormick, 1990). Although some infants without supplemental oxygen develop ROP, and multiple factors are thought to be associated with the disease, including early exposure of the immature retina to light (Fielder, Robinson, Shaw, Ng, & Moseley, 1992), oxygen is known to have toxic effects on immature retinal vessels (Friendly, 1994). Exposure to high levels of oxygen causes vasoconstriction of immature retinal vessels. Although this condition is initially reversible, continued vasoconstriction leads to irreversible adherence of the vessel walls and degenerative changes. The degree of vessel destruction appears to be proportional to at least three factors: (1) the degree of immaturity of the vessels, (2) the duration of oxygen therapy, and (3) the concentration of oxygen administered. Thus, early premature or LBW infants with a history of oxygen use are at the highest risk for developing ROP (Friendly, 1994).

ROP is staged and graded, using an international classification system, according to its severity as determined by findings on ophthalmologic examination. Proliferative phase changes are staged from I to IV; cicatricial phase changes are graded I through V (see glossary in Exhibit 23–1 for definitions of terms). The highest score, in the case of the proliferative phase fundus changes, Stage IV, and in the case of cicatricial phase fundus changes, Grade V, is the most severe (Friendly, 1994). ROP may subside and, in mild

Exhibit 23–1 Glossary of Terms

Anisometropia: unequal refractive state of the two eyes, one eye requiring a different lens correction from the other

Amblyopia: impaired vision without detectable organic lesion of the eye not correctable by refractive means

Astigmatism: differences in the curvature in different meridians of the refractive surfaces of the eye so that light rays are not sharply focused on the retina

Retinopathy of prematurity (ROP): a disease of the retina found predominantly in premature infants where severe vasoconstriction, usually due to the high oxygen necessary for survival, leads to hypoxia in vital structures of the eye

Proliferative phase of ROP: the growth of retinal capillaries into hypoxic areas of the eyes where vessels proliferate and dilate

Cicatricial phase of ROP: scarring of the retina and lens that follows the acute phase of ROP

Strabismus/squint: an abnormality of the eyes in which the visual axis of the eyes lacks parallelism; binocular vision is not present

Myopia: nearsightedness, too large an eye

Hyperopia: farsightedness, too small an eye

Visual acuity: clarity or clearness of vision; the degree to which smaller and smaller print can be resolved

cases, even regress over time. The extent of regression varies with the severity of the active phase, and many infants will be left with some degree of myopia in one or both eyes. Strabismus (an abnormality of the eye in which the visual axis of the eyes lacks parallelism) is another frequent complication (Page, Schneeweiss, Whyte, & Harvey, 1993). All individuals with cicatricial ROP can also experience retinal detachment and blindness. Retinal detachment and blindness can occur at any age in infants and children with severe ROP but they are most frequent in the first two decades of life and are directly related to the degree of myopia (Friendly, 1994).

Various types of treatment have been attempted for ROP. Vitamin E, an antioxidant, has been thought to have a therapeutic and protective effect. However, studies are conflicting, and the disadvantages to treatment with large doses of vitamin E include sepsis, necrotizing enterocolitis, and a poor cost benefit ratio. It has been recommended that until a consensus exists as to its efficacy, vitamin E levels in premature infants should be kept at physiologic levels (Friendly, 1994).

During the proliferative phase of ROP, cryotherapy using protocol-based criteria has demonstrated a 50% reduction in unfavorable retinal outcomes (The Cryotherapy for ROP Study Group, 1988). Laser therapy is now being evaluated, and preliminary results suggest that it is as effective as

cryotherapy with less stress on the infant (The Laser ROP Study Group, 1994). Vitreous surgery, for later retinal detachment, has been shown to have beneficial results, with some return of vision in 45% to 50% of cases. With successful surgical results, parents of a child with advanced ROP can expect the child to recognize faces and objects, to maneuver without assistance, and to watch television; any finer visual ability is unlikely (R.D. Reinecke, personal communication, November 29, 1994).

Other Visual Deficits

Other visual disorders found more often in preterm than full-term infants include strabismus (also called *squint*), poor visual acuity, anisometropia, and astigmatism. (See Exhibit 23–1.) As with ROP, the very low birth weight (VLBW) group is most susceptible (Glass, 1994). Two large studies of premature children at school age—one population based, the other using normal birth weight case controls—found that visual morbidity was significantly greater in the VLBW groups (Gallo & Lennerstrand, 1991; McGinnity & Bryars, 1992). There is increasing evidence that in addition to anatomically based visual deficits, children who were preterm also have difficulty with visually mediated tasks that influence cognition (Klein, 1988; Klein, Hack, & Breslau, 1989; Schraeder, Heverly, O'Brien, & McEvoy-Shields, 1992). Since even minor visual impairments can interfere with children's ability to process information and to learn to read fluently and easily, the early detection of visual deficits and attention to correction or remediation is critical.

EXAMINATIONS AND SCREENING

Periodic Ophthalmologic Examinations

Since any premature or LBW infant with a history of oxygen use is at risk for ROP, ophthalmologic evaluations should be performed before discharge from the hospital nursery or within 4 to 6 weeks after birth (Friendly, 1994). All children with any signs of ROP need regular, ongoing ophthalmic examinations. In fact, it recently has been recommended that all premature infants receive regular ophthalmic examinations through 2 years of age regardless of the results of early examination, because of the high incidence of optical abnormalities in this group (Page et al., 1993).

Vision Screening

Prior to vision screening, information should be obtained concerning oxygen use in the neonatal period (concentration and duration), previous findings on ophthalmic examinations, and any family history of visual deficits. While parents can be excellent informants, their understanding of information on oxygen exposure and ophthalmic examination results may not be complete. Accessing the child's medical record, with parental permission, increases the chance of obtaining a precise summary of vital information. In addition to the child's perinatal history, information should be elicited from parents about their observations and concerns related to the infant's visual abilities. An example of a documentation form for vision screening is provided in Appendix 23–A.

Vision screening should include a complete inspection of the external eye, including the lids, pupils, conjunctiva, and sclera. Lesions or discharge should be noted, as well as ptosis, pallor of the conjunctiva, and unequal or absent pupillary reaction to light. For testing the pupillary reaction to light, the room must be darkened. The examiner shines the penlight into one pupil while observing for pupillary constriction in the same and the opposite eye. The procedure is repeated on the other pupil.

The eyes should also be inspected for nystagmus and strabismus. Nystagmus is a rhythmic oscillation of the eyes that can be intermittent or continuous; eye movements may be vertical, horizontal, rotatory, or mixed. Strabismus can be detected by shining a penlight between the infant's eyes or above the nose. If the reflection does not come from corresponding parts of the cornea, strabismus is suspected. The cover–uncover test, described in other texts, may also be used in infants more than 12 months of age postterm.

In addition, the eyes should be inspected for the red reflex. An ophthalmoscope is used if available; alternatively, a penlight may be used. The light beam is directed at the pupil from 15° lateral and about 15 inches away while the pupils are focused straight ahead. A red-orange glow in the pupil is the expected finding.

A routine screening examination should also include observation for age-appropriate characteristics of visual development, as described in Table 23–1. Table 23–2 shows a timetable, screening method, and indicators that require further evaluation related to eye and vision examinations in primary care (Pediatric Evaluation Preferred Practice Pattern of the American Academy of Ophthalmology Quality of Care Committee, 1993).

PARENT EDUCATION AND SUPPORT

Anticipatory guidance and counseling are common needs of the parent of a high-risk infant who has potential or actual visual impairment. Parents can be taught to observe for major visual milestones, such as fixating and following, hand regard, and evidence of the development of eye–hand coordination. They may also be able to observe for signs of nystagmus and gross signs of eye muscle imbalance. However, these activities are not a substitute for eye examinations by an ophthalmologist. Parents must understand the importance of scheduling and keeping regular ophthalmic check-ups if vision problems are to be detected early enough for deficits to be remediated or to have their impact lessened.

Table 23–1 Chronology of Visual Development

Age	Level of development
Birth	Awareness of light and dark, infant closes eyelids in bright light.
Neonatal	Rudimentary fixation on near objects (3–30 inches).
2 weeks	Transitory fixation, usually monocular at a distance of roughly 3 feet.
4 weeks	Follows large, conspicuously moving objects.
6 weeks	Moving objects evoke binocular fixation briefly.
8 weeks	Follows moving objects with jerky eye movements. Convergence beginning to appear.
12 weeks	Visual following now a combination of head and eye movements. Convergence improving. Enjoys light objects and bright colors.
16 weeks	Inspects own hands. Fixates immediately on a 1-inch cube brought within 1–2 feet of eye. Vision 20/300–20/200 (6/100–6/70).
20 weeks	Accomodative convergence reflexes all organizing. Visually pursues lost rattle. Shows interest in stimuli more than 3 feet away.
24 weeks	Retrieves a dropped 1-inch cube. Can maintain voluntary fixation of stationary object even in the presence of competing moving stimulus. Hand-eye coordination appearing.
26 weeks	Will fixate on a string.
28 weeks	Binocular fixation clearly established.
36 weeks	Beginning of depth perception.
40 weeks	Marked interest in tiny objects. Tilts head backward to gaze up. Vision 20/200 (6/70).
52 weeks	Fusion beginning to appear. Discriminates simple geometric forms (squares and circles). Vision 20/180 (6/60).
12–18 months	Looks at pictures with interest.
18 months	Convergence well established. Localization in distance crude—runs into large objects.
2 years	Accommodation well developed. Vision 20/40 (6/12).
3 years	Convergence smooth. Vision 20/30 (6/9).
4 years	Vision 20/20 (6/6).

Source: Reprinted from *Current Pediatric Diagnosis & Treatment*, 8th ed., by C.H. Kemp et al. (Eds.), p. 25, with permission of Lange Medical Publications, Los Altos, CA, © 1984.

In the case of the child with a known visual impairment, the impact of the impairment on the parent–infant relationship should be assessed. Parents may need assistance both to notice the realms other than visual in which their infant does respond to them and to optimize communication through sound and touch. Parents also need referral to state and private agencies that specialize in services to the visually im-

Table 23–2 Eye and Vision Examination Recommendations for Primary Care Physicians

Age	Screening method	Indicators requiring further evaluation
Newborn to 3 months old	Red reflex Corneal light reflex Inspection	Abnormal or asymmetric Asymmetric Structural abnormality
6 months to 1 year old	Red reflex Corneal light reflex Differential occlusion Fix and follow with each eye Inspection	Abnormal or asymmetric Asymmetric Failure to object equally to covering each eye Failure to fix and follow Structural abnormality
3 years old (approximately)	Visual acuity[a] Red reflex Corneal light reflex/cover–uncover Stereoacuity[b] Inspection	20/50 or worse or two lines of difference between the eyes Abnormal or asymmetric Asymmetric/ocular refixation movements Failure to appreciate random dot or Titmus Stereogram Structural abnormality
5 years old (approximately)	Visual acuity[a] Red reflex Corneal light reflex/cover–uncover Stereoacuity[b] Inspection	20/30 or worse Abnormal or asymmetric Asymmetric/ocular refixation movements Failure to appreciate random dot or Titmus Stereogram Structural abnormality

[a]Allen figures, HOTV, Tumbling E, or Snellen.
[b]Optional, sometimes advocated in lieu of visual acuity; Random Dot E Game (RDE), Titmus Stereograms, Randot Stereograms.

Source: Reprinted with permission from the American Academy of Ophthalmology: *Comprehensive Pediatric Eye Evaluation, Preferred Practice Pattern,* American Academy of Ophthalmology, San Francisco, California, © 1992.

---

paired. Such agencies can provide emotional, educational, and financial support for their child's special needs.

DEVELOPMENTAL INTERVENTION

Attention to developmental intervention is important. Parents can be informed of services under Part H (See Special Issue, "Early Intervention For the High-risk Infant") and referred to local programs. For the visually impaired infant, stimulation should enhance tactile, proprioceptive (position, balance, and movement), auditory, and other sensory modes. To encourage appropriate gross motor development, which is closely tied to vision, programs of activities encouraging normal movement patterns are also important. Early intervention and parent instruction by trained therapists can optimize the developmental potential of the visually impaired infant.

REFERENCES

The Cryotherapy for ROP Study Group. (1988). Multicenter trial of cryotherapy for retinopathy of prematurity: Preliminary results. *Archives of Ophthalmology, 106,* 471.

Fielder, A., Robinson, J., Shaw, D., Ng, Y., & Moseley, M. (1992). Light and retinopathy of prematurity: Does retinal location offer a clue? *Pediatrics, 89,* 648–653.

Friendly, D. (1994). Eye disorders. In G. Avery, M.A. Fletcher, & M. MacDonald, (Eds.), *Neonatology: Pathophysiology and management of the newborn* (4th ed.). Philadelphia, PA: J.B. Lippincott.

Gallo, J.E., & Lennerstrand, G. (1991). A population-based study of ocular abnormalities in premature children aged 5 to 10 years. *American Journal of Ophthalmology, 111,* 539–547.

Gibson, N., Sheps, S., Uh, S.H., Schnechter, M., & McCormick, A. (1990). Retinopathy of prematurity—induced blindness: Birth weight specific survival and the new epidemic. *Pediatrics, 86,* 405–412.

Glass, P. (1994). The vulnerable neonate and the neonatal intensive care environment. In G. Avery, M.A. Fletcher, & M. MacDonald, (Eds.), *Neonatology: Pathophysiology and management of the newborn* (4th ed.). Philadelphia, PA: J.B. Lippincott.

Klein, N.K. (1988). Children who were very low birth weight: Cognitive abilities and classroom behavior at five years of age. *The Journal of Special Education, 22,* 41–54.

Klein, N., Hack, M., & Breslau, N. (1989). Children who were very low birth weight: Development and academic achievement at nine years of age. *Developmental and Behavioral Pediatrics, 10,* 32–37.

The Laser ROP Study Group. (1994). Laser therapy for retinopathy of prematurity. *Archives of Ophthalmology, 112,* 154–156.

McGinnity, F.G., & Bryars, J.H. (1992). Controlled study of ocular morbidity in school aged children born at preterm. *British Journal of Ophthalmology, 6,* 520–524.

Page, J., Schneeweiss, S., Whyte, H., & Harvey, P. (1993). Ocular sequelae in premature infants. *Pediatrics, 92,* 787–790.

Pediatric Evaluation Preferred Practice Pattern of the American Academy of Ophthalmology Quality of Care Committee. (1993, March). Comprehensive pediatric eye evaluation. *Abstracts of Clinical Care Guidelines,* 5–7.

Schraeder, B., Heverly, M., O'Brien, C., & McEvoy-Shields, K. (1992). Finishing first grade: A study of school achievement in very low birth weight children. *Nursing Research, 41,* 354–361.

Vision Assessment of the Infant

Name _____ Hosp # _____ DOB _____

HISTORY

1. Family member with visual defects

Explain _____ _____ yes _____ no

2. History of trauma to the eye

Describe _____ _____ yes _____ no

3. History of infections in the eye

Describe _____ _____ yes _____ no

4. Oxygen use in infancy

Concentration and duration _____ _____ yes _____ no

PARENT REPORT

Parental concerns _____

_____

_____

Previous vision or eye exams   Date   Type and result

Right	Left	External Exam	Indication for referral	Comment
___	___	Pupil (PERLA)[a]	unequal	___
___	___	Conjunctiva (clear)	pallor, lesions	___
___	___	Sclera (clear)	lesions	___
___	___	Lids (ptosis)	if positive	___
___	___	Lesions (describe)	if positive	___

Right	Left	Nystagmus	If present	Comment
___	___	vertical:	_____	_____
___	___	horizontal:	_____	_____
___	___	rotary:	_____	_____

Right	Left	Nystagmus	If present	Comment
_____	_____	mixed: _____		
_____	_____	intermittent: _____		
_____	_____	continuous: _____		
_____	_____			
_____	_____	Light reflections from center of pupil	if off-center/absent	_____

Right	Left	Developmental Skills	Indication for referral	Comment
_____	_____	red reflex (birth–1 yr)	if not red/not centered	_____
_____	_____	responsive smile (4 wks)	if behind chron/adju age	_____
_____	_____	follows 180° (4–12 wks)		_____
_____	_____	fixates easily (4–12 wks)		_____
_____	_____	inspects own hands (12–20 wks)		
_____	_____	fixates on objects up to 3 ft away (12–20 wks)		_____
_____	_____	hand-eye coordination developing (20–28 wks)		_____
_____	_____	rescues dropped blocks (20–28 wks)		_____
_____	_____	displays interest in tiny objects (28-44 wks)		_____
_____	_____	tilts head back to see up (28–44 wks)		_____
_____	_____	cover/uncover (toddler)	if objects to one eye being covered	_____
_____	_____	EOMS (toddler)	if not full in all directions	_____

Right	Left	Developmental Skills	Indication for referral	Comment
_____	_____	enjoys looking at picture books (toddler)	if no	_____
_____	_____	vision 20/40 with E cards at 20 ft. (3–5 yrs)	if less than 20/40	_____

Assessment _____

_____

_____

Plan _____

_____

_____

Signature of nurse completing assessment   Date

aPERLA = pupils equal, reactive to light, and accommodation.

Source: Courtesy of Children's Hospital National Medical Center, Home Health Care Services, Washington, D.C.

Part VII

Additional Concerns

Death in the Home:
Nurses' Roles and Responsibilities

Janice Miller-Thiel RN, BSN

Home care nurses expect to help children and families manage chronic and sometimes life-threatening illness. However, most home care nurses are not prepared for death in the home. Common questions nurses have about death in the home include the following: Who needs to be called? Can nurses pronounce death? What should be done for the child? Who calls the funeral home, and how soon must they come? What should be done for the siblings? What should the nurse tell the parents? When can the nurse leave the home? Then what does the nurse do?

The following overview will assist the nonhospice nurse to answer these questions and to increase his or her comfort in caring for a child with a "Do Not Resuscitate" order who has died in the home.

WHO NEEDS TO BE CALLED?

The first call the nurse makes when a child dies at home should be to the child's physician. Together, the nurse and physician can work out the details of pronouncement; talking with the funeral home, if desired; autopsy; organ donation; and other concerns.

Each state has its own requirements regarding notification of death. In the case of an expected death, many do NOT require 911 to be called. If the physician is willing and available to sign the death certificate, this may be considered adequate. Then the funeral home can come to the home and remove the body. In some states, the death certificate can be

signed the next day if the child is not being transported across state lines.

Burial assistance may be available to low-income families. However, some states will not authorize assistance if the child has already been provided service by a funeral home. Most funeral homes are aware of the state's requirements, and their on-call staff can share this information with the nurse and family.

CAN NURSES PRONOUNCE DEATH?

In most states, pronouncement of death consists of listening for both the heartbeat and respirations for a full minute and assessing for the presence of a blood pressure. Each state has different guidelines, but most authorize a *hospice* nurse (but not necessarily a home care or community health nurse) to pronounce for a patient enrolled in their program for whom death was expected. However, when death is unexpected, nurses usually may not pronounce, and the case becomes a medical examiner's case. An exception occurs when the physician determines that the death was reasonable and is willing to sign the death certificate.

WHAT SHOULD BE DONE FOR THE CHILD?

If the death was expected, neither an autopsy nor the medical examiner will be required, and the nurse may assist the family in any goodbye rituals that they may want to perform. Many parents do not know what they want to do or even what they can do.

Some options are the following:

- changing the clothes
- washing the body or hair
- taking a picture
- snipping a curl of hair
- holding the child
- singing a favorite song
- waking the siblings to say goodbye
- painting the nails.

The nurse should not remove any tubes unless authorized to do so by the physician. In hospice, and when no autopsy is being performed, it is permissible to remove nasogastric (NG) tubes and intravenous (IV) tubes.

WHO CALLS THE FUNERAL HOME, AND HOW SOON MUST THEY COME?

Not all families will choose to work with a funeral home; they may have alternative arrangements for burial. However, if a funeral home is to be contacted, the following guidelines apply.

In a nonhospice setting, the physician must make the initial call to the funeral home. The nurse or family can talk to the funeral home afterwards to arrange a time to come to the home. Some families want to wait until a grandparent arrives or until they have had a chance to hold their child for awhile. The funeral home can provide information about local practice. Usually, the child can remain in the home for a number of hours. This is especially important for some faith traditions: some parents will never see their child again because burial is immediate or there is a closed casket.

When the funeral home staff arrives, the nurse can both assist in answering their questions and can facilitate the family's decisionmaking. Some parents want the father to carry the child to the van. Others accept the use of a stretcher but want their child's face uncovered until inside the van. Some families request that the van or hearse be unmarked to help protect their privacy. Parents' level of anxiety and feelings of pain generally increase as their child leaves their home for the last time. This is a time for a nurse to offer hugs and support and to be present with the family to watch the van leave.

WHAT SHOULD BE DONE FOR THE SIBLINGS?

It is imperative to include siblings in events surrounding the child's death. For a brother or sister to wake up and find

their sibling gone is terrifying: it creates more long-term concerns than any involvement at the time of death. It is essential that nurses are aware of the developmental concepts of death for each age group. This will ensure appropriate guidance of the family in preparing the siblings.

Siblings may behave in ways that are confusing to adults: for example, poking at the dead child's body or, alternatively, simply refusing to stop playing. These behaviors may create stress for parents as they watch their surviving children behave in seemingly "unacceptable" ways. The nurse has an important role in explaining age-appropriate behavior to parents to help them to understand normal sibling reactions.

Nurses should also ask the parents what they want the sibling to be told and can offer assistance to parents as necessary in finding appropriate words. The best rule of thumb is to keep discussions very simple. As adults, we want to explain death in very long terms. However, for a child, it usually suffices to say "Johnny has died. You can come and say goodbye to him if you like." If there are visible changes, the siblings should be prepared for them, for example, "The last time you saw Johnny his lips were very blue, now they are pale."

WHAT SHOULD THE NURSE TELL THE PARENTS?

The nurse should first inform parents of whatever was observed at the time of death: any seizures, breathing changes, color changes, and so forth. However, it is not appropriate to explain or intimate what caused the death, as it is not possible to know the cause absolutely.

The nurse should prepare parents for the body secretions that are released, including bowel and bladder contents. At times, stomach and mouth contents can trickle from the mouth. Paents should be reassured that this does not mean that the child choked to death, rather that the relaxation of the muscles has allowed the secretions to be expelled.

Many people have been scared and caught off guard by what is sometimes called the "last sigh." This occurs when there is air trapped in the lungs that is released either on its own or when the child is moved. Parents should be prepared so that they can differentiate the last sigh from true respiration.

WHEN CAN THE NURSE LEAVE THE HOME?

Before leaving the home, the nurse needs to complete appropriate chart documentation. The agency may require the nurse both to remove the patient chart from the home and to call durable medical equipment (DME) and infusion companies so that they can remove equipment.

The nurse should stay until the child is removed from the home. It is not necessary to be doing something every minute while waiting. Perhaps sitting quietly in the kitchen with relatives or at the child's bedside is all that is needed.

THEN WHAT DOES THE NURSE DO?

After a death has occurred in the home, the nurse should review what happened with the nursing supervisor and talk over the situation with any other nurses on the case.

If the agency does not have policies to assist at the time of the death of a child, these should be developed. A local hospice may be helpful in this regard.

It is not unprofessional to go to the funeral or the wake. In fact, attending these rituals can be helpful to both the family and the nurse. After the funeral, nurses can link the family with community support for bereavement follow-up. A letter telling the family members a favorite memory of their child can be supportive. A call on the child's birthday can say, "Your child is not forgotten."

It can be difficult to know what to say to a bereaved family. Simply stating that one will never forget their child and that the family's love made a difference may be enough. A nurse who is comfortable with supporting a grieving family often shows this best by his or her quiet, calm, and listening manner. The simple offering of human compassion and pres-ence overrides the need for any statement intended to comfort. There is no one magic phrase that can make it all better for the family or the nurse. Yet, who better than the nurse who knew and cared for the child to share the family's pain and sorrow and to offer the assurance that they are not alone?

Nurses can be a source of strength and knowledge to families even when the nurse feels shaky and overwhelmed. It is not necessary to be the most knowledgeable professional. Simply staying close and being present is often gift enough.

SUGGESTED READING

Bluebond-Langner, M. (1978). *The private worlds of dying children.* Princeton, NJ: Princeton University Press.

Doka, K.J. (1995). *Children mourning, mourning children.* Washington, DC: Hospice Foundation of America.

Fitzgerald, H. (1992). *The grieving child: A parent's guide.* New York, NY: Simon & Schuster.

Johnson, C.J., & McGee, M.G. (1991). *How different religions view death and afterlife.* Philadelphia, PA: The Charles Press, Publishers.

Stein, S.B. (1974). *About dying: An open family book for parents and children together.* New York, NY: Walker & Co.

Tatelbaum, J. (1980). *The courage to grieve.* New York, NY: Harper & Row.

Wolfelt, A. (1983). *Helping children cope with grief.* Muncie, IN: Accelerated Development, Inc.

Chapter 24

Home Care of the Infant or Child with HIV Infection

Mary Rathlev, MSN, and Karen Patt Sachse, MSN, RN

Pediatric human immunodeficiency virus (HIV) infection poses special challenges as a chronic illness. Typically, the clinical signs of illness present earlier and its course is more acute when acquired in infancy than in adulthood. In the case of perinatal transmission, there is a period of uncertainty, when the infant's HIV infection is difficult to document because of the presence of maternal antibodies that may persist for up to 18 months. HIV infection poses an additional challenge in that it can also severely delay the process of growth and development in the young child.

Pediatric HIV infection is usually an intergenerational health problem, most prevalent among families of color. A majority of affected families have limited financial and health care resources. The Health Care Financing Administration, for example, reports that Medicaid funds pay for 90% of the care of children with HIV infection in the United States (Allbritten, 1990; Clark & Byrne, 1993).

ETIOLOGY AND DIAGNOSIS

Almost all HIV-infected children less than 13 years of age acquire the virus either vertically during pregnancy, and/or in the intrapartum period, as well as immediately postpartum via breast milk. Of those infected perinatally, more than half of the mothers are or were involved in intravenous (IV) drug use. While about 25% of infants born to HIV-infected women will become infected, all will be HIV antibody positive at birth. In addition, 50 cumulative cases of HIV infec-

tion from sexual abuse of children have been reported anecdotally (Parrott & Rathlev, 1993).

It is crucial to establish the diagnosis of HIV infection in an infant as soon as possible in order to begin prophylaxis against Pneumocystis carinii pneumonia (PCP) as well as treatment with antiretroviral therapy as indicated. Laboratory tests to demonstrate HIV infection include attempts to show antibody or antigen. The enzyme-linked immunosorbent assay (ELISA) and Western blot tests both detect antibody and are 99% specific for HIV infection in those greater than 18 months of age. Diagnosis in children less than 18 months of age, however, requires demonstrating the virus itself because of persistent maternal HIV antibody during this time. Among infected infants, the presence of the virus is ascertainable in 50% at birth, more than 90% by 3 months of age, and almost 100% by 6 months of age using HIV culture and/or polymerase chain reaction (PCR; Parrott & Rathlev, 1993).

SPECTRUM OF ILLNESS

Two classes of lymphocytes are important to the immune system: B-lymphocytes (B-cells) and T-lymphocytes (T-cells). There are three types of T-cells: T-suppressor cells, natural killer cells and T-helper cells, often called CD4+ cells. CD4+ cells essentially direct immune function. A key step in the pathogenesis of HIV infection is the attachment of the virus to the CD4+ cells of the immune system and its subsequent entry into these cells. Eventually, this entry leads to the replication of HIV, destruction of CD4+ cells, and release of the virus into the blood. Subsequently, immune functions begin to fail as HIV destroys more and more CD4+ cells. HIV also infects other cells, such as B cells that make antibody and the macrophages that transport the virus to organs and systems, including the digestive and central nervous systems.

As a result, HIV infection causes a wide spectrum of illness in children. Acquired immunodeficiency syndrome (AIDS) represents the most severe form of HIV illness. HIV can remain in the body for months or years before symptoms appear. As the epidemic has progressed, there is increasing evidence that the course of perinatal AIDS is bimodal (Duliege et al., 1992). One author reports 19% of infected infants with a short latency period with onset of symptoms by 4 months of age and 81% of infected infants with a long latency showing significant illness by 6 years of age (Wara, 1992).

The initial symptoms may be quite simple and nonspecific and include some of the following (Centers for Disease Control, 1994):

- lymphadenopathy
- hepatomegaly
- splenomegaly
- dermatitis
- parotid gland enlargement
- recurrent or persistent upper respiratory tract infection
- sinusitis
- otitis media.

Some moderate signs are characterized by their persistence or recurrence and include the following: fever, anemia, or neutropenia; diarrhea; oral candidiasis; varicella zoster infection; and herpes simplex (Centers for Disease Control, 1994). Two characteristics of children with AIDS are a serious pneumonia called lymphocytic interstitial pneumonia (LIP) and PCP. Some opportunistic infections in children with AIDS include esophageal candidiasis; cytomegalovirus (CMV) retinitis; encephalopathy; and wasting syndrome (Parrott & Rathlev, 1993).

PROPHYLAXIS AND TREATMENT

Treatments for children with HIV infection include those directed at preventing communicable diseases—immunizations; those designed to prevent secondary infections—prophylaxis; those aimed at inhibiting HIV replication—antiretroviral therapy; and the aggressive use of medications for longer periods of time than ordinary. (See Appendix 24–A.)

Children with HIV infection can and do respond to routine immunizations, although not as well as children with intact

immunity. In addition to diphtheria-pertussis-tetanus (DPT), hemophilus influenza conjugate (HbCV), and hepatitis B (HB) vaccines, the American Academy of Pediatrics, Committee on Infectious Diseases, (AAP; 1994a) recommends inactivated polio, measles-mumps-rubella (MMR) vaccine, the annual influenza vaccine, pneumococcal polysaccharide vaccine at age 2, varicella zoster immune globulin (VZIG) after chicken pox exposure, and immune serum globulin (IG) after measles exposure. At this time, the AAP does not recommend the attenuated varicella zoster vaccine for HIV-infected children.

New CDC guidelines recommend beginning PCP prophylaxis at 4 to 6 weeks of age for all children perinatally exposed to HIV; continuing prophylaxis through 12 months of age for children diagnosed as infected, and making decisions regarding prophylaxis for children greater than 12 months of age based on CD4+ counts and whether PCP previously has occurred (Centers for Disease Control, 1995).

Several antiretroviral drugs are in different stages of investigation, and two—Zidovudine (Zdv) and dideoxyinosine (ddI)—have been approved for use in certain children. Studies of HIV-infected children taking antiretroviral drugs demonstrate gains in height and weight, decreased signs and symptoms associated with HIV infection, improvements in immunological and neurological function, and a better short-term survival rate.

The care of common illnesses in children with HIV infection typically includes managing fevers; diarrhea; vomiting; ear, nose, and throat infections; and skin conditions. Because of the vulnerability of children with HIV infection to germs, physicians will often use antibiotics expectantly, while awaiting results of cultures (Parrott & Rathlev, 1993).

COLLABORATIVE CARE

While the primary health care provider—pediatrician, family physician, or nurse practitioner—is able to provide overall health supervision for a child with HIV infection, he or she will usually consult with a specialist about confirming the diagnosis, classifying the stage of the illness, entering into treatment protocols, and treating the complex sequelae of the disease. A nurse case-manager may help to coordinate services in order to keep appointments to a minimum and to ensure that both sets of health care providers share laboratory findings, growth and development measurements, and immunization records through timely phone calls and letters.

DISCHARGE PLANNING

While many infected women know their HIV status at the time of delivery, it is sometimes hard for them to believe that something may also be wrong with their infants. Women cope in many ways and often feel scared, angry, confused, or overwhelmed. The hospital discharge nurse may encourage a mother to find one person she trusts—someone who knows how to listen—with whom to share the diagnosis. It may be a relative, friend, clergy person, or another infected woman. It is essential to stress with the family that although it may be hard to think about sharing the diagnosis with others, health care team members, such as emergency department staff, do need to know the infant's HIV status so that they can make good medical decisions for the child.

At discharge from the nursery, the nurse will participate in assessing the potential effect of the mother's health on her ability to parent; review with the mother the AAP, Committee on Infectious Diseases, (1994b) recommendations for formula feeding; coordinate follow-up appointments for both mother and child; and request a home nursing visit to assess infection control practices and social service needs. For example, the social worker may need to arrange for a variety of entitlement programs, including Women's, Infant's, Children's (WIC) Program nutrition assistance.

THE FIRST HOME VISIT

During the first home visit, the community health nurse sets the stage for engaging the caregiver in a helping relationship. (See Appendix 24–B.) Any biases and judgments about the mode of transmission—especially if the mother used drugs—must be put aside, so they do not interfere with listening, supporting, and helping. If the caregiver is the mother, she may be distrustful of those associated with the health care system for fear they will report her to child protective services and take the infant away.

Assessment

At the first home visit, the diagnosis of HIV infection in the infant is probably uncertain. The results of definitive testing, such as HIV culture and PCR, may be pending. It could be 1 to 3 months until the infant has a follow-up appointment. Therefore, it is imperative that the community health nurse assess the child's growth and development according to the usual age-appropriate scales and complete a systems review with special attention to the following signs that may subtly suggest HIV disease progression:

- lymph nodes equal to or greater than 0.5 cm
- parotid gland enlargement
- acute or chronic otitis
- oral candidiasis and herpes stomatitis
- abdominal enlargement or distention
- changes in neurological function, that is, strength, tone, reflexes, and gait (Parrott & Rathlev, 1993).

The nurse should also ask about the mother's health: How is "Mom" feeling? Is she taking her own medications and keeping her own medical appointments?

Teaching

Because a child with HIV infection is vulnerable to germs in the environment, it is important for the community health nurse to emphasize how to keep the child healthy and prevent the spread of germs. The best way to prevent the spread of most germs is to wash hands with soap and warm water for 15 sec and then to dry them well (Ward-Wimmer & Riley, 1991). Along with good hand-washing, basic hygiene practices will prevent the spread of many germs found in body secretions and excretions while universal precautions will prevent the spread of germs found in blood and open sores. (See Table 24–1.) The nurse will want to check for the following in the home: warm running water, liquid soap, bleach, rubber gloves, and plastic bags. Written instructions describing how to care for a cut or bloody wound may be helpful for families to use with extended members or babysitters. (See Exhibit 24–1.)

The community health nurse should also review with the family the HIV-affected infant's immunization schedule. All infants who are at risk for HIV, and their siblings in the home, will receive the inactivated form of polio because of the theoretical risk of vaccine-associated polio transmission in the child or to the immunocompromised mother who is changing diapers. HIV-affected children and all household contacts will also receive the influenza vaccine each fall. Because measles and chicken pox (or shingles) can be potentially fatal to the immunocompromised child, the AAP (American Academy of Pediatrics, Committee on Infectious Diseases, 1994a, 1994b) recommends that caregivers should attempt to prevent exposures and notify the physician immediately of such exposures.

Although families try hard to keep children healthy, sooner or later, they get sick. It is essential for the community health nurse to teach the caregiver how to use and read a thermometer in order to tell the physician the child's temperature. Some children have unexplained fevers for varying lengths of time. The physician may ask: How long has the child had a fever? Does the fever come and go? Does the fever go down after giving Tylenol? How much Tylenol did you give? When was the last dose?

Infants with HIV infection sometimes need special or more concentrated formulas as well as a plan for introducing foods according to age and development. After calculating formula intake for the last 24 to 72 hr, the nurse should ask the caregiver to demonstrate how to reconstitute it. Some parents may inappropriately add additional water to make the formula last longer; others may add cereal to increase calories. (Chapter 9 discusses nutritional assessment and teaching in detail.)

Table 24–1 Infection Control at Home

Basic precautions	Universal precautions
Prevent contact	
Keep immunizations up to date	Complete the hepatitis-B vaccination series
Stay home when sick	
Turn away when someone coughs/sneezes	Do not share toothbrushes, toothpaste, pierced earrings, nail
Do not share cups, bottles, plates, utensils, food, drinks, or pacifiers	clippers or razors
Do not touch vomit, urine or stool	Do not touch blood
Do not kiss babies on the mouth	Discourage "blood brother" activities
Do not use fingers as a pacifier	
Discard unused refrigerated formula after 24 hours	
Change diapers away from food areas	Store toothbrushes/toothpaste separately
Dispose of trash daily	
Create barriers	
Cover mouth when coughing or sneezing	Leave scabs alone
Cover unused food/formula and refrigerate	Cover cuts with Bandaids
Cover vomit, urine and stool with a paper towel or newspaper before	Use barriers (gloves, tissues, towels) when caring for bloody
cleaning up	injuries/noses
Cover sand boxes when not in use	
Keep a bowl close by if you feel sick	
Fold soiled disposable diapers inward and tab	Bag blood-soiled disposable items and discard in a tightly covered,
Discard diapers in a tightly covered, plastic-lined container	foot-activated, plastic-lined container
Kill germs	
Wash hands with soap and water before eating and after using the	Wash hands with soap and water after touching blood
bathroom, wiping noses, changing diapers, cleaning up vomit or	
catching a sneeze	
Wipe secretions, stool, and urine from skin	Wash a cut with soap and water and apply disinfectants like
	Betadine
Use household cleaners to clean up vomit, urine, and stool	Remove blood from surfaces with paper towels, wash with any
	household cleanser such as Lysol, rinse with a 10% bleach
Wash soiled clothing/bedding	solution and air dry
Develop a family routine for cleaning	Rinse blood-soiled clothing with cold water or hydrogen peroxide

Source: Courtesy of Project CHAMP, Children's Hospital National Medical Center, Washington, DC.

The nurse can also teach good oral hygiene. The caregiver should feed the infant in an upright position and not prop a bottle or allow the infant to sleep with one, and he or she should clean the mouth after feeding with a cotton tip applicator moistened with warm water. During this procedure, the caregiver can look for white patches in the infant's mouth, suggesting candidiasis, or blisters or sores on the lips, mouth, or tongue, suggesting herpes. Recurrent and persistent candidiasis may make oral intake difficult or painful.

ROUTINE VISITS

The physician may make the diagnosis of HIV infection between 3 and 6 months of age if the child tests positive on two viral tests done at two different times. The children who test negative on two tests—about 75%, also called *serorevertors*—and show no clinical or immunological signs of

infection, will no longer need home nursing care for risks due to HIV.

Assessment

The frequency of routine home visits depends on several factors. These include whether or not the infant is showing evidence of immunosuppression or clinical symptoms of HIV infection and the overall health and coping ability of the mother as primary caregiver. A woman living with HIV infection must acknowledge her emotions as they significantly influence her child's future as well as the family's overall quality of life.

During routine visits, the nurse again assesses the child's growth and development and completes a systems review as described in the first home visit. Because the HIV-infected child is susceptible to organisms that attack the respiratory,

Exhibit 24–1 Helpful Tips for the Babysitter

Important Phone Numbers	
Police	
Fire	
Ambulance	
Poison Center	
Hospital	

IN AN EMERGENCY, DIAL 911

Tips for Caring for Our Child

Feeding routines.	
If our child gets sick. (vomiting, diarrhea, fever)	

Giving Medicines

Child receiving this medicine _____ Time to be given _____

The medicine can be found _____

Amount to be given and how _____

Special instructions:

First Aid

Cuts	**To care for a cut properly:** • Wash your hands first. • Use a cloth or a paper towel to apply pressure and stop bleeding. (A child can often do this himself while you're washing your hands.) • Do not touch blood; blood can have germs. • Wash the cut with soap and water using a cloth or paper towel. • Apply a bandage. Wash your hands.
	To clean bloody surfaces: • Wipe up blood with a paper towel. • Wash surface with soap and water. • Rinse the surface with bleach and water. (1:10 dilution). • Wrap bloody things in newspaper or a plastic bag and discard. • Wash your hands.
Nosebleed	• Sit the child upright with head bent forward. • Do not touch blood; blood can have germs. • Pinch nostrils against the bridge of the nose for 5 minutes. • Repeat if necessary. Wash hands.

Source: Adapted from *Caring at Home: A Guide for Families* by D. Ward-Wimmer and M.W. Riley, The Child Welfare League of America, pp. 35–37, with permission of Children's Hospital National Medical Center, Washington, D.C., © 1991.

gastrointestinal, and integumentary systems, the nurse should pay special attention to any breathing difficulties, coughs, vomiting, diarrhea, and rashes. Finally, all children get cranky or tired. Caregivers soon learn what is normal for their children. The community health nurse may ask if the child has been irritable or fussy for long periods of time, has trouble eating or going to sleep, or seems to be in pain.

Teaching

Infants diagnosed with HIV infection will begin on trimethoprim/sulfamethoxazole (TMP-SMX) for PCP prophylaxis. Those who are symptomatic may begin Zdv, ddI, or a combination of both. When treatment protocols are offered, the community health nurse may help families consider the pros and cons of standard treatment versus protocol, if they have the support of other family members and friends, and whether or not they can accept the changes the protocol may make on family routines (Parrott & Rathlev, 1993). Sometimes, for example, it will be necessary for families participating in a protocol to give antiretroviral medications every 4 to 6 hr, even at night; to record side effects, such as nausea and vomiting, in a log; and to bring the child for laboratory tests every 2 to 4 weeks.

It is important that the community health nurse review the action and side effects of all medications and have the caregiver demonstrate administration when possible. It is a good idea for the caregiver to keep a written log of these medications specifying amount and frequency. The nurse may check the log as well as the amount of medication in the container to assess for compliance. Compliance can be a problem for HIV-infected mothers who may use denial because of the guilt associated with the transmission mode.

If an infant with HIV infection has oral candidiasis, then the community health nurse will need to teach how to administer antifungal agents such as nystatin. Specifically, the caregiver cleans the infant's mouth after eating with a cotton swab and warm water and then applies the medication with another cotton swab to the inside of the cheeks and mouth. The infant then should not eat or drink for at least 30 min.

Skin care is also important. If an infant with HIV infection has dry skin, the caregiver should use mild soaps, oatmeal baths, and lubricating lotions like Eucerin or Aveno. Sometimes baby oil to a dry scalp will minimize cradle cap. It is best to avoid tight braids and plats. The community health nurse should also encourage families to change diapers as soon as they become wet. They should avoid vaseline and cornstarch that can be a breeding ground for germs. Finally, if a rash persists or a candida infection develops, then the child will require special care such as soaking in a sitz bath, leaving the bottom open to air, and applying prescribed medications.

The nurse should also encourage the caregiver to keep the telephone numbers of the pediatrician and specialist close at hand and call for advice if the child has any of the following:

- fever over 101° F
- vomiting and diarrhea
- decreased appetite, difficultly swallowing, or drooling
- rashes, bumps, lumps, or skin sores
- coughing, chest congestion, difficult or painful breathing
- dizziness or shaking of a hand, leg, or foot
- painful, frequent urination
- ear pain, pulling on ears, or drainage of ears
- wounds that will not heal
- exposure to chicken pox or measles (Nieboer, 1992).

Taking the child to the physician is real work for most families. Yet, it is important for families to keep scheduled appointments and think ahead about how to get to the physician for routine and emergency care. In addition, the nurse can prepare families for what happens during blood tests, radiographs, scans, and special procedures. It is important to emphasize to parents that even toddlers understand simple explanations. The nurse or case manager may also arrange for volunteers to provide transportation to appointments and offer respite care to families.

SUBSEQUENT VISITS

As the child becomes severely immunocompromised, and AIDS-defining illnesses develop, the number of physician's appointments multiply, and hospitalizations begin. With repeat visits and hospitalizations, medications are added or changed.

Assessment

During routine visits, the nurse continues to regularly conduct a complete systems review as described in the first home visit with special attention to how comfortable or uncomfortable the child is, to respiratory illnesses, and to changes in growth and development.

As the child experiences more symptoms, pain and discomfort sometimes become a problem. Caregivers are primary interpreters of their children's pain, reporting when and how often it occurs, how long it lasts, what makes it worse, and what makes it better. As the child's condition deteriorates, the use of medical equipment, such as a nebulizer, oxygen, or a feeding pump, may become necessary. The nurse continually assesses the child as well as the caregiver's ability to perform procedures, especially in the following areas:

- *Respiratory illness*—Severe distress with fever, tachypnea, rhonchi, rales, and wheezing may necessitate albuterol via nebulizer and treatment with intravenous antibiotics or prophylaxis with monthly intravenous immune globulin (IVIG) using a heparin lock or indwelling catheter.
- *Growth*—Continued loss or failure to gain weight, as well as dehydration from vomiting and diarrhea may result in alternative feeding methods, such as nasogastric tube (NG), gastrostomy tube (GT), or total parenteral nutrition (TPN).
- *Development*—Failure to attain or loss of milestones may result in changes in treatments or protocols as well as referral to physical or occupational therapy (PT/OT).

Teaching

Often children receive nutrition by alternative means to supplement oral feedings. Many times, alternative feeds are given at night while the child sleeps. If the infant has a NG tube, then the nurse must teach the caregiver how to pass it, check for placement, and administer the feeding slowly. Feedings may be bolus or continuous. If the child has a GT, the nurse must also teach site care. (Chapter 10 discusses enteral feedings in detail.)

Many physicians avoid prescribing TPN because of costs, little or no reimbursement by payers, and associated complications. When TPN is ordered, teaching should center around the daily set-up, take-down, and monitoring of the infusion, and signs and symptoms of hypo- or hyperglycemia. (Chapter 11 discusses parenteral feedings in detail.)

A child who requires intravenous medications at home may have a heparin lock or an indwelling subcutaneous catheter. The community health nurse can demonstrate how to remove the old dressing, clean the insertion site with betadine using clean technique, and apply a new dressing to an indwelling catheter. The nurse should also teach the family how to flush external catheters with heparin or saline (according to agency policy). The caregiver will need to observe the site for tenderness, redness, leakage, or swelling.

A second type of indwelling catheter, such as a port-a-cath, is implanted under the skin. No site care is necessary; however, the family must observe the area for redness or swelling. How much responsibility is expected of the caregiver in catheter maintenance and medication administration is individual and is a decision the nurse makes during teaching and return demonstration.

With some respiratory conditions, the physician may order chest physical therapy (chest PT), oxygen, and aerosols or nebulizer treatments in the home. Chest PT is usually done once or twice a day. The affected lung segment will dictate how to position the child. Often, the caregiver can place the child over his or her knees and gently bounce during the procedure. A television can be a good distraction. The nurse shows the family how to cup hands. Usually, the child wears a thin T-shirt to protect the skin. (Chapter 12 includes a diagram illustrating chest PT.)

If the physician orders an aerosol or nebulizer treatment in conjunction with chest PT, it is given first to open up the bronchial passages and loosen secretions. The nurse teaches the family how to mix and administer aerosol medications via a nebulizer. The nebulizer pieces are cleaned with warm water and left to air dry after each treatment; they are soaked in white vinegar and water for 30 minutes, rinsed with warm water and left to air dry at the end of each day.

During each home visit, the nurse checks the settings on the oxygen to ensure the correct liter flow as ordered, the nasal cannula for correct placement, and the nares for irritation. Periodic equipment maintenance checks are done by the nurse and the durable medical equipment (DME) provider. The nurse continually reinforces fire and electrical safety during oxygen therapy. (Chapters 12 through 16 discuss respiratory care and teaching in detail.)

Infants with developmental delay may need OT and PT at home to maximize and build on abilities. The nurse should encourage caregivers to incorporate what is learned from the therapist into everyday activities. (Chapters 19 and 20 address developmental issues in detail.)

Finally, children should not have to be in pain. There is always something that can be done to lessen pain. The nurse can teach families how to give recommended over-the-counter medicines or stronger prescription drugs when indicated. It also is important to allow for periods of uninterrupted rest. The following tips may be helpful:

- Give older children an active role in controling pain: deep breathing, relaxation, visualization, music, stories, television.
- Keep the environment as calm as possible: speak quietly; keep lights dim; move carefully.
- Make the child comfortable: line the bed with pillows; alternate positions using the palms of the hands; apply gentle heat or use warm baths (Ward-Wimmer & Riley, 1991).

ONGOING CONCERNS

As a significant number of perinatally infected children with HIV are living longer and even into their teens, some of the following issues emerge.

Telling the Child

Parents often say children are not "old enough" to know about HIV. The reluctance to tell an infected child may derive from the fear that the child will tell others the diagnosis. Parents are also concerned that the child will be curious about how the mother became infected. Unlike other illnesses, HIV infection is associated with taboo sex- and drug-related practices. For infected parents, discussing the child's illness equates with discussing "my own infection," which equals guilt. Acknowledgement of HIV infection also brings death into consciousness, while avoidance keeps the illness and its consequences at bay.

Children, quite normally, have an interest in their illness and treatments that they often do not put into words. They may try to listen to conversations with physicians, hint or ask other caregivers about their condition, or otherwise indicate curiosity or partial knowledge.

There is no single or right approach to whether, when, or how to tell a child about HIV. Letting the child know can be a continuum with secrecy at one end and full disclosure at the other (Tasker, 1992). Some parents will pick a specific moment to tell the child. Others may "feed" information over time. Many families will enlist the help of a trusted professional, who may offer to be with them when they talk with the child about HIV infection. It is important for parents to think through how they will respond to questions. The nurse can encourage family members to be honest with the child and siblings about physician's visits and planned procedures as well as in response to questions asked. Additionally, the nurse can role play or "practice" with the caregiver the process of telling the child.

Entry into Day Care or School

Because HIV does not transmit through everyday casual contact, children with HIV infection can attend day care and schools and participate in athletic events (American Academy of Pediatrics, Committee on Sports Medicine and Fitness, 1991; American Academy of Pediatrics, Task Force on Pediatric AIDS, 1991, 1992). They are entitled to all the rights, privileges, and services other children receive. A child with HIV, however, may be immunocompromised, which increases the risks of experiencing severe complications from varicella, tuberculosis, measles, cytomegalovirus, and herpes simplex. Child care providers, teachers, and coaches do not need to know a child's HIV status in order to protect their own health or that of other children. Rather, staff should follow universal precautions at all times. If the family does decide to tell the school, the community health nurse will have the opportunity to shape attitudes about HIV infection. Such efforts serve to strengthen the rights of children with special needs to participate in the normal developmental events of childhood.

HIV-affected Youth

Because children with HIV infection are living into their teens, it is important that they know the facts. The community health nurse may share written materials with families that describe for youth HIV transmission, protection, and prevention (including abstinence and safer sex practices; Rathlev & Riley, 1993). Laws about HIV differ from state to state. Infected teens will need to know their legal rights with regard to testing and future opportunities. In addition, youth will want to know about services that may be available specifically for them. The community health nurse can help youth assess resources for friendliness, accessibility, fee schedule, and privacy.

Alternative Care

It is important for infected women to begin planning for their children's future while they are still healthy. Many want the opportunity to build or strengthen a relationship with the potential caregivers before the children are placed with them. All want their children to be loved and supported emotionally. Some want brothers and sisters to remain together. Often, however, children with HIV infection have special needs, which means that one family cannot take care of all children. The community health nurse can help the mother explore placement options such as standby guardianship, kinship care, and foster and adoptive families. The nurse can also help the mother think about how she wants to share information about her life so that the children will have memories of the family (Merkel-Holguin, 1994).

Loss

While children with HIV infection are living longer, they will eventually develop AIDS and die. Sometimes, families will need to make difficult decisions about a child's care. Should aggressive treatment continue, or should the physicians simply make the child more comfortable? Most of the time, these decisions are not made quickly. The child's condition may change gradually. The nurse working with the family can encourage them to talk with the physician first, to be sure they fully understand the medical realities, expectations, and options. Sometimes, it is hard for families to listen to what the physician says about the disease progression because what they want to hear is that the child is getting well.

The community health or home care nurse may be someone families can trust to help with making the difficult decisions about how to provide comfort, access hospice, and make funeral arrangements. This may seem difficult, because the death of a child is incomprehensible. Fortunately, the skills required in supporting a family are merely a willingness to listen, a commitment to be with them in whatever they are feeling, and caution not to allow personal feelings to usurp the feelings of the family (Rathlev, Riley, & Jones, 1992).

REFERENCES

Allbritten, D.J. (1990). *Children with HIV/AIDS: A sourcebook for caring.* Alexandria, VA: Stone Webb Print Communications Company.

American Academy of Pediatrics, Committee on Infectious Diseases. (1994a). Active and passive immunization. In G. Peter (Ed.), *1994 Red book.* Elk Grove Village, IL: American Academy of Pediatrics.

American Academy of Pediatrics, Committee on Infectious Diseases. (1994b). Recommendations for care of children in special circumstances. In G. Peter (Ed.), *1994 Red book.* Elk Grove Village, IL: American Academy of Pediatrics.

American Academy of Pediatrics, Committee on Sports Medicine and Fitness. (1991). Human immunodeficiency virus (acquired immunodeficiency syndrome—AIDS) in the athletic setting. *Pediatrics, 88*(3), 640–641.

American Academy of Pediatrics, Task Force on Pediatric AIDS. (1991). Education of children with human immunodeficiency virus infection. *Pediatrics, 88*(3), 645–648.

American Academy of Pediatrics, Task Force on Pediatric AIDS. (1992). Guidelines for human immunodeficiency virus (HIV)-infected children and their foster families. *Pediatrics, 89,* 681–683.

Centers for Disease Control. (1994, September). Revised classification system for HIV infection in children, 13 years of age. *Morbidity and Mortality Weekly Report, 43*(RR-12), 1–10.

Centers for Disease Control. (1995, April 28). Revised guidelines for prophylaxis against PCP for children infected with or perinatally exposed to HIV. *Morbidity and Mortality Weekly Report, 44*(RR-4).

Clark, P.J., & Byrne, M.W. (1993). A step from home: Enhanced care for medically complex HIV. *Maternal and Child Health Nursing, 18,* 94–98.

Duliege, A.-M., Messiah, A., Blanche, S., Tardieu, M., Griscelli, C., & Spira, A. (1992). Natural history of human immunodeficiency virus 1 infection in children; prognostic value of laboratory tests on bimodal progression of the disease. *Pediatrics, 11,* 630–635.

Merkel-Holguin, L.A. (1994). *Because you love them: A parent's planning guide.* Washington, DC: The Child Welfare League of America.

Nieboer, N. (1992). *My child's care.* Washington, DC: State of the Art, Inc.

Parrott, R.H., & Rathlev, M. (1993). *Access to primary health care for children with HIV: A guide for pediatricians, family physicians and nurse practitioners.* Washington, DC: Children's National Medical Center.

Rathlev, M., & Riley, M.W. (1993). *Youth and HIV, it's up to you and me. A reference guide for service providers.* Washington, DC: Children's National Medical Center.

Rathlev, M., Riley, M.W., & Jones, S.J. (1992). *Caring in the community for children with HIV: A guide for child care providers, foster families, home health aides, and volunteers.* Washington, DC: The Child Welfare League of America.

Tasker, M. (1992). *How can I tell you?* Bethesda, MD: The Association for the Care of Children's Health.

Wara, D. (1992). Address at the annual meeting of the American Academy of Pediatrics.

Ward-Wimmer, D., & Riley, M.W. (1991). *Caring at home: A guide for families.* Washington, DC: The Child Welfare League of America.

Common Medications for Children with HIV Infection

Name/description/route	Proper use	Precautions	Side effects
Acetaminophen, oral (Tylenol, Panadol, Tempra & store brands) Relieves pain and lowers fevers.	Check directions on bottle. Give with plenty of fluids.	If child is under 12 years old: • do not give more than 5 times a day. • do not give for more than 10 days without doctor's direction. Call a doctor if the pain or fever gets worse.	• diarrhea, nausea or vomiting • stomach cramps or pain in stomach area • loss of appetite • increased sweating
Acyclovir, oral Treats certain viral infections.	Take with meals or snack. Give only the dose ordered.	Do not give a double dose, even if a dose is missed.	• diarrhea, nausea or vomiting • dizziness • headaches • joint pain • loss of appetite
Acyclovir, ointment Treats herpes. Does not cure it.	Apply to cleaned skin. Use a disposable glove to apply the ointment. Turn it inside out before throwing in the trash. Wash hands well.	Do not use near the eyes. If it gets in the eyes, flush right away with lots of cold water and call the doctor.	• mild pain, burning or stinging • itching • skin rash
Dapsone, oral (DDS) Prevents pneumocystis carinii pneumonia (PCP).	Usually given once a day. Give as soon as possible if you miss a dose. If child is also taking ddI, dapsone must be given 2 hours before or 2 hours after ddI dose. Please call the nurse or doctor before you give any other medicines with dapsone (including over the counter).	May cause low blood counts or liver function changes. Be sure to take your child for all scheduled blood tests.	• fever • weakness and fatigue • nausea and vomiting • rashes • numbness or tingling in hands or feet
Videx, oral (ddI) Treats the HIV virus; does not cure it.	Must be given at specific intervals (every 12 hours). Give as soon as possible if you miss a dose. Give 1 hour before or 2 hours after meals.	Call the doctor right away if child has: • stomach discomfort • severe nausea or vomiting • blurred vision • numbness, tingling or pain in hands or feet	• stomach discomfort • nausea or vomiting • diarrhea • numbness, tingling, or pain in hands or feet • constipation
Fluconazole, oral (Diflucan®) Treats serious fungal infections.	Keep liquid form in the refrigerator. Shake well. Keep giving the medicine for as long as the doctor ordered. Do not double doses.	Call the doctor right away if you see: • yellow skin or eyes • dark urine • loss of appetite • red, blistered, or loose skin	• diarrhea • headache • nausea • stomach pain • vomiting

(Continued on next page)

Name/description/route	Proper use	Precautions	Side effects
Retrovir, oral (Zidovudine) Treats the HIV virus, but does not cure it.	Must be given at specific intervals; you may need to set an alarm clock. May be given with food.	Can cause low blood counts. Be sure to take your child for all scheduled blood tests.	• nausea or vomiting • headaches • muscle aches
Rifabutin, oral (Mycobutin) Prevents mycobacterium avium complex (MAC).	Take with food if stomach upset occurs. Can be mixed with food, like applesauce.	May cause low blood counts. Be sure to take your child for all scheduled blood tests.	• rash • nausea or vomiting • diarrhea • body fluids, skin and stool may be colored brown-orange
Gancyclovir, oral Treats CMV (cytomegalovirus) infection—does not cure it.	Give on a regular schedule to keep a constant amount in the body.	May lower the number of platelets in the blood that are needed for clotting. Call the doctor if you notice: • bleeding or bruising • black, tarry stools • blood in urine or stools • pinpoint red spots on skin. Be careful using a toothbrush, dental floss, or toothpick. Check with the doctor before having any dental work done.	• mood changes • skin rash • tiredness • loss of appetite
Ketoconazole, oral (Nizoral®) Treats fungal infections.	Be careful when breaking tablet into smaller pieces for younger children. Never make up missed doses. Give *only* the exact dose. If patient also taking ddI, Ketoconazole should be taken 2 hours before or 2 hours after dose of ddI.	Call the doctor right away if you see: • dark or amber urine • pale stools • unusual tiredness or weakness • yellow skin or eyes	• diarrhea • headache • skin rash or itching • eye sensitivity to light
Nystatin, oral Treats fungal infections in the mouth.	Use right after eating. Clean mouth before applying. Apply with a swab—rub on white patches in mouth. Do not give food or drink for 30 minutes after applying.		• nausea or vomiting • diarrhea
Nystatin, ointment or powder Treats fungal infections on the skin.	Apply to cleaned skin. Apply *thin* layer wearing a glove. Do not wrap or apply a barrier unless instructed.	Call the doctor if swelling or redness appears where medicine was applied.	
Steroids, oral (Prednisolone, Prednisone, Prelone, Pediapred) Reduces inflammation (swelling).	Take with food. If you miss a dose and the dosing schedule is: • one dose a day—do *not* double the next dose. • several doses a day—double the next dose. Always check these instructions with the doctor. Doses will be reduced gradually—check directions carefully.	Call the doctor right away if the child has: • blurred vision • increased thirst or urination • persistent abdominal pain Do not stop the medicine without checking with the doctor.	• may slow growth in children and adolescents if taken for a long time. • stomach upset • increased appetite • general facial puffiness • acne or other skin problems

(Continued on next page)

Name/description/route	Proper use	Precautions	Side effects
Trimethoprim sulfa, oral (Bactrim®, Septra®) Treats infection. It may also be given IV (by vein) in the hospital. Helps prevent PCP.	When used to ***treat*** an infection, is given every day. When used to ***prevent*** an infection, is usually given 3 days per week. Use ***exactly*** as directed.	Some children are allergic to this. Call the doctor right away if the child gets a rash. Don't give any more doses without the doctor's instructions.	• upset stomach • low blood counts • nausea or vomiting • diarrhea

Source: Adapted from *Caring at Home: A Guide for Families,* by D. Ward-Wimmer and M.W. Riley, The Child Welfare League of America, pp. 43–45, with permission of Children's Hospital National Medical Center, Washington, D.C., © 1991.

Home Care Plan: The Infant or Child Who Is HIV Positive

Date _____   Case manager _____

Name _____ Hosp # _____ DOB _____

PROBLEM: **HIV**

GOALS/OBJECTIVES	METHODS	STAFF/REVIEW
The family will share the diagnosis of HIV infection with health professionals who need to know and one significant person for support.	Assess in what stage of disclosure the family is. Encourage the family members to share the diagnosis with health care professionals—primary health caregivers, specialists, and emergency department (ED) staff— so they can make the best decisions for the child. Help the family members to name one person with whom they can share the diagnosis; use role play. Help the family decide who else needs to know the child's diagnosis— extended family, babysitters, child care providers. Accept the use of denial for periods of emotional respite. Identify support groups when the family is ready. Refer to a psychiatric social worker as appropriate.	
The child will be free of infections.	Assess the child for signs of infection. Administer IVIG as ordered; monitor for side effects. Teach families about • basic infection control, universal precautions, PCP, and prophylaxis • how to measure/give antibiotics and actions and side effects • how to take a temperature/read a thermometer • when to give antipyretics • when to call the physician	

GOALS/OBJECTIVES	METHODS	STAFF/REVIEW
The child's immunizations will be up to date.	Review the child's immunization record. Encourage families to keep well-child and immunization appointments. Teach the families that HIV-affected children also need the following: • inactivated polio (also siblings) • annual influenza (also household members) • pneumovax at age 2 • VZIG following chicken pox exposure • IG following measles exposure.	
The child will take in adequate calories to meet metabolic and growth needs.	Compare changes in height, weight, abdominal, and head circumference to previous visit. Review caloric intake for 72 hr and compare to norms. Inquire about urine and stool output. Examine mouth for lesions including milky patches. Teach families about culturally acceptable foods that are high in protein, vitamins, minerals, and calories and how to give supplements. Encourage families to offer six small meals/nutritious snacks per day. Suggest the following if the child has sores in the mouth: • licks of popsicles or ice before eating • soft bland foods at room temperature • a straw for older children. Teach families how to pass a nasogastric (NG) tube and give feedings through an NG, gastrostomy (GT), or central line as appropriate. Refer to a nutritionist as appropriate.	
The child will have clear breath sounds and pulse and respiratory rate for age.	Auscultate chest for rales, rhonchi, decreased breath sounds, retractions, nasal flaring, and grunting. Assess characteristics of cough and sputum. Check oxygen equipment for setting, flow, and filter change. Check the nebulizer for filter change.	

GOALS/OBJECTIVES	METHODS	STAFF/REVIEW
	Teach families how to perform chest physiotherapy, coughing, and deep breathing exercises and give nebulizer treatments (clean after each use). Refer to physical therapist as appropriate.	
The child's skin will be clean, dry, and intact.	Examine the skin for redness, breakdown, and dryness as well as white patchy areas. Teach families how to care for open sores: • Clean with mild soap and warm water. • Apply a thin layer of antifungals and other agents as ordered. • Cover with a pad. • Watch for signs of infection. Teach families the following about diaper care: • Change diapers as soon as they are wet. • Clean the diaper area with warm water; squeeze water from a wet rag if skin is sore. • Pat or air day. Teach families central line and GT site care.	
The child's mouth will be free of sores.	Teach families the following about mouth care: • Clean teeth 2–3 times a day with a soft brush or cotton swab. • Apply antifungals as ordered with a swab. • Do not give food or medication for 30 minutes after giving antifungals.	
The child will attain developmental milestones.	Complete developmental assessment as appropriate. Teach families how to measure/give antiretrovirals and what their actions and side effects are. Review and reinforce antiretroviral protocol requirements with families. Assist families with completing protocol paperwork; encourage them to keep monthly laboratory appointments.	

GOALS/OBJECTIVES	METHODS	STAFF/REVIEW
	Teach families about safe, age-appropriate toys; reinforce how families can integrate what they learn into activities of daily living (ADL) and play. Refer to OT as appropriate.	
The child will be comfortable.	Listen to the family when they say the child is in pain; compare with vital signs. Teach families when to give analgesics and what common side effects are. Review some other pain management techniques with families: • Line the bed with soft blankets. • Alternate positions. • Lift child using palms of hands. • Apply gentle heat or use warm baths. • Use distraction—imagining, television, music, stories.	
The family will make decisions about providing comfort versus care and funeral arrangements.	Continuously clarify with the family treatment options for mother, child, and other affected family members. Encourage the family members to share their grief. Support the family members when they choose comfort versus treatment as their goal. Refer to the legal department, ethics committee, or hospice as appropriate. Assist the family with funeral plans; determine with them what else needs to be done.	

Chapter 25

Assessment and Management of Genetic Problems in the Home Setting

Lynette Wright, RN, MN

Nurses practicing in the community health or home care setting should recognize dysmorphic features, problems in growth, or delays in development in infants, children, or adults within the family unit. Many such problems have a specific genetic cause. Early identification of genetic problems has benefits ranging from saving a life (e.g., galactosemia); to ensuring appropriate supportive services (e.g., Down syndrome); to encouraging genetic testing and counseling for uncertain signs, symptoms, and family patterns.

This chapter begins with a discussion of the importance of genetics in pediatric nursing practice, provides both a review of genetic principles and a general introduction to causes of genetic disorders, and outlines the role of the home care and community health nurse with regard to genetic conditions. Additionally, the chapter provides an in-depth discussion, an example, and nursing implications for the various categories of genetic disorders: chromosomal, single gene (autosomal dominant, autosomal recessive, X-linked dominant, X-linked recessive), and multifactorial disorders. (See Appendix 25–A for definitions of these and other genetics terms.)

GENETICS AND PEDIATRIC NURSING PRACTICE

In the past, many nurses have thought of genetics as a collection of a few exotic disorders that were fascinating and challenging but not a part of their daily practice. This is partly because it was not until recent decades that genetic intervention strategies developed. In 1956, the correct number of chromosomes was identified, and by the late 1950s, Down syndrome was shown to be caused by an extra chromosome (Thompson, McInnes, & Huntington, 1991). During the 1960s, chromosome testing expanded, and biochemical techniques had advanced to the point that a few rare recessive disorders could be identified and treated; by the end of the decade, population-based newborn screening for phenylketonuria (PKU) was beginning. The early 1970s ushered in amniocentesis as a prenatal diagnostic technique that became a major strategy in identifying serious genetic disorders. Newborn screening expanded to include a variety of disorders, and carrier screening for Tay-Sachs and sickle cell anemia was instituted across the country. In the 1980s, prenatal diagnosis expanded to include sophisticated ultrasound and other high-technology early diagnostic techniques, and screening for spina bifida and Down syndrome from maternal blood samples became widespread. In the 1990s, both molecular techniques that analyze genetic problems at the DNA level and the beginning of gene therapy emerged (Thompson et al., 1991).

In this decade and into the 21st century, genetics must become more than a disease model. Each person's individual genetic pattern forms the outside framework upon which all health and illness interacts. Genetic patterns determine the degree of our ability to adapt to specific environmental alterations, including how long we will live and whether we will develop infections or malignancies. Our genetic self reaches far beyond prenatal and neonatal variations. Techniques are being developed, as part of the ongoing worldwide Human Genome Project, that will include strategies to identify not only the genetic problems of childhood but also most of the predisposing genes for adult-onset disorders (Cook-Deegan, 1991). In this generation, delivery of health services will be adapted to account for individual genetic variation and predisposition, and almost all of these screening services will take place in community or home settings. As we move into the 21st century, such advances will prevent death and disability, foster the development of new and more effective therapeutic techniques, and make actual cures for lethal genetic disorders possible (Cook-Deegan, 1991). Genetic assessment and early intervention will be an essential step if we are to be effective in instituting therapies and cures for previously untreatable genetic disorders.

Even with current techniques, recognizable genetic problems are not rare. Genetic problems account for over 60% of all pregnancy losses, with 50% occurring due to identifiable chromosome errors (Centers for Disease Control, 1988). Of live born children, 15% to 16% have genetic problems that can be identified by 1 year of age. Birth defects are the leading cause of infant mortality and the fourth leading cause of diminished life span. Genetic disorders account for 30% to 50% of pediatric hospital admissions in developed countries (Centers for Disease Control, 1989). However, except for Down syndrome, fewer than 3% of patients with known genetic disorders receive genetic counseling while hospitalized (Hall, 1990). With early hospital discharge becoming the normal procedure, many genetic problems and birth defects will be missed. Only the most serious structural defects will be identified at birth, and virtually all children will be discharged before the cardiac, metabolic, and other systems have completed their normal newborn adjustments. Therefore, nurses in community and home health practices must be well grounded in genetic principles and basic counseling techniques if they are to be able to recognize genetic problems, provide support, make appropriate referrals, provide case management, and prepare patients for testing and/or genetic counseling.

CLASSIFICATION OF GENETIC DISORDERS

Many nurses have not completed a genetics course. Biological principles taught in science courses and in the clinical setting may not have been connected to genetics. Therefore, basic biological principles must be reviewed if the home health nurse is to grasp the profound new scientific discoveries that are revealing the mechanisms by which healthy and disease-producing genes work. (See Appendix 25–A for a glossary of terms and Exhibit 25–1 for a concise review of concepts.)

Genes control both the development of every body structure and the regulatory processes that account for normal growth, development, and maintenance throughout the life span. Basically, genetic information is carried in the chromosomes of human cells, packaged into tightly wound coils of DNA. The genetic information carried on DNA codes for the production of proteins that have structural, circulatory, metabolic, hormonal, or transport functions and, thus, determine structural, functional, and developmental traits of the individual.

The human cell contains 46 chromosomes (23 pairs). One pair will include the X or Y sex chromosome. Traits coded for by genes included on these sex chromosomes are called *sex-linked*, or *X-linked*, traits. Traits coded for by genes on any of the other 22 pairs (called *autosomal pairs*) are called *autosomal traits*. Some traits are dominant, which means they can manifest any time the gene coding for that trait is present in the cell. Other traits are recessive and only manifest if two genes in the cell (one from each parent) both code for the trait (e.g., two genes code for blue eyes). A separate pattern of inheritance occurs in X-linked inheritance, which is discussed later in this chapter.

While genetic variation is the source of variety and adaptability in the human race (see detailed explanation in Exhibit 25–1), some variations or mutations in the genes can lead to problems. Genetic problems range from minor malformations or dysmorphisms (e.g., an extra digit) to major syndromes (e.g., Down syndrome) and ultimately fatal disorders (e.g., Tay-Sachs disease).

Traditionally, geneticists and other health care providers have classified genetic disorders into three major groups, as follows:

1. *Chromosome disorders*—include variations in chromosome number, deletions of chromosome material, and chromosomal rearrangements.
2. *Single gene disorders*—include syndromes that are inherited in an autosomal dominant, autosomal recessive, or X-linked pattern of inheritance.
3. *Multifactorial disorders*—include malformations and diseases that occur because of interaction between several interactive liability genes and one or more negative environmental influences.

These three categories account for most malformations, syndromes, and childhood illnesses, including allergies and response to infection. Only problems resulting from childhood accidents or prenatal teratogenic exposure would be exempt from some level of genetic causation or interaction. These groups of genetic disorders will be more thoroughly defined and described, with examples, later in the chapter. Understanding these genetic disorders will prepare the nurse to answer questions that families inevitably ask, such as: Why did this happen? What is the chance this will happen again?

Exhibit 25–1 A Review of General Concepts in Genetics

Fundamentally, human genetics is not entirely predictable. Interaction occurs within the genome itself and between genes and the environment. While our understanding of less traditional concepts is just emerging, review of major concepts is essential if we are to understand the "new genetics" and apply it to nursing practice in the home setting.

REVIEW OF CELL FUNCTIONS

Understanding heredity begins with a review of the individual cell and cell cycle. Within the nucleus of each human cell lies the entire genetic code. When the cell is not dividing, it performs biological functions. During this portion of the cell cycle, the genetic material is spread out in loose strands, somewhat like a plate of spaghetti. When the cell prepares to divide, the genetic material replicates (makes a complete copy of itself) and then condenses into discrete bodies called *chromosomes,* which contain precise sequences of tightly coiled DNA. At this point, we can count 46 individual chromosomes in the human species. These 46 chromosomes (23 pairs) house over 80,000 genes made up of 6 billion base pairs that form DNA strands. Being tightly coiled during cell division is essential to ensure that the precise amount of DNA information on each chromosome will be transmitted to the new cell. This type of cell division, which ensures that daughter cells receive the appropriate set of genetic information, is called *mitosis.* It is during the stage of mitosis called *metaphase* that the chromosomes become compact enough to be individually identified under the ordinary microscope. The ability to see individual chromosomal bodies makes modern chromosome analysis possible (Thompson et al., 1991).

Meiosis is the special two-step process of cell division by which gametes (eggs and sperm) are formed. Meiosis I, or reduction division, is a complex series of steps in which the DNA replicates, and the 46 chromosomes are matched in homologous pairs and then divided so that the egg or sperm (only 23 chromosomes each) will have one of each chromosome pair in its reduced number. Genetic information is also exchanged between chromatids (individual chromosome strands) during this pairing. During meiosis II, the already replicated chromatids are divided without further replication, producing 4 gametes with 23 chromosomes each.

Many errors can occur in both types of cell division, meiosis and mitosis, but certain stages of meiosis I are prone to cell division irregularities that can lead to chromosome abnormalities in offspring.

MICROPACKAGING INFORMATION

A major concept in understanding human genetics is micropackaging. The most sophisticated computer does not begin to house the amount of information found in the human cell: six billion base pairs are compacted into 80,000+ genes that are arranged on DNA strands spun into 46 chromosomes that are packaged into the nucleus of each cell. Within the nucleus of each cell in the body is contained almost all of the genetic information for an entire individual. The genetic information is housed on linear strands of DNA. The DNA is made up of individual base pairs arranged in a precise order. Small groups of these base pairs make up individual genes that code for specific proteins that have many functions in the body, including structural, circulatory, enzymatic, transport, and hormonal (Mange & Mange, 1994). Genetic traits are the structural or functional outcomes or manifestations of the action of these proteins.

To encode an enormous amount of information into a single-cell nucleus, DNA strands are twisted into a double helix, super coiled onto spools of protein, and arranged like beads on a string. The coiled DNA becomes the basic structural unit, called *chromatin,* which is then supercoiled again. Micropackaging into coiled units does more than confine information into a small space. Packaging DNA in precise ways appears to provide control over which genes are expressed and at what time. Perhaps this partially explains why a differentiated cell such as bone or muscle "knows" to perform only certain functions, even though the entire genome is present in the nucleus of each cell (Thompson et al., 1991).

GENETIC VARIATION

Genes code for the production of specific structural, circulatory, metabolic, or transport proteins. These proteins, through their action in the human body, determine structural, functional, and developmental traits or characteristics of an individual. Thus, variations in genes ultimately lead to variations in the manifestation of human traits. Genes code for traits as varied as hair color and blood type. Of course, some traits, such as age, height, weight, and disease risk are understood to have both genetic and environmental influences. The wide range of gene–environment interactions is only beginning to be appreciated.

In fact, the key to genetic health lies in the vast variability and adaptive capacity of the human species. Put simply, hybrids are more healthy than inbreds. Therefore, over evolutionary time, biological species have developed a number of ways to ensure variability. In fact, several natural mechanisms encourage genetic variations: crossing over (recombination), assortment, and mutation.

Crossing over, or *recombination,* occurs during meiosis when the pairing of maternal and paternal chromosomes, and the point-to-point exchange of small segments between chromatids, bring new combinations of genes to the subsequent gametes. While crossing over is a healthy event, an error such as a microdeletion of genetic material can be introduced any time an exchange occurs. In addition, the presence of a recombination event can be a source of confusion when one is attempting to track a particular gene within a family unit.

Assortment, one of the major principles described by Gregor Mendel in 1865, is the random distribution of different combinations of maternal and paternal chromosomes during the process of gamete formation (Thompson et al., 1991).

(continues)

Exhibit 25–1 Continued

Mutation means any permanent change in the DNA. At a practical level, mutation is a change in the message or code that indicates what type of protein should be produced. Once a mutation occurs, it is transmitted as part of the DNA code to subsequent generations.

Not all mutations or other variations are harmful. Alternative forms of genetic information at a particular gene location are called *alleles*. Many genes have only one healthy version, but other genes have many forms. One of the oldest and best examples of healthy allelic variations are those found in human blood groups, such as the ABO and Rh systems.

On the other hand, mutations can have serious consequences. Genes code for specific proteins that dictate our structural characteristics and control our regulatory functions. Even a minute variation in the sequence of the bases in the DNA or a loss of a small fraction of chromosomal material can have profound biological consequences. Faulty transmission of genetic information can result in a variety of genetic disorders.

ROLE OF THE NURSE

Genetic assessment of the newborn includes a battery of newborn screening tests that are designed to identify treatable disorders that can cause death or mental retardation in the first few weeks of life. (See galactosemia model later in the chapter.) Neonatal screening tests are regulated by public health authorities, and required tests vary from state to state. The nurse should be familiar with state regulations and the types of tests provided before hospital discharge. Some tests may need to be provided or repeated after discharge. In regard to screening tests, the nurse should be able to educate families about the reasons for neonatal testing, the types of tests provided, the difference between a screening test and a diagnostic test, and ways to access test results.

The community health or home care nurse has several other important roles related to the assessment of genetic disorders. These include obtaining a family history and completing an assessment of the infant or young child. A basic genetic assessment should include the following:

- obtaining a three-generation family history or reviewing an existing history
- conducting a physical assessment, which should include growth parameters, a description of any unusual features, and minor or major malformations
- conducting age-appropriate neurological and developmental assessments.

When combined with objective data from the child's physical assessment, the family genetic history (and the resulting pedigree chart, if developed) will provide the basis both for determining if other family members need assessment or information and for making recommendations to the family regarding their need for a comprehensive genetic evaluation.

In addition to participating in the assessment of genetic disorders, the community or home health nurse has important roles to play in providing family support, direct nursing care, family education, and care coordination.

Family History

Obtaining and analyzing a family history is part of the nursing role regardless of clinical setting. Its purpose is to assess genetic risk within a family unit. Obtaining a comprehensive genetic family history assists in making an appropriate diagnosis; clarifies the natural history of the disorder; provides insight into the medical and social burden; and establishes the reliability of the parent, relative, or other caregiver who is providing the information. Important information that should be obtained routinely as part of the genetic family history is listed in Exhibit 25–2.

While a narrative family history may be adequate for most purposes, only a pedigree can illustrate the relationships between relatives that then allows the nurse or the genetic specialist to calculate risks for specific disorders. The pedigree lays out in diagram form the medical, health, social, and ethnic background information obtained in the genetic family history of the individual and family. All first-degree relatives (parents, siblings, and children) who are one step away from the identified patient and second-degree relatives (grandparents, aunts, uncles, nieces, nephews, and grandchildren) who are two steps away should be included. The family may have an informal historian who can supplement information provided by the parent. A sample pedigree chart is included in Appendix 25–B.

Exhibit 25–2 Genetic Family History

1. Centers around an identified client (index case)
2. Includes at least first- and second-degree relatives
3. Identifies ethnicity
4. Defines potential risks by asking about:
   - recurrent spontaneous abortions (miscarriages)
   - stillbirths
   - children born with malformations
   - children who have died
   - conditions occurring more than once in a family
   - any known genetic disorder

Assessment of the Infant and Young Child

A referral may have been made for home nursing follow-up of a newborn because serious chromosomal problems, such as Down syndrome, trisomy 18, or trisomy 13, were identified or suspected or because meconium ileus was present in the newborn nursery, raising a suspicion of cystic fibrosis. Obvious variations, such as cleft lip or polydactyly, may have been noted in the nursery. More often, however, specific concerns may not have been noted in the hospital, and the nurse in the home picks up on subtle signs, such as poor muscle tone, ineffective sucking, or minor malformations, that should lead to further genetic evaluation.

Assessment of the infant or young child has several components. First, the nurse should conduct both a systems review and a thorough physical assessment, obtain growth parameters, and chart a description of any unusual features, including minor or major malformations. Minor malformations are generally subtle structural differences or characteristics that, in themselves, do not have medical implications. Examples of minor malformations are included in Exhibit 25–3. Major malformations include either the more noticeable structural characteristics, such as an extra digit, or structural characteristics with functional or medical implications, such as cleft lip and palate. In addition to a physical assessment, age-appropriate neurological and developmental assessments are part of a thorough assessment for genetic disorders.

Because early detection and intervention may prevent complications and reduce the severity of some disorders, the nurse should consider a genetic referral whenever major abnormalities or more than two minor anomalies are detected. Specific symptom checklists can be used to assist the nurse in completing a thorough assessment when there is reason to suspect or rule out particular genetic disorders. (See Appendix 25–C for an example.)

During the first month of life, the home care or community health nurse has a crucial role in early identification of both congenital heart and metabolic disorders. Because of early hospital discharge, many forms of congenital heart disorders will not be identified in the newborn nursery and may first be identified by the nurse in the home. Additionally, many metabolic problems will become apparent over the course of the infant's first month of life. In this regard, the nurse should be alert for any history of vomiting, lethargy, or apnea following feeding or any unusual odors or coloration that might suggest a metabolic problem. Seizures at any age are a concern, but early onset seizures can suggest a metabolic cause that may be treatable. Similarly, either hypotonia or spasticity should make one "think genetic." For example, Prader-Willi syndrome and congenital myotonic dystrophy are characterized by hypotonia that can be extreme. Children with untreated maple syrup urine disease have severe spasticity and dysarthria that are indistinguishable from cerebral palsy.

Exhibit 25–3 Examples of Minor Malformations or Dysmorphic Features

Variation	Significance
Low-set ears	May indicate craniofacial problems, small head or small brain, developmental delay
2 crown hair whirls	Underlying brain variation from 10 weeks gestation
Hyperpigmented spots	Usually abnormal: cafe au lait, ash leaf, shagreen patch, midline nevus flammeus, etc.
Pectus excavatum or carinatum	May indicate underlying cardiac malformations
Hairy or pigmented base of spine	May indicate underlying spinal malformations
Eye slant	May be familial or may be associated with a variety of syndromes (i.e., upslant in Down syndrome, downslant in Turner syndrome)
Micrognathia (receding chin)	Familial, teratogen influences, or associated with over 60 different syndromes, such as Treacher Collins syndrome or trisomy 18
Flat nasal bridge	May be a normal variant in some ethnic groups; also associated with over 50 syndromes, including achondroplastic dwarfism, Down syndrome, and osteogenesis imperfecta

By 1 month of age, most autosomal chromosome disorders (though not disorders of sex chromosomes) will have been identified. Multifactorial conditions such as pyloric stenosis, congenital dislocated hips, and club feet should also be identified by this time.

By 2 to 4 months of age, other forms of genetic conditions such as sickle cell anemia and cystic fibrosis can be identified. Many disorders that are recognizable early on have dysmorphic craniofacial features or bony abnormalities. Children with several forms of genetic illness do not grow well, and failure to thrive during the first months of life may be a marker for some genetic disorders. In this regard, the single most important genetic assessment tool for the nurse working with the infant and young child is a tape measure. Assessment of height, weight, and head circumference is critical at this stage, and their measurement should not be delegated to less qualified personnel.

Speech and language delays are also clues to genetic disorders. Girls with XXX syndrome have specific delays in language even when general development is near normal.

Speech delays and unusual language patterns have previously been noted in individuals with fragile X. Hearing loss, which may be dominant, recessive, or X-linked, is associated with speech delays. The nurse should be alert to genetic causes during both hearing and vision screening evaluations.

Any child with developmental delay should be assessed for physical features such as multiple hair whirls or microcephaly, which identify the central nervous system insult as prenatal rather than a result of birth trauma. Mental retardation and developmental disabilities have a genetic cause in many children. Some such disorders are chromosomal, such as Down syndrome, trisomy 18 or 13. Others are ultimately fatal autosomal recessive disorders, such as Tay-Sachs disease or adrenoleukodystrophy. All children with significant developmental delay should have a referral to a geneticist and a developmental specialist for in-depth assessments. Since genetic problems tend to recur in families, precise diagnosis is essential in order to both determine the most appropriate treatment plan and to provide appropriate genetic counseling. Children with genetically based developmental delay do not "outgrow it," although early intervention is significant in maximizing their potential.

Family Support

Family members may need particular support when a child is first diagnosed with a genetic disorder. Denial, anger, and bargaining responses are common and are part of the grief process. This is especially true when the condition has lifelong implications or is lethal. Parental depression, guilt, overprotectiveness of the child, and anxiety regarding reproductive options are frequent responses. Guilt for having "passed on" an abnormal gene may affect several generations of family members.

The nurse cannot solve all the family's problems but can help in several ways. Caring communications, including holding or touching the child, will help the family feel less alone. Active listening, in which the nurse is nonjudgmental but interprets and reflects communications back to the family for clarification, assists family members to explore feelings, work through emotional reactions, and consider options (Bauer & Hill, 1986; Gordon, 1970). The nurse can also support the family by providing information about the diagnosis, available services, and parent-support and advocacy organizations. (Two of the most widely known organizations providing information and support are the local chapters of March of Dimes and the Alliance of Genetics Support Groups at 1-800-336-4363.)

Direct Care and Family Education

Nurses may be called upon to assist families over time with the various direct care needs of the child with a genetic condition. These may include hygiene, medications, fluid and nutrition management, pain relief, comfort measures, and periodic examinations. Direct care provides an opportunity for assessing parental educational needs and for providing instruction as appropriate.

Coordination of Care

Genetic disorders are complex and require a team approach that may include a variety of agencies and specialists such as geneticists; genetic counselors; nutritionists; physical, occupational, and speech therapists; and special education services staff. The nurse can assist the family in case management tasks (see Chapter 6) including arranging appointments, gathering information, and ensuring communication between the numerous professionals and agencies.

The nurse working with a child having a genetic problem should also recognize that genetics is a fast-moving field and should be alert for new developments, tests, and therapies that are rapidly becoming available. The nurse and family should further be aware that if the child's medical situation changes, an additional genetic evaluation may be warranted.

UNDERSTANDING CHROMOSOME DISORDERS

A chromosome disorder is any clinical presentation in which there is an identifiable alteration in chromosome number or arrangement. This may involve either a whole chromosome or a small segment of a particular chromosome. Chromosome disorders result from nondisjunction in gamete formation (the failure of chromosomes to separate during cell division), mosaicism (a nondisjunction occurring after a normal egg and sperm have joined), translocation (when chromosomes break and are rearranged during cell division), and duplications and deletions of genetic material (occurring during cell division or as a result of exposure to mutagens). Maternal age can increase the risk of nondisjunction.

Causes of Chromosome Disorders

Nondisjunction

The mechanism by which most variations in chromosome number occur is called *nondisjunction* because one or more chromosomes fail to "disjoin" or separate during cell division. The most common live-born example of nondisjunction results in gametes (sperm or egg cells) that will have one extra chromosome (trisomy). Pregnancies involving a fetus with a missing chromosome (monosomy) most commonly result in miscarriage. Nondisjunction is usually an accident of cell division and not an inherited characteristic, so chromosome problems resulting from nondisjunction events rarely recur in subsequent pregnancies. However, there is evidence that suggests that some families are predisposed to nondisjunction. In these cases, one might find a variety of chromosome problems scattered throughout the family history. Additionally, because of this, the home health nurse should note any miscarriages or previous chromosomal disorders as part of the health history.

Mosaicism

Even if the gametes (sperm or egg cells) have the appropriate chromosome number, and fertilization proceeds normally, a chromosome problem can still be introduced by a nondisjunction error in subsequent cell division. This is called *mosaicism* and results when an error of cell division (mitosis) in early embryonic development causes some cells within an individual to have an extra chromosome, some cells to have a missing chromosome, and some cells to be normal all within the same individual. Most of the time, the monosomy (missing chromosome) cell line will not survive, but the trisomy cells may persist along with the normal cells producing a clinically observable condition. Mosaic children are usually more mildly affected than children with full trisomy conditions, but this will vary depending on the proportion of normal and abnormal cells. Genetically normal parents have no increased recurrence risk for mosaicism; but a parent who is even mildly mosaic has a greatly increased risk for children with full trisomy. Genetic counseling is warranted for these families.

Translocations

Another type of chromosome disorder results from rearrangements, also called *translocations.* Chromosome rearrangements are called translocations because in either meiosis or mitosis, chromosomes can be broken and reattached (translocated) to other chromosomes. Translocations are permanent attachments and can be passed on to subsequent generations. A person who has a chromosome rearrangement without extra or missing chromosome material is called a *balanced translocation carrier* and is physically and mentally normal. However, when translocation carriers produce gametes, it is possible to transmit chromosome combinations with extra or missing chromosome material. Some of these combinations are always lethal, whereas others produce children with recognizable chromosome syndromes. Other combinations are balanced like the parent or entirely normal. Parents who are balanced translocation carriers have a significant risk for producing chromosomally abnormal offspring. Therefore, any child with a chromosome abnormality should have chromosome analysis to determine if the cause was a trisomy or a translocation. If a translocation is noted, both parents should be studied to determine if either parent is a balanced carrier or if the orig-

inal translocation occurred in the child (de novo translocation). Expert genetic counseling is essential whenever a translocation is suspected.

Duplications or Deletions

Structural changes in the chromosome can also result from duplications or deletions. Causes can include errors during mitosis and meiosis or exposure to radiation or chemical mutagens. Large deletions have been associated with known syndromes, such as cri du chat syndrome (chromosome 5p-) with mental retardation, growth retardation, dysmorphic facial features, and an abnormal cry, or Prader-Willi syndrome (chromosome 11q-) in which children present with marked hypotonia and are poor feeders but become grossly obese, short, and mentally retarded. Recent molecular techniques have uncovered microdeletions and molecular duplications that account for numerous other syndromes with previously unknown causes. Deletions may be inherited or may arise in a particular zygote. Therefore, careful genetic evaluation is essential for any couple who delivers a child with a chromosome problem, and prenatal diagnosis is available for reassurance in subsequent pregnancies.

Maternal Age

Another important factor contributing to the presence of chromosomal disorders is maternal age. Each month during ovulation, the individual ovum must complete meiosis as it proceeds down the Fallopian tube. Any woman has only one set of ova that were established during her fetal life, and these eggs are subject to the effects of aging, influences of illness, background radiation, or whatever else has occurred to her. These factors increase the chance for nondisjunction to occur in the ova or during meiosis in an older female, particularly after age 30. This is true whether it is a first or subsequent pregnancy. While the individual risk for nondisjunction increases with maternal age, chromosomal errors do occur in young mothers as well. Counseling regarding prenatal diagnosis options is typically considered for any woman over 35 years of age and should also be available to a woman of any age who has had a child with a chromosomal error. Males are not at an increased risk for nondisjunction until much later in life, as a new supply of sperm is made every 64 days (Hook & Cross, 1979).

Chromosome Analysis

Extra or missing chromosome material can be identified in chromosomes during the metaphase of mitosis. Therefore, to complete a chromosome analysis, cells must be cultured, cell division suspended, metaphases identified, and nuclei visually inspected under the microscope. Chromosomes are then counted in each metaphase, photographed, and paired for analysis in a standard karyotype format.

Chromosome studies take 1 to 3 weeks to complete. Therefore, most infants with possible chromosome disorders are sent home from the hospital before the results are available. The nurse providing home follow-up may find some families quite anxious and upset about the long wait for study results and other families denying that the infant has problems. Understanding chromosome analysis and possible causes of chromosome disorders will help the nurse support the family, establish early intervention strategies, and assuage problems in the home setting.

Example: Down Syndrome

Because of its frequency, Down syndrome is a useful example of a chromosome disorder to discuss in detail. The chromosomal cause of Down syndrome was identified in 1959, although the first clinical description was published by John Langdon Down in 1866 (Stine, 1989; Thompson et al., 1991). Down syndrome is common, occurring throughout the world in all races and both sexes with a frequency of at least 1 per 1,000 live births (Stine, 1989). It is also frequently identified in studies of spontaneous abortions (Stine, 1989).

Genetics

Approximately 95% of Down syndrome cases are due to trisomy 21 (Stine, 1989). In these cases, an accident of cell division occurred in the egg or sperm or at fertilization resulting in a zygote with an extra number 21 chromosome. All other chromosome pairs are normal. Parents of children with trisomy 21 have about a 1% chance for recurrence of this problem in subsequent pregnancies, and prenatal diagnosis may be used to reassure these parents (Stine, 1989).

Some forms of Down syndrome are inherited. Some normal-appearing persons have chromosomes that have misaligned and have become abnormally attached to each other. These translocations cause about 4% of the Down syndrome cases (Stine, 1989). It is critical to identify translocation carrier parents as they have a significant recurrence risk. Translocation causes should be considered whenever there are multiple chromosomal disorders in a family.

Parental mosaicism for Down syndrome accounts for only about 1% of Down syndrome cases (Stine, 1989). Mosaicism (described earlier) occurs when fertilization is correct but a chromosomal error occurs during the first few cell divisions. Parents who are mosaic and who are mildly affected may be undiagnosed for this condition and may be reasonably functional. However, they have a greatly increased chance of producing multiple cases of fully expressed Down syndrome children. The Down syndrome checklist (Appendix 25–C) is useful during the home visit if a parent has features or delays that suggest Down syndrome or mosaicism for that condition (Stine, 1989).

Identification

Down syndrome is often identified prenatally because ultrasound reveals a short femur length or an increased nuchal fold. Subsequent amniocentesis and chromosome analysis can confirm the diagnosis before birth. Many parents who learn that their infant will have Down syndrome continue the pregnancy and need information and support from the nurse during the first home visit after birth. When the diagnosis is known, nurses should obtain medical, social, and referral information prior to visiting the home.

When not identified prenatally, Down syndrome is identifiable at birth because of the characteristic dysmorphic facial features, hand and feet findings, and hypotonia (poor muscle tone) that is almost always present in Down syndrome infants. However, the combination of initial edema, cranial molding, and early hospital discharge may cause some of these infants to be missed in the newborn nursery. While approximately 40% of children with Down syndrome will have significant heart lesions (Jones, 1988), including ventricular septal defects, transposition of great vessels, tetrology of Fallot, hypoplastic left heart, and other severe structural heart lesions, significant cardiac findings also may not be present in the first few days of life.

Down syndrome should be considered following any newborn or childhood assessment in which there is developmental delay, hypotonia, and facies with features including the following:

- a flat occiput
- a flattened profile appearance
- upslanting eyes
- flat nasal bridge
- small nose and mouth
- white specks in the irises (Brushfield spots)
- protruding tongue
- low-set ears with overfolded helices.

Hands and feet should also be examined for transverse palmar creases, incurving fifth fingers, a gap between the great toe and the other toes, and unusual fingerprints. Documentation of height, weight, head circumference (typically small), and heart sounds is an essential part of the initial evaluation. Since no one symptom is diagnostic of Down syndrome, the nurse should complete a checklist (see Appendix 25–C) including minor anomalies and then consider the constellation of findings in these infants. Any significant pattern of findings should be immediately referred for a complete genetic evaluation and chromosome analysis (Jones, 1988).

All forms of Down syndrome look clinically identical. Therefore, all children with Down syndrome should have immediate chromosomal analysis. A family history should be obtained. If either parent has other affected relatives or unexplained short stature, a history of developmental delay, school problems, or mild dysmorphic features, a parental Down syndrome checklist should be completed (Appendix 25–C) and referral for chromosomal analysis considered.

Prognosis

With infant stimulation programs and the proper support systems, children with Down syndrome may progress well during infancy and young childhood. They will learn at a slower pace but will develop in the same sequence as chromosomally normal children. Short stature, speech problems, and mental retardation (IQ scores usually in the range of 50–70) are universal findings (Stine, 1989).

Since children with Down syndrome have variations in their immune system, upper respiratory problems and other infections are extremely frequent. They are at an increased risk for diabetes, the incidence of leukemia is close to 1%, and thyroid disorders are fairly common (Jones, 1988). There are variations in the pelvis and other bony structures. The shape of the foramen magnum and vertebral changes may place some Down syndrome children at risk for spinal cord compromise. Girls with Down syndrome are fertile, and there are numerous cases of effected females delivering live born children. The theoretical risk for chromosomally abnormal offspring is 50%, but the actual number of abnormal births has been about 20% (Stine, 1989). Spontaneous abortion of abnormal fetuses may account for this discrepancy. Down syndrome males are usually infertile.

Individuals with Down syndrome age rapidly and are subject to premature senility. Families should be assisted during the childhood years to make appropriate plans for as much independent living as is possible during young adulthood and for supportive care as their child ages. It is essential that these plans be developed during the early years, as many children with Down syndrome outlive their parents, and placement options for adults with Down syndrome are limited and often have long waiting lists.

UNDERSTANDING SINGLE GENE DISORDERS: OVERVIEW

A single gene disorder is any condition that is caused by a variant allele or a pair of variant alleles at a particular location along a chromosome. A single gene variation can sufficiently alter the protein produced by that gene so that a clinical effect is manifest without interaction of other genes or environmental influences. While genes themselves are not dominant or recessive, traits and inheritance of traits can be described that way. Single gene disorders can occur by autosomal dominant, autosomal recessive, X-linked dominant, or X-linked recessive inheritance.

Distinguishing the mode of transmission for single gene traits, through identifying the pattern of inheritance, allows the nurse or other health care provider to predict the chance that a disorder will occur in an offspring or other relatives (see Figure 25–1). Since chromosomes come in pairs, genes on the chromosomes also come in pairs. For any particular trait, an individual should inherit one gene from the mother and one from the father. The type of trait will determine whether activity from one or both genes is necessary to produce a specified effect. If a person inherits the same allele for both of the gene pairs, he or she is said to be homozygous for that trait. If the alleles are different, the person is said to be heterozygous for that trait. It is possible to have many alleles for a given trait in the world's population. For example, there are over 400 different alleles coding for hemoglobin, even though the normal hemoglobin A is the most frequent (Bowman & Murray, 1990). While many different combinations are possible, in a given individual most traits are coded for by a pair of alleles. In a few cases, multiples pairs of alleles are needed to code for a particular trait.

Understanding Autosomal Dominant Inheritance

A trait is dominant if it is determined by a gene from only one of the two parents. That is, it is expressed whenever a single copy of the gene is transmitted. Dominantly inherited traits (see examples in Table 25–1) have the following characteristics in common: they are frequently structural defects, such as six fingers and toes; variations in bones, such as osteogenesis imperfecta or some forms of dwarfism; craniofacial syndromes; and other changes that can be noted externally, such as neurofibromatosis and tuberous sclerosis. Even when the dominant gene is transmitted within the same family group, there will be wide variation of expression. Therefore, whenever any suspected dominant feature is identified in an individual, other family members should be examined for mild expression of the disorder. Many mildly affected persons reach adulthood without being diagnosed, yet their offspring may be more profoundly affected.

If a parent is heterozygous (which means that they have one copy of a normal gene and one copy of an altered gene), there is a "heads or tails risk"—one chance in two—that he or she will transmit the altered gene in a particular egg or sperm. If the altered gene is transmitted, the child will be affected, even if the other parent is normal for this trait. Thus, if a person carries the gene for the dominant trait, the risk of passing this gene to each offspring is 50%. This risk is the same regardless of the degree of expression in the carrier: mildly affected individuals can have severely affected offspring, and persons with severe manifestations can have mildly affected children. The degree of expression depends on interaction with other genes and the prenatal environment and cannot be predicted. A more serious condition occurs when two parents carry the same gene for a dominant trait: homozygous affected offspring will be profoundly affected.

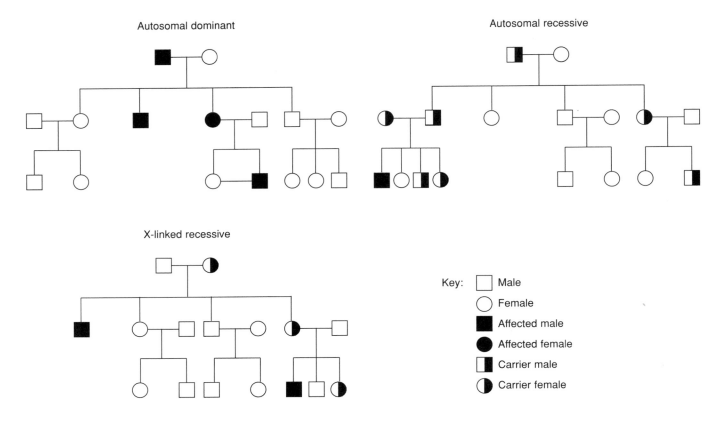

Figure 25–1 Modes of Inheritance of Single Gene Disorders (X-linked Dominant not shown)

Source: Office of Technology Assessment, 1992.

Example: Craniosynostosis

In any newborn assessment, the focus is on the head and face. The shape and size of the head are particularly important, and resources to confirm normal measurements are widely available. Skull variations can have a number of causes; however, premature closure of the bones of the skull (craniosynostosis) is a primary cause for small or unusually shaped heads. Sutures fuse and fontanels close as a result of skull ossification that continues from infancy to adulthood. Timing of skull closure is an important genetically controlled developmental step. We now know that some genes that control for premature fusion of the skull sutures are located on chromosome 7 and on the X chromosome (Mange & Mange, 1994) and even isolated primary craniosynostosis of a single suture may have a genetic basis.

Most cases of craniosynostoses are associated with other malformations or well-described genetic syndromes. Most of these, including Apert and Crouzon syndromes, are inherited as autosomal dominant traits. In Crouzon syndrome, the condition is limited to craniosynostosis, which causes skull malformation and facial dysmorphic features such as ocular proptosis (bug eyes), hypertelorism (widely spaced eyes),

and frontal bossing (a very prominent forehead). Conductive hearing loss may also be present. The nurse should note ridging of the coronal, lambdoid, and saggitta sutures. Only 3% of children with Crouzon syndrome exhibit mental delay, and there are no limb abnormalities (Jones, 1988). Apert syndrome, however, includes irregular craniosynostosis, especially of the coronal suture, and a characteristic "mitten hand" malformation with fusion of the fingers and sparing of the thumb. Mental retardation or delay is a frequent, but not universal, feature. There is midface hypoplasia with flat facies, shallow orbits, hypertelorism, downslanted eyes, small chin, and narrow palate. There many be a cleft palate or bifid uvula.

Primary craniosynostosis usually occurs without other developmental anomalies, and many mild cases are missed in infancy and childhood. Therefore, whenever premature closure of sutures is observed, other family members should also be examined for head size, shape, and mild dysmorphic facial features.

In any infant, it is very important to assess for premature closure of the skull: premature closure and suture ossification can lead to restricted brain growth as well as increased intracranial pressure leading to irreversible brain damage.

Table 25–1 Examples of Autosomal Dominant Conditions

Condition	Manifestation
Achondroplasia	Most common form of short-limbed dwarfism
Amyotrophic lateral sclerosis	Degeneration of nerve cells
Brachydactyly	Hand malformation, shortened fingers
Dimples	Indentations of the chin or cheeks
Earlobes	Unattached are dominant over attached
Freckles	Pigmented spots on the skin
Holt Oram syndrome	Hand and heart problems, narrow shoulders
Hypercholesterolemia	Elevated blood cholesterol
Hyperlipidemia	Raised level of fats
Hypospadius (some forms)	Abnormal placement of penile opening
Lobster claw deformity	Clefting abnormalities of the hands and feet
Marfan syndrome	Affects bone, muscle, and heart
Myotonic dystrophy	Congenital form has severe hypotonia; respiratory distress
Osteogenesis imperfecta	Brittle bones and blue sclerae
Neurofibromatosis	Cafe au lait spots, tumors and scoliosis
Polycystic kidney disease	Cysts on the kidneys leading to kidney destruction
Retinitis pigmentosa	Common cause of blindness
Right eye preference	Use of right eye over left
Treacher Collins syndrome	Jaw and facial malformations; deafness

The posterior fontanel and the anteriorlateral fontanels (created by the sagittal and lambdoidal sutures and the frontal, parietal, temporal, and shenoid bones) should close at about 2 to 3 months of age. The anterior fontanel is formed by the intersection of coronal and sagittal sutures and should close by 12 to 18 months of age. By 2 years of age, the posterior-lateral fontanel formed by the parietal, occipital, and temporal bones should be closed. While there may be some variation in timing in the premature infant, the order of closure should be the same (Betz, Hunsberger, & Wright, 1994).

Understanding Autosomal Recessive Inheritance

A trait is recessive if it is determined only by being transmitted from both parents. That is, the trait is expressed only when the individual receives two copies (a "double dose") of the variant allele. An individual with a normal allele and a recessive variant allele will be a carrier for that trait, but

should be clinically healthy. If both parents are carriers for a given trait, with each pregnancy, the child has a 25% chance for manifesting the disorder, a 50% chance for being a healthy carrier, and a 25% chance for being genotypically normal for this particular allele.

Most commonly, autosomal recessive disorders are due to variations in enzymes that affect metabolic pathways or circulatory proteins. Thus, most recessive disorders reflect biochemical rather than structural changes. There are over 1,500 identified autosomal recessive disorders (McKusick, 1992). Common recessive examples include cystic fibrosis, sickle cell anemia, PKU, galactosemia, congenital adrenal hyperplasia, and occasionally storage disorders such as Tay-Sachs disease or Hurler syndrome.

Most states screen for four to eight conditions that are either metabolic or hemoglobin problems. The most common autosomal disorders for which screening is conducted are described in Table 25–2. One should "think metabolic" whenever there is a history of unexplained vomiting, seizures, lethargy, or neurological deterioration. Some cases of sudden infant death syndrome (SIDS) may be misdiagnoses of metabolic disorders. The single most important action that can be taken to diagnose serious recessive disorders in the home setting is to repeat the state newborn screening tests.

Example: Galactosemia

Galactosemia is an important metabolic condition that is being added to many state metabolic screening programs. Galactosemia is caused by the reduced or absent activity of galactose-phosphate-1-uridyl-transferase, which is the enzyme that converts the milk sugar galactose to glucose. When the enzyme is missing, galactose accumulates in the blood, brain, liver, and kidneys and is converted to several toxic products. Other rare variant forms also exist, and all forms are inherited as recessive traits.

Affected infants appear normal at birth and will be routinely discharged by 48 hours of age. If a newborn screening test is not obtained on the 2nd or 3rd day of life, or if the state does not screen for this condition, affected children will become very ill by 7 to 10 days of life, and many will die. If the correct diagnosis is not made, the cause of death will likely be listed as sepsis or dehydration, and the parents will not know that they have a 25% chance of recurrence in subsequent offspring.

In the newborn infant, symptoms of galactosemia include vomiting and diarrhea leading to extreme dehydration, infection (particularly E. coli sepsis), and liver pathology with severe jaundice. Infants who survive will become mentally retarded and may be blind. Some children are born with existing cataracts, a sign that may be lifesaving in states that do not routinely screen for this disorder. Even in older treated children, there is considerable risk for speech problems as well as premature ovarian failure in females.

Table 25–2 Newborn Screening: Summary of Common Conditions

Disorder	Early symptoms	Incidence	Treatment	Follow-up needs
PKU (classic)	Severe mental retardation, eczema, seizures, behavior disorders, decreased pigmentation, distinctive "mousey" odor	1:10,000 to 1:15,000 More common in Northern European groups	Low phenylalanine diet Possible tyrosine supplementation	Lifelong dietary management; careful monitoring of PKU variants; careful management and preconception counseling and intervention for PKU women in the reproductive years
Congenital hypothyroidism (primary)	Mental and motor retardation, short stature, coarse, dry skin and hair, hoarse cry; constipation	Overall 1:4,000 with ethnic variation 1:12,000 African-Americans 1:1,000 Native American	Replacement of L-thyroxine	Maintain L-thyroxine levels in upper half of normal range; periodic bone age to monitor growth
Galactosemia (transferase deficiency)	Neonatal death from severe dehydration, sepsis or liver pathology; mental retardation, jaundice, blindness, cataracts	1:10,000 to 1:90,000	Eliminate galactose and lactose from the diet Soy formula in infancy Lactose-free solid foods	Provide early monitoring for speech and neurological problems; educate parents about hidden sources of lactose; monitor females for secondary ovarian failure; avoid medications with lactose fillers
Maple syrup urine (MSUD)	Acidosis; hypertonicity and seizures, vomiting, drowsiness, apnea, coma; infant death or severe mental retardation and neurological impairment; behavioral disorders	1:90,000 to 1:200,000	Diet low in leucine, isoleucine, and valine Thiamine supplement if responsive	Educate family and friends regarding strict dietary regimen; social and education evaluation; behavioral counseling; neurological monitoring; prompt treatment of illness to minimize acidosis
Congenital adrenal hyperplasia (CAH)	Hyponatremia, hypo-kalemia, hypoglycemia, dehydration and early death; ambiguous genitalia in females; progressive virilization in both sexes	Overall 1:15,000 to 1:18,000 1:3,000 native Eskimos	Replace corticosteroids Plastic surgery to correct ambiguous genitalia	Maintain adequate corticosteroids; elevate doses or give injectable doses in times of stress; periodic bone age to monitor adequate treatment; maintain pediatric endocrinology follow-up appointments
Sickle cell anemia	Overwhelming bacterial infections, sudden massive enlargement of liver and spleen, shock, painful swelling of the hands and feet, abdominal pain, anemia, stroke	1:400 African-Americans Elevated incidence in Southern European, Asian, and Middle-Eastern groups	Penicillin prophylaxis beginning with newborn (250 mg BID) Maximize fluids Careful hygiene Green leafy vegetables and folic acid supplements	Maintain adequate dosage of penicillin; maximize fluid intake; monitor for pain and infections; regular follow-up by a specialty center; parental education

Source: Copyright Lynette Wright, RN, MN. Reprinted by permission.

Treatment should be instituted immediately whenever there is a possibility of galactosemia; a delay of even a few hours can result in death. Treatment consists of a dietary plan that eliminates lactose (milk sugar) from the diet. This includes breast milk and any milk-based formula. Substitution is easy in infancy since there are a number of commercially available soy formulas. Once the child begins to eat table food, however, treatment becomes more challenging. Almost all powdered or packaged foods have a lactose filler, and milk, cheese, and yogurt are frequently incorporated into casseroles and many other combined dishes. Even ampicillin, a drug frequently used to treat bacterial infections, has a lactose filler in the pediatric suspension form (Wright, Brown, & Davidson-Mundt, 1992). Affected children need lifelong management through a metabolic center, and parents need specific dietary education and support.

Notification of a positive newborn screen for galactosemia should be considered a medical emergency and should require an immediate home visit or transport to a physician. A nurse making a home visit for a positive newborn screen should complete the following tasks:

1. Examine the infant.
2. If the child is ill or responds poorly, transport immediately to the nearest hospital emergency department and contact the child's pediatrician. Describe galactosemia and the likelihood of E. coli sepsis. Do not assume that the local physician is familiar with this condition.
3. Contact the state metabolic newborn screening center to obtain a referral to a metabolic specialist who is familiar with the management of this disorder. Many will have contracts with the state and will provide telephone consultation to the local physician or will see the child in a metabolic center.
4. If the child is not ill, obtain a heel stick blood sample and mail it to the state so that the screening test can be repeated. Inform parents that prematurity, metabolic immaturity, samples mailed during hot weather, and bacterial contamination can all cause false positives. Some infants who carry a single copy of the galactosemia gene will be initially positive but not be ill. With a few weeks' maturation, enough enzyme is made so that repeat tests are normal.
5. Obtain a three-generation family history, and ask specifically about early or sudden infant infections, jaundice, or deaths in previous children or any family history of infant deaths or mental retardation.

Understanding X-linked Inheritance

Sex-linked, commonly called X-linked, inheritance is a special case of single gene inheritance and refers to any trait that is carried on the X or Y chromosome and not on one of the 22 autosomal pairs. The Y chromosome contains relatively few genes, primarily those associated with maleness. The X chromosome, on the other hand, carries many genes related to traits other than sex. Thus, a male is hemizygous, which means that he does not have a corresponding gene for many of the X chromosome loci. However, because there are no clinical examples of Y-linked diseases, the term *sex-linked* usually refers to X-linked disorders. X-linked disorders can be dominant or recessive.

Understanding X-linked Recessive Inheritance

In an X-linked recessive condition, two mutant genes, or one mutant gene and a missing corresponding gene, are necessary for a trait to express itself.

Typically, males are affected when they receive a mutant X from their mother and the Y has no corresponding gene to counteract its effects. Females who receive an altered X from their mother and also receive a normal X from their father are usually healthy carriers. Rarely a female is affected: it requires receiving a mutant gene from an affective father and a second mutant gene from a carrier mother. The gene is never transmitted directly from father to son since males have received the Y chromosome. It is transmitted by affected males to every female offspring who must receive the variant X since her father has only one to pass on. Thus, all daughters of affected males are carriers. The gene is also transmitted through carrier females to sons who are affected 50% of the time (depending on which X is transmitted) and daughters who are carriers 50% of the time. Thus, for most X-linked recessive conditions, males are affected with the disorder, and carrier females are clinically asymptomatic. If females show some evidence of the trait, the expression is milder, unless a second condition exists, such as a deleted or missing X, which causes the gene to be fully manifested. In taking a history, X-linked inheritance should be considered whenever there is an excess of affected males in the family.

Example: Duchenne Muscular Dystrophy. Duchenne muscular dystrophy is an X-linked recessive disorder affecting 1 in 3,000 male births (Stine, 1989; Thompson et al., 1991). Multiple mutations can occur in the large gene that codes for dystrophin, a protein of muscle cells. When dystrophin is absent or disrupted, the muscle fibers atrophy, and muscle cells fail to regenerate. Creatinine phosphokinase (CPK) is markedly elevated in the early stages, and muscle biopsies and electromyograms will be abnormal at an early age.

The most consistent feature of Duchenne muscular dystrophy in young boys is delayed walking, usually later than 18 months. They may "toe walk," and most are never able to run. The muscle fibers are affected beginning early in life. The pelvic girdle appears to be affected first, and weak hip extensors cause delayed walking and frequent stumbling. The lower leg muscles are rapidly deteriorating even in infancy and are being replaced by fatty tissue. This eventually results in the common finding of pseudohypertrophied calves. Lordosis, which is characteristic for normal toddlers, persists in these boys because of weakened adductors and gluteal muscles. Eventually, shoulder and arm muscles are affected, and in the late stages, cardiac muscle involvement is a universal finding (Betz et al., 1994).

The nurse should check for strength and muscle tone and compare upper and lower limbs. Affected young children have difficulty climbing stairs and typically pull themselves up with their arms. It is difficult to imagine how such a child could be missed until 6 or 7 years of age if a thorough history and assessment were completed. Any male child older than age 2 years should be asked to sit "Indian style" and then get up without support. If the child cannot do this or uses his arms to "walk up his legs" to an upright position, an immediate referral should be made.

A careful family history is also important as related females may be undiagnosed carriers with a 50% risk for producing affected sons. By using molecular techniques, it is possible to diagnose female relatives precisely, offer prenatal diagnosis for families at risk, and confirm difficult clinical diagnoses at an earlier stage. Supportive care has improved both the quality of life and the life span for boys with this fatal disease. Nevertheless, even with the best of care, affected boys rarely survive beyond age 30. Great progress has been made in dystrophin research, and it is hoped that a gene therapy approach will provide a cure for this progressive and lethal disorder.

Understanding X-linked Dominant Inheritance

As with an autosomal dominant disorder, an X-linked dominant disorder requires only one mutant gene for the trait to be manifested. This determines the pattern of inheritance because affected females transmit to both male and female offspring. A child of either sex has a 50% chance of inheriting the mutant gene from an affected female. Affected males, who have only one X, will transmit the mutant X gene to all of their daughters and none of their sons. Thus, on average, there are twice as many females as males affected by X-linked dominant disorders. Expression is variable but tends to be milder in affected females. Some conditions may be fully penetrant and also lethal in males. Therefore, X-linked dominance should be considered when the family history demonstrates an excess of affected females or when all affected persons are female.

Example: Familial Hypophosphatemic Rickets. An important X-linked dominant disorder for the nurse to be familiar with is familial hypophosphatemic rickets. Because nutritional rickets is rare in the United States, a metabolic cause is likely and a genetics consult is essential when rickets is encountered. The condition is treatable if detected and addressed early.

UNDERSTANDING MULTIFACTORIAL INHERITANCE

Most differences in human beings are due to complex interactions between genes and environment. These types of traits are called *multifactorial* because they are determined by the additive effects of many genetic and environmental factors. There is a spectrum of expression for any given multifactorial trait that reflects a continuous variation. Height and IQ are excellent examples of traits that are influenced by a combination of genetic and environmental factors. We see a continuous variation from short to tall in height or from less to more verbal, math, or performance skills, with most people falling somewhere in the middle range. The same principles apply to malformations or diseases that are multifactorial. The clinical expression will range from mild to severe along a continuum.

Important clinical examples include isolated malformations such as cleft lip or cleft lip and palate, congenital dislocated hips, club feet, almost all isolated congenital heart malformations, and neural tube defects such as spina bifida and anencephaly. Important multifactorial diseases include insulin-dependent juvenile diabetes, allergies, and immune deficiency disorders. It is also important to note that most cancers, adult onset stroke, heart disease, and many psychiatric disorders fall into a multifactorial classification with significant genetic input.

The most important concept for multifactorial expression is the threshold effect. That is the point at which the additive effects of genetic and environmental influences exceed the ability of the body to adapt, and malformations or diseases become expressed. Close to the threshold, one may see minor anomalies that may indicate underlying malformations or may be clinically insignificant but indicate a need for careful evaluation and counseling regarding risk for future offspring. Once the threshold is exceeded, one would expect to see a spectrum of clinical expression.

Because it is assumed that more than one gene locus contributes to the genetic variation and that environment also plays a prominent role, multifactorial inheritance is more difficult to predict than the single gene modes of inheritance. Multifactorial traits tend to cluster in families, but there is no clear pattern of inheritance. However, by analyzing many families with multifactorial disorders, certain principles for recurrence within families have emerged. These principles are significantly different from those governing single gene inheritance and are important to review:

- The incidence of any particular multifactorial trait varies with ethnicity, for example, the extremely high rate of congenital dislocated hips in Navajo Indians and the world's highest rate of spina bifida occurring among the Irish.
- The more severe the defect, the greater the risk of recurrence. The risk also increases as the number of affected relatives increases.

- If no other relatives have expressed the disorder, and a couple has one affected child, the recurrence risk is in the range of 3% to 5% (Thompson et al., 1991).
- There is an altered sex ratio. For example, pyloric stenosis and cleft lip without cleft palate is more frequent in males. Congenital dislocated hips are more frequent in females.

Example: Neural Tube Defects. The neural tube is one of the earliest organs to form and closes between the 23rd and 28th day after fertilization. If proper closure does not occur, the result is usually anencephaly or spina bifida. The incidence of neural tube malformations in the United States is about 1 in 1,000 with many racial and geographic variations (Thompson et al., 1991). About half of these malformations are spina bifida, and the other half are anencephaly. Although some neural tube malformations are due to single gene syndromes or chromosomal abnormalities, most neural tube defects are multifactorial in origin.

Anencephaly is characterized by lack of skull closure and poor brain development and generally results in miscarriage or a stillborn infant. Spina bifida, on the other hand, is characterized by incomplete closure of one or more vertebrae and protrusion of meninges and possibly the spinal cord into a sac-like structure. The amount of physical and mental impairment in spina bifida depends on the size and location of the defect and the amount of disruption to the flow of cerebrospinal fluid. Individuals with spina bifida occulta may be asymptomatic, and closed defects may have a better prognosis. However, 80% to 90% of spina bifida are open defects (personal communication, Robert Best, 1993) and are associated with paralysis, lack of skin sensation below the lesion, hydrocephalus, and, in extreme cases, severe mental retardation, stillbirth, or perinatal death.

Around the world, persons of Irish decent have the highest rate of neural tube defects, and there is also an increased rate among some Mexican groups. In the United States, the rate is highest in Appalachia and increased in Mexican immigrant groups who have migrated to all parts of the United States. African Americans have a decreased risk for these types of malformations. Incidence rates vary seasonally with the greatest risk occurring when conception occurs during months associated with a high incidence of viral illness. The incidence decreases in all ethnic groups as the socioeconomic status improves. When a couple has had one child with a neural tube defect, the recurrence rate is about 3% and rises to 10% if a second affected child is born; however, 95% of all cases occur in families with no history of neural tube defects (Thompson et al., 1991).

Because there is a spectrum of spinal anomalies, the nurse in a home setting should evaluate the child for scoliosis; lower limb strength; and any dimples, pigmentation, or hairy patches. These minor anomalies usually signal an underlying malformation. Only mongolian spots (blue-grey pigmentation seen in many darker skinned individuals)

should be considered normal. Any other lower spine changes should receive careful follow-up. For example, if a child has an attached spinal cord, the child will seem perfectly normal as an infant. The only sign may be hair or pigmentation over the site of attachment. As the child grows, however, the cord will stretch, and scoliosis, loss of sensation, and paralysis will occur unless the cord is surgically released. Once nerve damage occurs, it cannot be repaired.

Many fetuses with anencephaly or spina bifida are diagnosed prenatally by either ultrasound or through alpha fetoprotein screening and amniocentesis. While hydrocephalus can be monitored by ultrasound, there is no prenatal correction for spina bifida, and the degree of damage cannot be predicted by ultrasound techniques. At present, families must wrestle with the difficult choice of ending the pregnancy early or anticipating the birth of a child with a significant abnormality. The genes that control this important step in development are being characterized, and several important environmental factors have been discovered. The most important negative environmental influence is deficiency of folic acid. It is believed that 50% to 70% of spina bifida can be prevented if all women of reproductive age have adequate levels of folic acid at the time of conception. Any nurse making a home visit should inquire about vitamin supplements and can specifically recommend folic acid supplements and green leafy vegetables for women who have any possibility of becoming pregnant (Centers for Disease Control and Prevention, 1992). The Centers for Disease Control and Prevention (CDC) and the Food and Drug Administration (FDA) recently agreed that as of 1998 cereals and bread must be fortified with folic acid. Until this is implemented, supplementation with pills and dietary choices will be the best preventative measure

REFERENCES

Betz, C.L., Hunsberger, M. & Wright, S. (1994). *Family centered nursing care of children* (2nd ed.) Philadelphia, PA: W.B. Saunders.

Bowman, J.E. & Murray, R.F. (1990). *Genetic variation and disorders in peoples of African origin.* Baltimore, MD: The Johns Hopkins University Press.

Centers for Disease Control. Contribution of birth defects to infant mortality: United States. *Morbidity and Mortality Weekly Report, 28*(27), 823–826.

Centers for Disease Control. (1989). Contribution of birth defects to infant mortality: United States, 1986. *Morbidity and Mortality Weekly Report, 38,* 633–636.

Centers for Disease Control and Prevention. (1992, September 11). Recommendations for the use of folic acid to reduce the number of cases of spina bifida and other neural tube defects. *Morbidity and Mortality Weekly Report, 41*(RR-14) pp. 1–5.

Cook-Deegan, R.M. (1991). The Human Genome Project: The formation of federal policies in the United States, 1986–1990. K.E. Hanna (Ed.), *In Biomedical Politics.* Washington, DC: National Academy Press.

Hall, J.G. (1990, December). Nontraditional inheritance. *Growth: Genetics and Hormones 7*(4), 1–3

Hook, E.B. & Cross, P.K. (1979). *American Journal of Human Genetics, 31,* 137A.

Jones, K.W. (1988). Smith's recognizable patterns of human malformation (4th ed.). Philadelphia, PA: W.B. Saunders Co.

Mange, E.J. & Mange, A.P. (1994). Basic human genetics. Sunderland, MA: Sinauer Associates.

McKusick, V. (1992). *Mendalian inheritance in man* (10th ed.). Baltimore, MD: The Johns Hopkins University Press.

Stine, G.J. (1989). *The new human genetics.* Dubuque, IO: Wm. C. Brown Publishers.

Thompson, M.W., McInnes, R.R. & Huntington, W.F. (1991). *Genetics in medicine* (5th ed.). Philadelphia, PA: W.B. Saunders.

Wright, L., Brown, A. & Davidson-Mundt, A. (1992, February). Newborn screening: The miracle and the challenge. *J Peds Nursing, 7*(1), 26, 31–33.

ADDITIONAL RESOURCES

Teratology, (1993, December) *48*(6), 545–709.

Gordon, T. (1970). *PET: Parent effectiveness training.* New York, NY: Peter H. Wyden.

Bauer, B.B. & Hill, S.S. (1986). Essentials of mental health care: Planning and interventions. Philadelphia, PA: W.B. Saunders.

Appendix 25–A

Glossary of Common Genetics Terms

Allele Alternative forms of a gene occurring in the same place on a chromosome. For example, alleles for eye color.

Autosome Any of the chromosomes other than the sex chromosomes.

Autosomal A trait which is located on any of the 22 pairs of autosomes. For example, having freckles is an autosomal dominant trait.

Base pairs Adenine, thymine, guanine and cytosine are the 4 bases which make up units which form genes. These are precisely paired by hydrogen bonds. For example, Adenine (A) is always paired with thymine (T) and guanine (G) with cytosine (C). Changes at the base pair level produce mutations in the DNA.

Chromatid One of the two structurally distinguishable subunits of a metaphase chromosome.

Chromosome A self-reproducing unit in the cell nucleus which contains a set of linked genes along strands of coiled DNA. Individual chromosomes are visible only when they condense and prepare to divide.

Crossing over The exchange of genetic material that occurs between members of a pair of homologous chromosomes during the synapse phase of meiosis.

Cytoplasm The portion of the cell that surrounds the nucleus.

DNA Abbreviation for a double helix made up of two deoxyribose-phosphate backbones joined together by hydrogen bonded base pairs; Deoxyribonucleic acid.

Dominant The trait that is expressed when two different alleles are present, eg: blue allele and brown allele will yield a brown eyed individual who might pass on either blue or brown.

Gametes Eggs or sperm which should have 23 chromosomes each.

Gene A biological unit of hereditary information which is normally transmitted unchanged from one generation to the next; a segment of DNA which codes for one functional polypeptide chain.

Homologous Chromosomes or genes which are complementary to its other pair. For example, each of the two number 21 chromosomes would be homologous to each other. Each one will be quite similar, but not genetically identical since they were inherited from different parents.

Interphase The period of cell growth and metabolism which occurs between cell divisions. This is when the "work" of the cell takes place.

Karyotype An arrangement of chromosomes by size and shape which pairs homologous chromosomes for systematic counting and structural analysis.

Liability gene A gene which may predispose one to the expression of a harmful trait. Such genes usually interact with other genes and with negative environmental influences before expression can occur.

Meiosis The form of cell division which produces gametes (eggs and sperm) with 23 individual chromosomes.

Metaphase The stage of cell division during which a chromosome is tightly condensed and can be viewed under a light microscope. This is the only time that chromosomes can be accurately counted.

Minor malformations Variations found in 8–11% of newborns which do not have serious consequences in themselves but may indicate the presence of more serious underlying malformations.

Mitosis Cell division that gives rise to two cells with identical chromosomes and genotypes. This is the body's method for growing and for replacing old or dead cells.

Nucleus A membrane bounded structure of the cell which houses the chromosomes which contain the genetic material, DNA.

Pedigree A diagram of at least 3 generations of a family history (grandparents, parents and children with appropriate siblings) often showing the expression of one or more genetic traits among family members.

Recessive An allele that is expressed only when two copies are present and the person is homozygous for the trait. For example, blue eyes are recessive to the darker eye colors. They are only expressed when each parent transmits a blue allele to a given child.

Reduction division Meiosis I or the stage in which the number of chromosomes are reduced from 46 to 23.

X-linked A gene which is carried on the X chromosome. The traits which are expressed, such as hemophilia, are also said to be X-linked.

Source: Copyright Lynette Wright, RN, MN. Reprinted by permission.

Appendix 25–B

Developing a Pedigree

Step I

- Use pencil
- Start in the middle of the page
- Start 2/3 of the way down the page

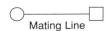

Mating Line

Step II

- Add children
- Identify index case with an arrow

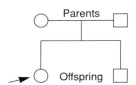

Parents

Offspring

Step III

- Do mother's side first
- Ask about each family member individually

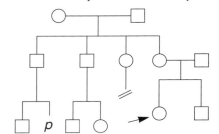

Step iV

- Add the father's side

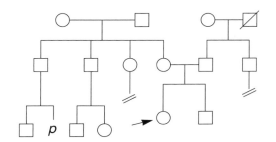

Step V

- Complete with ages, generation numbers and legend

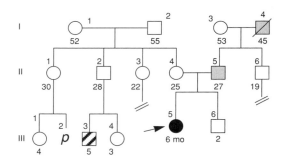

Legend:
I, 4-died following MI
  ↑ Cholesterol
  ↑ BP
II, 3-mild MR
II, 5- ↑ Cholesterol
III, 2-LMP, 5/3/89
III, 3-Pyloric Stenosis repaired @ 6 wks
III, 5-Index Case: Down Syndrome
   Chromosomes confirm Trisomy 21

▨ = **Pyloric Stenosis**
● = **Down Syndrome**
▨ = **↑ Cholesterol**

Legend for Pedigrees:

□, ○ : Square symbol for male, circle for female

→○ : Arrow indicates the index case

▨ : Deceased indicated by slash line

□─○ : Mating line

□⁽³⁾○ : Multiple matings

□═○ : Consanguinous mating (inbred couple)

▮ : Miscarriage or spontaneous abortion

(□) : Adoption

◑, ◪ : (Presumed) carrier for an autosomal recessive trait

⊙ : Obligate carrier female for an X-linked recessive trait

●, ■ : Condition expressed

□△□ : Twins

p : Pregnant

III : Roman numeral = generation

²○ : Superscript = position in pedigree

□₃₆ : Subscript = age in years

Source: Copyright © Lynette Wright, RN, MN. Reprinted by permission.

368

Checklist for Down Syndrome

NAME_____   MATERNAL AGE AT CHILD'S BIRTH _____

HOSPITAL # _____   PATERNAL AGE AT CHILD'S BIRTH _____

DATE OF EXAMINATION _____

CRANIOFACIAL
Large or accessory fontanel (infancy)
Open fontanel (beyond 1/2 yrs)
Flat occiput
Microcephaly (mild)
Flat facial profile and nasal bridge

EYES
Upslanting palpebral fissures
Inner epicanthal folds
Speckling of iris (Brushfield's spots)
Fine lens opacities
Strabismus

EARS
Small
Overfold of superior helix
Small or absent lobes

MOUTH
Protruding tongue
High arched palate
Dysplastic teeth
Low, hoarse voice

HANDS
Short
Clinodactyly of 5th fingers
Single flexion crease of 5th fingers
Single horizontal palmar creases

FEET
Increased gap between toes 1 and 2
Planter furrow

DERMATOLOGIC
Cutis marmorata
Straight pubic hair
Fine sparse hair

GENITALIA
Underdeveloped male genitalia
Cryptorchidism
Delayed puberty
Menstrual irregularities

NEUROLOGIC
Developmental delay
Mental retardation
Hypotonia

NECK
Redundant or loose skin
Appears short

CARDIOVASCULAR
Congenital heart disease
TYPE _____

GASTROINTESTINAL
Umbilical hernia
Diastasis recti
Duodenal artresia
Other organ abnormalities

MUSCULOSKELETAL
Relatively short stature
Hyperflexibility of joints

OTHER
Frequent infections
Thyroid dysfunction
Leukemia (1%)

SPECIAL STUDIES
X-rays:
    Hypoplastic iliac wings
    Shallow acetabilar angle
    Double ossification centers in
      manubrium sterni
    Vertebral body or rib abnormality

DERMATOGLYPHICS
Distal palmar axial triradii
Ulnar loops on digits (especially 1–3)
True patterns in palmar 3rd interdigital
Arch tibial or narrow loop in plantar
    hallucal areas

Index

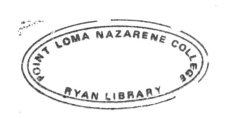